HEALTH AND HUMAN RIGHTS
Basic International Documents

Edited by
Stephen P. Marks

Published by Harvard University
François-Xavier Bagnoud Center for Health and Human Rights

Harvard Series on Health and Human Rights

Distributed by Harvard University Press
Cambridge, Massachusetts
London, England
2004

Copy Editing, Production, and Photo Research: Lynn Martin

Design, Layout, and Copy Editing: Catlin Rockman

Proofreading: Aparna Kollipara

Cover Photos:

Stephen P. Marks, IPPNW, WHO, John Mottern, International Tribune for the former Yugoslavia

Printed in the United States of America on Recycled Paper

Library of Congress Control Number: 2004117297
Data available at www.loc.gov
ISBN: 0-674-01809-5

CONTENTS

i

III. PROTECTION OF EXISTENCE AND PHYSICAL INTEGRITY

IV. HEALTH ASPECTS OF THE RIGHT TO AN ADEQUATE STANDARD OF LIVING
(OTHER THAN THE RIGHT TO HEALTH)

INTRODUCTION

This collection of texts is designed to provide the practitioner, scholar, and advocate easy access to the most basic instruments of international law and policy that express the values of human rights for advancing health. The selection is deliberately limited so that this book may be used with maximum facility. The collection is thus similar in scope and purpose to the compilations published by the Center for the Study of Human Rights of Columbia University relating to several other aspects of human rights.[1]

The reader in need of more complete and thorough documentation is fortunate to be able to refer to a volume by Alfredsson and Tomaševski published in 1998 containing 629 pages, including not only the text of numerous conventions, declarations, guidelines and policy statements, but also a chronological list with full references and an alphabetical index.[2] Several important documents have been issued since that publication, and it is not always convenient to keep such a voluminous reference work at hand. The present collection is therefore designed to be less exhaustive than the excellent *Guide to Documents on Health and Human Rights*.

In addition, there are nearly unlimited resources on health and human rights available on the Internet. Most human rights issues are thoroughly covered at the website of the Office of the High Commissioner for Human Rights (www.unhchr.ch). Health-related information, including explicit references to human rights, are available at the website of the World Health Organization (www.who.org). The François-Xavier Bagnoud Center and Global Lawyers and Physicians for Human Rights have collaborated in the preparation of a reader called *Perspectives in Health and Human Rights*.[3] That publication is accompanied by a special website containing links to documents, organizations, and other references on health and human rights.[4] The University of Minnesota Human Rights Collection also provides a valuable list of retrievable documents on bioethics.[5]

The chapter headings and criteria for inclusion and exclusion require some explanation. The collection in is eight parts. The first two relate to the areas that are likely to come immediately to mind for the health professional seeking human rights documents, namely professional ethics and the right to health. The next two parts relate to the two principal categories of human rights that determine capabilities of enjoying the right to health, namely, rights relating to physical integrity and rights relating to social and economic conditions. The remaining parts contain human rights texts that have addressed four areas where standard setting has been particularly relevant to health and human rights: vulnerable populations, health policy, biotechnology, and the environment. The identification of these eight parts has been more inductive than deductive in that they do not reflect a theoretical articulation of the relationship between health and human rights but rather a practical enumeration of the areas where the most relevant standard setting has occurred.

It is particularly important to clarify the selection in Part I on health and medical professions. This part begins with sections on professional ethics and research and experimentation. For many, there remains some confusion on the relationship between ethics or bioethics and human rights. A brief allusion to history may help clarify how these fields converge and diverge. In response to the atrocities committed during the Second World War, the organized international community began in the 1940s to define norms of behavior relating to both human rights, exemplified in the Universal Declaration of Human Rights of 1948, and the specific field of medical experimentation and responsibilities of health practitioners, exemplified by the Nuremburg Code, included in the judgment on the Nazi doctors in 1947. The progeny of the Nuremburg Code has included codes of ethics for doctors and nurses, as well as detailed principles relating to research and experimentation. Many of these texts are of a technical nature and are not strictly speaking human rights texts. Representative ones are included in Part I of this compilation because they expand on some basic norms that are included among internationally recognized human rights, such as the prohibition of medical or scientific experimentation without the free consent of the person concerned. Others are included because they relate the responsibilities of health practitioners explicitly invoking human rights, such as the declaration on nurses and human rights. The section in Part I on treatment of prisoners and detainees contains texts that relate to the role of health professionals, while the more general questions of torture are covered in Part II B. Part I ends with a declaration on patients' rights.

Part II contains the core international and regional texts on the right to health and concludes with two general texts on health and human rights. Part III covers five areas where international human rights norms prohibit violations of physical integrity, while Part IV deals with four aspects of the rights to the social and economic conditions necessary for health.

Part V provides the main human rights texts of relevance to the health of women, children, people with disabilities, older persons, and refugees and displaced persons. The quantity of human rights texts applicable to these categories is quite vast and many omissions and abridgements were necessary. For example, extracts from the Declaration on the Elimination of Violence Against Women are included but not the General Recommendation (No. 19) of the Committee on the Elimination of Discrimination Against Women on violence against women, which can be consulted on the website of the High Commissioner for Human Rights. The convention on the worst forms of child labor is included but not the protocol to the Convention on the Rights of the Child dealing with child soldiers, also available on the High Commissioner's website.

Part VI on health policy begins with infectious diseases. One of the most important international texts on this topic is the International Health Regulations, recently updated by WHO in response, in part, to the experience with the outbreak of severe acute respiratory syndrome (SARS). However, this text is not included because it does not deal explicitly with human rights, although issues, such as the right to information, were among the human rights concerns surrounding the SARS cases. The text may be consulted on the WHO website. The section on infectious diseases is limited to two texts on HIV/AIDS and a resolution on access to medication, while the remaining texts in Part VI concern intellectual property and occupational health. Parts VII and VIII deal respectively with biotechnology and the environment. Each of these areas has been the subject of considerable international standard setting and only the most basic texts focusing on human rights are included.

A final word is in order on the legal nature of the texts selected. Human rights instruments normally consist of formal treaties and declarations drafted by human rights bodies, such as the

United Nations Commission on Human Rights, as well as authorized interpretations of these instruments, such as general comments by treaty bodies. These are the normal reference documents of human rights lawyers. Where such documents do not exist or do not adequately cover the concerns by the international community, documents by professional organizations and by major international conferences and summits have been included. Such documents, while not carrying the same legal authority as law-making instruments, are nevertheless invaluable to understanding the normative issues involved in the relationship between health and human rights and to elaborating policies and programs in this field. Two documents are not in final form because negotiations were not completed when this edition went to press, namely, the draft UN conventions on persons with disabilities and on human cloning. Because of the importance of these two texts for health and human rights, the most current draft is included and the reader will be able to locate the final version when available. Readers should note that the draft convention on cloning represents only one of two major approaches, namely to ban all forms of cloning, and that the alternative approach, namely to let states decide how to deal with non-reproductive cloning, also has many supporters.

I wish to thank my colleagues, especially George Annas, Michael Grodin, Sofia Gruskin, Jennifer Leanning, Mindy Roseman and Daniel Wikler, for their invaluable advice. I am also indebted to Jason Cunningham, Lynn Martin, Catlin Rockman, and Aparna Kollipara for their tireless efforts in the preparation of this publication.

This publication is the first in a Harvard Series on Health and Human Rights published by the François-Xavier Bagnoud Center at the Harvard School of Public Health and distributed by Harvard University Press. As this collection of basic texts will be updated regularly, suggestions by readers to improve the selection and eliminate inaccuracies are welcome.

Stephen P. Marks
Director
François-Xavier Bagnoud Center for Health and Human Rights

Notes
1. Center for the Study of Human Rights, *25+ Human Rights Documents,* 2001; *Women and Human Rights: The Basic Documents*, 1996; *Religion and Human Rights: Basic Documents,* 1998.
2. Gudmundur Alfredsson and Katarina Tomaševski, *A Thematic Guide to Documents on Health and Human Rights*: *Global and Regional Standards Adopted by Intergovernmental Organizations, International Non-Governmental Organizations and Professional Associations*, The Hague: Martinus Nujhoff Publishers, 1998.
3. Sofia Gruskin, Michael Grodin, Stephen Marks, and George Annas, *Perspectives on Health and Human Rights,* New York: Routledge/Taylor and Francis, 2005.
4. http://www.glphr.org/resources/appendix.
5. See http://www1.umn.edu/humanrts/links/bioethics.html.

François-Xavier Bagnoud Center
for Health and Human Rights

The François-Xavier Bagnoud Center for Health and Human Rights was founded at the Harvard School of Public Health in January 1993. The Center considers the promotion and protection of health and the promotion and protection of human rights to be inextricably linked. The Center is dedicated to exploring the conceptual dimensions and practical applications of this critical relationship. Through its concentrated focus on the intersection of health and human rights, the Center also seeks to help revitalize the field of public health and broaden human rights thinking and practice.

 ## Harvard School of Public Health

The Harvard School of Public Health includes more than 200 faculty members working in various disciplines of public health. The overriding mission of the School — to advance the public's health through learning and discovery — comprises four objectives: to educate scientists, professionals, and leaders in public health; to foster new discoveries and develop better technologies for improved health of individuals and populations; to inform and influence debate on key public health issues; and to strengthen capacities and services that meet health needs in the community.

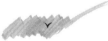

Association François-Xavier Bagnoud

The Association François-Xavier Bagnoud currently supports worldwide programs in humanitarian assistance, aerospace research for the benefit of people, and community life in the Swiss canton of Valais. Humanitarian assistance focuses on children's rights — especially the right to medical care — of children who are orphaned, abandoned, or sick, many of whom have AIDS or are HIV-infected. Projects are located in Thailand, India, Switzerland, Kenya, Uganda, Uruguay, Colombia, and the United States. The Association François-Xavier Bagnoud bears the name of a young Swiss helicopter rescue pilot who died in a helicopter accident while flying over the desert in Mali in 1986.

1. HEALTH AND MEDICAL PROFESSIONS
A. Professional Ethics

Declaration of Geneva (1948, 1968, 1983, 1994)

Adopted by the 2nd General Assembly of the World Medical Association, Geneva, Switzerland, September 1948 and amended by the 22nd World Medical Assembly, Sydney, Australia, August 1968, the 35th World Medical Assembly, Venice, Italy, October 1983 and the 46th WMA General Assembly, Stockholm, Sweden, September 1994. [Available at http://www.wma.net/e/policy/c8.htm]

PHYSICIAN'S OATH

At the time of being admitted as a member of the medical profession:

I solemnly pledge myself to consecrate my life to the service of humanity;

I will give to my teachers the respect and gratitude which is their due;

I will practice my profession with conscience and dignity;

The health of my patient will be my first consideration;

I will respect the secrets which are confided in me, even after the patient has died;

I will maintain by all the means in my power, the honor and the noble traditions of the medical profession;

My colleagues will be my sisters and brothers;

I will not permit considerations of age, disease or disability, creed, ethnic origin, gender, nationality, political affiliation, race, sexual orientation, or social standing to intervene between my duty and my patient;

I will maintain the utmost respect for human life from its beginning even under threat and I will not use my medical knowledge contrary to the laws of humanity;

I make these promises solemnly, freely and upon my honor.

World Medical Association International Code of Medical Ethics (1919, 1968, 1983)

Adopted by the 3rd General Assembly of the World Medical Association, London, England, October 1949 and amended by the 22nd World Medical Assembly, Sydney, Australia, August 1968 and the 35th World Medical Assembly, Venice, Italy, October 1983. [Available at http://www.wma.net/e/policy/c8.htm]

DUTIES OF PHYSICIANS IN GENERAL

A physician shall always maintain the highest standards of professional conduct.

A physician shall not permit motives of profit to influence the free and independent exercise of professional judgement on behalf of patients.

A physician shall in all types of medical practice, be dedicated to providing competent medical service in full technical and moral independence, with compassion and respect for human dignity.

A physician shall deal honestly with patients and colleagues, and strive to expose those physicians deficient in character or competence, or who engage in fraud or deception.

The following practices are deemed to be unethical conduct:

a) Self advertising by physicians, unless permitted by the laws of the country and the code of ethics of the national medical association.

b) Paying or receiving any fee or any other consideration solely to procure the referral of a patient or for prescribing or referring a patient to any source.

A physician shall respect the rights of patients, of colleagues, and of other health professionals and shall safeguard patient confidences.

A physician shall act only in the patient's interest when providing medical care which might have the effect of weakening the physical and mental condition of the patient.

A physician shall use great caution in divulging discoveries or new techniques or treatment through non-professional channels.

A physician shall certify only that which he has personally verified.

DUTIES OF PHYSICIANS TO THE SICK

A physician shall always bear in mind the obligation of preserving human life.

A physician shall owe his patients complete loyalty and all the resources of his science. Whenever an examination or treatment is beyond the physician's capacity he should summon another physician who has the necessary ability.

A physician shall preserve absolute confidentiality on all he knows about his patient even after the patient has died.

A physician shall give emergency care as a humanitarian duty unless he is assured that others are willing and able to give such care.

DUTIES OF PHYSICIANS TO EACH OTHER

A physician shall behave towards his colleagues as he would have them behave towards him.

A physician shall not entice patients from his colleagues.

A physician shall observe the principles of the Declaration of Geneva approved by the World Medical Association.

Nurses and Human Rights (1998)
Adopted in 1998 by the International Council of Nurses.
[Replaces previous ICN Position: "The Nurse's Role in Safeguarding Human Rights",
adopted 1983, updated 1993.]
[Available at www.icn.ch/pshumrights.htm]

ICN POSITION

Human rights in health care involve both recipients and providers. The International Council of Nurses (ICN) views health care as a right of all individuals, regardless of financial, political, geographic, racial or religious considerations. This right includes the right to choose or decline care, including the right to accept or refuse treatment or nourishment; informed consent; confidentiality, and dignity, including the right to die with dignity.

HUMAN RIGHTS AND THE NURSE'S ROLE

Nurses have an obligation to safeguard people's health rights at all times and in all places. This includes assuring that adequate care is provided within the resources available and in accordance with nursing ethics. As well, the nurse is obliged to ensure that patients receive appropriate information prior to consenting to treatment or procedures, including participation in research.

ICN advocates inclusion of human rights issues and the nurses' role in all levels of nursing education programmes.

As professionals, nurses are accountable for their own actions in safeguarding human rights. National nurses' associations have a responsibility to participate in the development of health and social legislation related to patient rights.

NURSES' RIGHTS

Nurses have the right to practice in accordance with the nursing legislation of the country in which they work and to adopt the ICN Code for Nurses or their own national ethical code. Nurses also have a right to practice in an environment that provides personal safety, freedom from abuse and violence, threats or intimidation.

National nurse's associations need to ensure an effective mechanism through which nurses can seek confidential advice, counsel, support and assistance in dealing with difficult human rights situations.

Madrid Declaration on Ethical Standards for Psychiatric Practice (1996, 2002)

Approved by the General Assembly on August 25, 1996, and amended by the General Assembly in Yokohama, Japan, in August 2002.
[Available at: http://www.wpanet.org/generalinfo/ethic1.html.]

DECLARATION OF MADRID

In 1977, the World Psychiatric Association approved the Declaration of Hawaii, setting out ethical guidelines for the practice of psychiatry. The Declaration was subsequently updated in Vienna in 1983. To reflect the impact of changing social attitudes and new medical developments on the psychiatric profession, the World Psychiatric Association has once again examined and revised some of these ethical standards.

Medicine is both a healing art and a science. The dynamics of this combination are best reflected in psychiatry, the branch of medicine that specializes in the care and protection of those who are ill and infirm, because of a mental disorder or impairment. Although there may be cultural, social and national differences, the need for ethical conduct and continual review of ethical standards is universal.

As practitioners of medicine, psychiatrists must be aware of the ethical implications of being a physician, and of the specific ethical demands of the specialty of psychiatry. As members of society, psychiatrists must advocate for fair and equal treatment of the mentally ill, for social justice and equity for all.

Ethical behavior is based on the psychiatrist's individual sense of responsibility towards the patient and their judgment in determining what is correct and appropriate conduct. External standards and influences such as professional codes of conduct, the study of ethics, or the rule of law by themselves will not guarantee the ethical practice of medicine.

Psychiatrists should at all times keep in mind the boundaries of the psychiatrist-patient relationship, and be guided primarily by the respect for patients and concern for their welfare and integrity.

It is in this spirit that the World Psychiatric Association approved at the General Assembly on August 25th, 1996, the following ethical standards that should govern the conduct of psychiatrists worldwide.

1. Psychiatry is a medical discipline concerned with the provision of the best treatment for mental disorders, with the rehabilitation of individuals suffering from mental illness and with the promotion of mental health. Psychiatrists serve patients by providing the best therapy available consistent with accepted scientific knowledge and ethical principles. Psychiatrists should devise therapeutic

interventions that are least restrictive to the freedom of the patient and seek advice in areas of their work about which they do not have primary expertise. While doing so, psychiatrists should be aware of and concerned with the equitable allocation of health resources.

2. It is the duty of psychiatrists to keep abreast of scientific developments of the specialty and to convey updated knowledge to others. Psychiatrists trained in research should seek to advance the scientific frontiers of psychiatry.

3. The patient should be accepted as a partner by right in the therapeutic process. The psychiatrist-patient relationship must be based on mutual trust and respect to allow the patient to make free and informed decisions. It is the duty of psychiatrists to provide the patient with relevant information so as to empower the patient to come to a rational decision according to personal values and preferences.

4. When the patient is incapacitated and/or unable to exercise proper judgment because of a mental disorder, or gravely disabled or incompetent, the psychiatrists should consult with the family and, if appropriate, seek legal counsel, to safeguard the human dignity and the legal rights of the patient. No treatment should be provided against the patient's will, unless withholding treatment would endanger the life of the patient and/or those who surround him or her. Treatment must always be in the best interest of the patient.

5. When psychiatrists are requested to assess a person, it is their duty first to inform and advise the person being assessed about the purpose of the intervention, the use of the findings, and the possible repercussions of the assessment. This is particularly important when the psychiatrists are involved in third party situations.

6. Information obtained in the therapeutic relationship should be kept in confidence and used, only and exclusively, for the purpose of improving the mental health of the patient. Psychiatrists are prohibited from making use of such information for personal reasons, or financial or academic benefits. Breach of confidentiality may only be appropriate when serious physical or mental harm to the patient or to a third person would ensue if confidentiality were maintained; as in case of child abuse in these circumstances, psychiatrists should, whenever possible, first advise the patient about the action to be taken.

7. Research that is not conducted in accordance with the canons of science is unethical. Research activities should be approved by an appropriately constituted ethical committee. Psychiatrists should follow national and international rules for the conduct of research. Only individuals properly trained for research should undertake or direct it. Because psychiatric patients are particularly vulnerable research subjects, extra caution should be taken to safeguard their autonomy as well as their mental and physical integrity. Ethical standards should also be applied in the selection of population groups, in all types of research including epidemiological and sociological studies and in collaborative research involving other disciplines or several investigating centers.

GUIDELINES CONCERNING SPECIFIC SITUATIONS

The World Psychiatric Association Ethics Committee's recognizes the need to develop a number of specific guidelines on a number of specific situations. The first five were approved by the General Assembly in Madrid, Spain, on August 25, 1996, and the last by the General Assembly in Hamburg, Germany, on August 8, 1999.

Euthanasia

A physician's duty, first and foremost, is the promotion of health, the reduction of suffering, and the protection of life. The psychiatrist, among whose patients are some who are severely incapacitated and incompetent to reach an informal decision, should be particularly careful of actions that could lead to the death of those who cannot protect themselves because of their disability. The psychiatrist should be aware that the views of a patient may be distorted by mental illness such as depression. In such situations, the psychiatrist's role is to treat the illness.

Torture

Psychiatrists shall not take part in any process of mental or physical torture, even when authorities attempt to force their involvement in such acts.

Death Penalty

Under no circumstances should psychiatrists participate in legally authorized executions nor participate in assessments of competency to be executed.

Selection of Sex

Under no circumstances should a psychiatrist participate in decisions to terminate pregnancy for the purpose of sex selection.

Organ Transplantation

The role of the psychiatrist is to clarify the issues surrounding organ donations and to advise on religious, cultural, social and family factors to ensure that informed and proper decisions be made by all concerned. The psychiatrists should not act as a proxy decision maker for patients nor use psychotherapeutic skills to influence the decision of a patient in these matters. Psychiatrists should seek to protect their patients and help them exercise self-determination to the fullest extent possible in situations of organ transplantation.

Psychiatrists Addressing the Media

The media has a key role in shaping the attitudes of the community. In all contacts with the media psychiatrists shall ensure that people with mental illness are presented in a manner which preserves their dignity and pride, and which reduces stigma and discrimination against them. An important role of psychiatrists is to advocate for those people who suffer from mental disorders. As the public perception of psychiatrists and psychiatry reflects on patients, psychiatrists shall ensure that in their contact with the media they represent the profession of psychiatry with dignity. Psychiatrists shall not make announcements to the media about presumed psychopathology on any individuals. In presenting research findings to the media, psychiatrists shall ensure the scientific integrity of the information given and be mindful of the potential impact of their statements on the public perception of mental illness and on the welfare of people with mental disorders.

Psychiatrists and Discrimination on Ethnic or Cultural Grounds

Discrimination by psychiatrists on the basis of ethnicity or culture, whether directly or by aiding others is unethical. Psychiatrists shall never be involved or endorse, directly or indirectly, any activity related to ethnic cleansing.

Psychiatrists and Genetic Research and Counseling

Research on the genetic bases of mental disorders is rapidly increasing and more people suffering from mental illness are participating in such research. Psychiatrists involved in genetic research or counseling shall be mindful of the fact that the implication of genetic information are not limited to the individual from whom it was obtained and that its disclosure can have negative and disruptive effects on the families and communities of the individuals concerned. Psychiatrist shall therefore ensure that:

• People and families who participate in genetic research do so with a fully informed consent;

• Any genetic information in their possession is adequately protected against unauthorized access, misinterpretation or misuse;

• Care is taken in communication with patients and families to make clear that current genetic knowledge is incomplete and may be altered by future findings.

• Psychiatrists shall only refer people to facilities for diagnostic genetic testing if that facility has:

— Demonstrated satisfactory quality assurance, procedures for such testing;

— Adequate and easily accessible resources for genetic counseling.

Genetic counseling with regard to family planning or abortion shall be respectful of the patients' value system, while providing sufficient medical and psychiatric information to aid patients to make decisions they consider best for them.

FOUR ADDITIONAL SPECIFIC ETHICAL GUIDELINES

1) Ethics of Psychotherapy in Medicine

Medical treatments of any nature should be administered under the provisions of good practice guidelines regarding their indications, effectiveness, safety, and quality control. Psychotherapy, in its broadest sense, is an accepted component of many medical interactions. In a more specific and restricted sense, psychotherapy utilizes techniques involving verbal and non-verbal communication and interaction to achieve specified treatment goals in the care of specific disorders. Psychiatrists providing specific forms of psychotherapy must have appropriate training in such techniques. The general guidelines that apply to any medical treatment also apply to specific forms of psychotherapy in regard to its indications and outcomes, positive or negative. The effectiveness of psychotherapy and its place in a treatment plan are important subjects for both researchers and clinicians. Psychotherapy by psychiatrists is a form of treatment for mental and other illnesses and emotional problems. The treatment approach utilized is determined in concert by the doctor and patient and/or the patient's family and/or guardians following a careful history and examination employing all relevant clinical and laboratory studies. The approach employed should be specific to the disease and patient's needs and sensitive to personal, familial, religious and cultural factors. It should be based on sound research and clinical wisdom and have the purpose of removing, modifying or retarding symptoms or disturbed patterns of behavior. It should promote positive adaptations including personal growth and development.

Psychiatrists and other clinicians responsible for a patient have to ensure that these guidelines are fully applied. Therefore, the psychiatrist or other delegated qualified clinician, should determine the indications for psychotherapy and follow its development. In this context the essential notion is that the treatment is the consequence of a diagnosis and both are medical acts performed to take care of an ill person. These two levels of decisions, interventions and responsibilities are similar to other situations in clinical medicine, however this does not exclude other interventions such as rehabilitation which can be administered by non-medical personnel.

1. Like any other treatment in medicine, the prescription of psychotherapy should follow accepted guidelines for obtaining informed consent prior to the initiation of treatment as well as updating it in the course of treatment if goals and objectives of treatment are modified in a significant way.

2. If clinical wisdom, long standing and well-established practice patterns (this takes into consideration cultural and religious issues) and scientific evidence suggest potential clinical benefits to combining medication treatment with psychotherapy this should be brought to the patient's attention and fully discussed.

3. Psychotherapy explores intimate thoughts, emotions and fantasies, and as such may engender intense transference and counter-transference. In a psychotherapy relationship the power is unequally shared between the therapist and patient, and under no circumstances shall the psychotherapist use this relationship to personal advantage or transgress the boundaries established by the professional relationship.

4. At the initiation of psychotherapy, the patient shall be advised that information shared and health records will be kept in confidence except where the patient gives specific informed consent for release of information to third parties, or where a court order may require the production of records. The other exception is where there is a legal requirement to report certain information as in the case of child abuse.

2) Conflict of Interest in Relationship with Industry

Although most organizations and institutions, including the WPA, have rules and regulations governing their relationship with industry and donors, individual physicians are often involved in interactions with the pharmaceutical industry, or other granting agencies that could lead to ethical conflict In these situations psychiatrists should be mindful of and apply the following guidelines.

1. The practitioner must diligently guard against accepting gifts that could have an undue influence on professional work.

2. Psychiatrists conducting clinical trials are under an obligation to disclose to the Ethics Review Board and their research subjects their financial and contractual obligations and benefits related to the sponsor of the study. Every effort should be made to set up review boards composed of researchers, ethicists and community representatives to assure the rights of research subjects are protected.

3. Psychiatrists conducting clinical trials have to ensure that their patients have understood all aspects of the informed consent. The level of education or sophistication of the patient is no excuse for bypassing this commitment. If the patient is deemed incompetent the same rules would apply in obtaining informed consent from the substitute decision maker. Psychiatrists must be cognizant that covert commercial influence on the trial design, promotion of drugs trials without scientific value, breach of confidentiality, and restrictive contractual clauses regarding publication of results may each in different ways encroach upon the freedom of science and scientific information.

3) Conflicts Arising with Third Party Payers

The obligations of organizations toward shareholders or the administrator regarding maximization of profits and minimization of costs can be in conflict with the principles of good practice. Psychiatrists working in such potentially conflicting environments, should uphold the rights of the patients to receive the best treatment possible.

1. In agreement with the UN Resolution 46/119 of the "Principles for the Protection of Persons with Mental Illness," psychiatrists should oppose discriminatory practices which limit their benefits and entitlements, deny parity, curb the scope of treatment, or limit their access to proper medications for patients with a mental disorder.

2. Professional independence to apply best practice guidelines and clinical wisdom in upholding the welfare of the patient should be the primary considerations for the psychiatrist. It is also the duty of the psychiatrist to protect the patient privacy and confidentiality as part of preserving the sanctity and healing potential of the doctor-patient relationship.

4) Violating the Clinical Boundaries and Trust Between Psychiatrists and Patients

The psychiatrist-patient relationship may be the only relationship that permits an exploration of the deeply personal and emotional space, as granted by the patient. Within this relationship, the psychiatrist's respect for the humanity and dignity of the patient builds a foundation of trust that is essential for a comprehensive treatment plan. The relationship encourages the patient to explore deeply held strengths, weaknesses, fears, and desires, and many of these might be related to sexuality. Knowledge of these characteristics of the patient places the psychiatrist in a position of advantage that the patient allows on the expectation of trust and respect. Taking advantage of that knowledge by manipulating the patient's sexual fears and desires in order to obtain sexual access is a breach of the trust, regardless of consent. In the therapeutic relationship, consent on the part of the patient is considered vitiated by the knowledge the psychiatrists possess about the patient and by the power differential that vests the psychiatrist with special authority over the patient. Consent under these circumstances will be tantamount to exploitation of the patient.

The latent sexual dynamics inherent in all relationships can become manifest in the course of the therapeutic relationship and if they are not properly handled by the therapist can produce anguish to the patient. This anguish is likely to become more pronounced if seductive statements and inappropriate non-verbal behavior are used by the therapist. Under no circumstances, therefore, should a psychiatrist get involved with a patient in any form of sexual behavior, irrespective of whether this behavior is initiated by the patient or the therapist.

B. Research and Experimentation

Nuremberg Code (1947)

Trials of War Criminals before the Nuremberg Military Tribunals under Control Council Law No. 10. Nuremberg, Germany, October 1946-April 1949.
Washington, D.C.: U.S. G.P.O, 1949-1953, Vol. 2, pp. 181-182.
Available at http://ohsr.od.nih.gov/guidelines/nuremberg.html

PERMISSIBLE MEDICAL EXPERIMENTS

The great weight of the evidence before us is to the effect that certain types of medical experiments on human beings, when kept within reasonably well-defined bounds, conform to the ethics of the medical profession generally. The protagonists of the practice of human experimentation justify their views on the basis that such experiments yield results for the good of society that are unprocurable by other methods or means of study. All agree, however, that certain basic principles must be observed in order to satisfy moral, ethical and legal concepts:

1. The voluntary consent of the human subject is absolutely essential.

This means that the person involved should have legal capacity to give consent; should be so situated as to be able to exercise free power of choice, without the intervention of any element of force, fraud, deceit, duress, over-reaching, or other ulterior form of constraint or coercion; and should have sufficient knowledge and comprehension of the elements of the subject matter involved as to enable him to make an understanding and enlightened decision. This latter element requires that before the acceptance of an affirmative decision by the experimental subject there should be made known to him the nature, duration, and purpose of the experiment; the method and means by which it is to be conducted; all inconveniences and hazards reasonably to be expected; and the effects upon his health or person which may possibly come from his participation in the experiment.

The duty and responsibility for ascertaining the quality of the consent rests upon each individual who initiates, directs or engages in the experiment. It is a personal duty and responsibility which may not be delegated to another with impunity.

2. The experiment should be such as to yield fruitful results for the good of society, unprocurable by other methods or means of study, and not random and unnecessary in nature.

3. The experiment should be so designed and based on the results of animal experimentation and a knowledge of the natural history of the disease or other problem under study that the anticipated results will justify the performance of the experiment.

4. The experiment should be so conducted as to avoid all unnecessary physical and mental suffering and injury.

5. No experiment should be conducted where there is an *a priori* reason to believe that death or disabling injury will occur; except, perhaps, in those experiments where the experimental physicians also serve as subjects.

6. The degree of risk to be taken should never exceed that determined by the humanitarian importance of the problem to be solved by the experiment.

7. Proper preparations should be made and adequate facilities provided to protect the experimental subject against even remote possibilities of injury, disability, or death.

8. The experiment should be conducted only by scientifically qualified persons. The highest degree of skill and care should be required through all stages of the experiment of those who conduct or engage in the experiment.

9. During the course of the experiment the human subject should be at liberty to bring the experiment to an end if he has reached the physical or mental state where continuation of the experiment

seems to him to be impossible.

10. During the course of the experiment the scientist in charge must be prepared to terminate the experiment at any stage, if he has probable cause to believe, in the exercise of the good faith, superior skill and careful judgment required of him that a continuation of the experiment is likely to result in injury, disability, or death to the experimental subject.

International Covenant on Civil and Political Rights
Adopted and opened for signature, ratification and accession by General Assembly Resolution 2200A (XXI) of 16 December 1966.
Entered into force 23 March 1976.
[Available at http://www.unhchr.ch/html/menu3/b/a_ccpr.htm]

* * *

Article 7

No one shall be subjected to torture or to cruel, inhuman or degrading treatment or punishment. In particular, no one shall be subjected without his free consent to medical or scientific experimentation.

* * *

Human Rights Committee General Comment 20 (1992)
Human Rights Committee, General Comment 20, Article 7 (Forty-fourth session, 1992), Compilation of General Comments and General Recommendations.
Adopted by Human Rights Treaty Bodies. U.N. Doc. HRI\GEN\1\Rev.1 at 30 (1994).
[Available at http://www.unhchr.ch/tbs/doc.nsf/0/6924291970754969c12563ed004c8ae5?]

* * *

Article 7 expressly prohibits medical or scientific experimentation without the free consent of the person concerned. The Committee notes that the reports of States parties generally contain little information on this point. More attention should be given to the need and means to ensure observance of this provision. The Committee also observes that special protection in regard to such experiments is necessary in the case of persons not capable of giving valid consent, and in particular those under any form of detention or imprisonment. Such persons should not be subjected to any medical or scientific experimentation that may be detrimental to their health.

* * *

Declaration of Helsinki: Ethical Principles for Medical Research Involving Human Subjects (1964, 1975, 1983, 1996, 2000, 2002)

Adopted by the 18th WMA General Assembly, Helsinki, Finland, June 1964, and amended by the 29th WMA General Assembly, Tokyo, Japan, October 1975
35th WMA General Assembly, Venice, Italy, October 1983
41st WMA General Assembly, Hong Kong, September 1989
48th WMA General Assembly, Somerset West, Republic of South Africa, October 1996
and the 52nd WMA General Assembly, Edinburgh, Scotland, October 2000.
Note of Clarification on Paragraph 29 added by the WMA General Assembly, Washington 2002.
[Available at http://www.wma.net/e/policy/b3.htm]

A. AN INTRODUCTION

1. The World Medical Association has developed the Declaration of Helsinki as a statement of ethical principles to provide guidance to physicians and other participants in medical research involving human subjects. Medical research involving human subjects includes research on identifiable human material or identifiable data.

2. It is the duty of the physician to promote and safeguard the health of the people. The physician's knowledge and conscience are dedicated to the fulfillment of this duty.

3. The Declaration of Geneva of the World Medical Association binds the physician with the words, "The health of my patient will be my first consideration," and the International Code of Medical Ethics declares that, "A physician shall act only in the patient's interest when providing medical care which might have the effect of weakening the physical and mental condition of the patient."

4. Medical progress is based on research which ultimately must rest in part on experimentation involving human subjects.

5. In medical research on human subjects, considerations related to the well-being of the human subject should take precedence over the interests of science and society.

6. The primary purpose of medical research involving human subjects is to improve prophylactic, diagnostic and therapeutic procedures and the understanding of the aetiology and pathogenesis of disease. Even the best proven prophylactic, diagnostic, and therapeutic methods must continuously be challenged through research for their effectiveness, efficiency, accessibility and quality.

7. In current medical practice and in medical research, most prophylactic, diagnostic and therapeutic procedures involve risks and burdens.

8. Medical research is subject to ethical standards that promote respect for all human beings and protect their health and rights. Some research populations are vulnerable and need special protection. The particular needs of the economically and medically disadvantaged must be recognized. Special attention is also required for those who cannot give or refuse consent for themselves, for those who may be subject to giving consent under duress, for those who will not benefit personally from the research and for those for whom the research is combined with care.

9. Research Investigators should be aware of the ethical, legal and regulatory requirements for research on human subjects in their own countries as well as applicable international requirements. No national ethical, legal or regulatory requirement should be allowed to reduce or eliminate any of the protections for human subjects set forth in this Declaration.

B. BASIC PRINCIPLES FOR ALL MEDICAL RESEARCH

10. It is the duty of the physician in medical research to protect the life, health, privacy, and dignity of the human subject.

11. Medical research involving human subjects must conform to generally accepted scientific principles, be based on a thorough knowledge of

the scientific literature, other relevant sources of information, and on adequate laboratory and, where appropriate, animal experimentation.

12. Appropriate caution must be exercised in the conduct of research which may affect the environment, and the welfare of animals used for research must be respected.

13. The design and performance of each experimental procedure involving human subjects should be clearly formulated in an experimental protocol. This protocol should be submitted for consideration, comment, guidance, and where appropriate, approval to a specially appointed ethical review committee, which must be independent of the investigator, the sponsor or any other kind of undue influence. This independent committee should be in conformity with the laws and regulations of the country in which the research experiment is performed. The committee has the right to monitor ongoing trials. The researcher has the obligation to provide monitoring information to the committee, especially any serious adverse events. The researcher should also submit to the committee, for review, information regarding funding, sponsors, institutional affiliations, other potential conflicts of interest and incentives for subjects.

14. The research protocol should always contain a statement of the ethical considerations involved and should indicate that there is compliance with the principles enunciated in this Declaration.

15. Medical research involving human subjects should be conducted only by scientifically qualified persons and under the supervision of a clinically competent medical person. The responsibility for the human subject must always rest with a medically qualified person and never rest on the subject of the research, even though the subject has given consent.

16. Every medical research project involving human subjects should be preceded by careful assessment of predictable risks and burdens in comparison with foreseeable benefits to the subject or to others. This does not preclude the participation of healthy volunteers in medical research. The design of all studies should be publicly available.

17. Physicians should abstain from engaging in research projects involving human subjects unless they are confident that the risks involved have been adequately assessed and can be satisfactorily managed. Physicians should cease any investigation if the risks are found to outweigh the potential benefits or if there is conclusive proof of positive and beneficial results.

18. Medical research involving human subjects should only be conducted if the importance of the objective outweighs the inherent risks and burdens to the subject. This is especially important when the human subjects are healthy volunteers.

19. Medical research is only justified if there is a reasonable likelihood that the populations in which the research is carried out stand to benefit from the results of the research.

20. The subjects must be volunteers and informed participants in the research project.

21. The right of research subjects to safeguard their integrity must always be respected. Every precaution should be taken to respect the privacy of the subject, the confidentiality of the patient's information and to minimize the impact of the study on the subject's physical and mental integrity and on the personality of the subject.

22. In any research on human beings, each potential subject must be adequately informed of the aims, methods, sources of funding, any possible conflicts of interest, institutional affiliations of the researcher, the anticipated benefits and potential risks of the study and the discomfort it may entail. The subject should be informed of the right to abstain from participation in the study or to withdraw consent to participate at any time without reprisal. After ensuring that the subject has understood the information, the physician should then obtain the subject's freely-given informed consent, preferably in writing. If the consent cannot be obtained in writing, the non-written consent must be formally documented and witnessed.

23. When obtaining informed consent for the research project the physician should be particularly cautious if the subject is in a dependent relationship with the physician or may consent under

duress. In that case the informed consent should be obtained by a well-informed physician who is not engaged in the investigation and who is completely independent of this relationship.

24. For a research subject who is legally incompetent, physically or mentally incapable of giving consent or is a legally incompetent minor, the investigator must obtain informed consent from the legally authorized representative in accordance with applicable law. These groups should not be included in research unless the research is necessary to promote the health of the population represented and this research cannot instead be performed on legally competent persons.

25. When a subject deemed legally incompetent, such as a minor child, is able to give assent to decisions about participation in research, the investigator must obtain that assent in addition to the consent of the legally authorized representative.

26. Research on individuals from whom it is not possible to obtain consent, including proxy or advance consent, should be done only if the physical/mental condition that prevents obtaining informed consent is a necessary characteristic of the research population. The specific reasons for involving research subjects with a condition that renders them unable to give informed consent should be stated in the experimental protocol for consideration and approval of the review committee. The protocol should state that consent to remain in the research should be obtained as soon as possible from the individual or a legally authorized surrogate.

27. Both authors and publishers have ethical obligations. In publication of the results of research, the investigators are obliged to preserve the accuracy of the results. Negative as well as positive results should be published or otherwise publicly available. Sources of funding, institutional affiliations and any possible conflicts of interest should be declared in the publication. Reports of experimentation not in accordance with the principles laid down in this Declaration should not be accepted for publication.

C. ADDITIONAL PRINCIPLES FOR MEDICAL RESEARCH COMBINED WITH MEDICAL CARE

28. The physician may combine medical research with medical care, only to the extent that the research is justified by its potential prophylactic, diagnostic or therapeutic value. When medical research is combined with medical care, additional standards apply to protect the patients who are research subjects.

29. The benefits, risks, burdens and effectiveness of a new method should be tested against those of the best current prophylactic, diagnostic, and therapeutic methods. This does not exclude the use of placebo, or no treatment, in studies where no proven prophylactic, diagnostic or therapeutic method exists. [See footnote.]

30. At the conclusion of the study, every patient entered into the study should be assured of access to the best proven prophylactic, diagnostic and therapeutic methods identified by the study.

31. The physician should fully inform the patient which aspects of the care are related to the research. The refusal of a patient to participate in a study must never interfere with the patient-physician relationship.

32. In the treatment of a patient, where proven prophylactic, diagnostic and therapeutic methods do not exist or have been ineffective, the physician, with informed consent from the patient, must be free to use unproven or new prophylactic, diagnostic and therapeutic measures, if in the physician's judgement it offers hope of saving life, reestablishing health or alleviating suffering. Where possible, these measures should be made the object of research, designed to evaluate their safety and efficacy. In all cases, new information should be recorded and, where appropriate, published. The other relevant guidelines of this Declaration should be followed.

Footnote: Note of clarification on paragraph 29 of the WMA Declaration of Helsinki.

The WMA hereby reaffirms its position that extreme care must be taken in making use of a placebo-controlled trial and that in general this methodology should only be used in the absence of existing proven therapy. However, a placebo-controlled trial may be ethically acceptable, even if proven therapy is available, under the following circumstances:

• Where for compelling and scientifically sound methodological reasons its use is necessary to determine the efficacy or safety of a prophylactic, diagnostic or therapeutic method; or

• Where a prophylactic, diagnostic or therapeutic method is being investigated for a minor condition and the patients who receive placebo will not be subject to any additional risk of serious or irreversible harm.

All other provisions of the Declaration of Helsinki must be adhered to, especially the need for appropriate ethical and scientific review.

International Ethical Guidelines for Biomedical Research Involving Human Subjects (2002)

Prepared by the Council for International Organizations of Medical Sciences (CIOMS) in collaboration with the World Health Organization (WHO), Geneva, Switzerland, 2002. [Available at http://www.cioms.ch/frame_guidelines_nov_2002.htm]

BACKGROUND

The new text, the 2002 text, which supersedes that of 1993, consists of a statement of general ethical principles, a preamble and 21 guidelines, with an introduction and a brief account of earlier declarations and guidelines. Like the 1982 and 1993 Guidelines, the present publication is designed to be of use, particularly to low-resource countries, in defining national policies on the ethics of biomedical research, applying ethical standards in local circumstances, and establishing or redefining adequate mechanisms for ethical review of research involving human subjects …

Not specifically concerned with biomedical research involving human subjects but clearly pertinent … are international human rights instruments. These are mainly the Universal Declaration of Human Rights, which, particularly in its science provisions, was highly influenced by the Nuremberg Code; the International Covenant on Civil and Political Rights; and the International Covenant on Economic, Social and Cultural Rights. Since the Nuremberg experience, human rights law has expanded to include the protection of women (Convention on the Elimination of All Forms of Discrimination Against Women) and children (Convention on the Rights of the Child). These and other such international instruments endorse in terms of human rights the general ethical principles that underlie the CIOMS International Ethical Guidelines.

GENERAL ETHICAL PRINCIPLES

All research involving human subjects should be conducted in accordance with three basic ethical principles, namely respect for persons, beneficence and justice. It is generally agreed that these principles, which in the abstract have equal moral force, guide the conscientious preparation of proposals for scientific studies. In varying circumstances they may be expressed differently and given different moral weight, and their application may lead to different decisions or courses of action. The present guidelines are directed at the application of these principles to research involving human subjects.

Respect for persons incorporates at least two fundamental ethical considerations, namely:

a) respect for autonomy, which requires that those who are capable of deliberation about their personal choices should be treated with respect for their capacity for self-determination; and

b) protection of persons with impaired or diminished autonomy, which requires that those who are dependent or vulnerable be afforded security against harm or abuse.

Beneficence refers to the ethical obligation to maximize benefits and to minimize harms. This principle gives rise to norms requiring that the risks of research be reasonable in the light of the expected benefits, that the research design be sound, and that the investigators be competent both to conduct the research and to safeguard the welfare of the research subjects. Beneficence further proscribes the deliberate infliction of harm on persons; this aspect of beneficence is sometimes expressed as a separate principle, non-maleficence (do no harm).

Justice refers to the ethical obligation to treat each person in accordance with what is morally right and proper, to give each person what is due to him or her. In the ethics of research involving human subjects the principle refers primarily to distributive justice, which requires the equitable distribution of both the burdens and the benefits of participation in research. Differences in distribution of burdens and benefits are justifiable only if they are based on morally relevant distinctions between persons; one such distinction is vulnerability. "Vulnerability" refers to a substantial incapacity to protect one's own interests owing to such impediments as lack of capability to give informed consent, lack of alternative means of obtaining medical care or other expensive necessities, or being a junior or subordinate member of a hierarchical group. Accordingly, special provision must be made for the protection of the rights and welfare of vulnerable persons.

Sponsors of research or investigators cannot, in general, be held accountable for unjust conditions where the research is conducted, but they must refrain from practices that are likely to worsen unjust conditions or contribute to new inequities. Neither should they take advantage of the relative inability of low-resource countries or vulnerable populations to protect their own interests by conducting research inexpensively and avoiding complex regulatory systems of industrialized countries in order to develop products for the lucrative markets of those countries.

In general, the research project should leave low-resource countries or communities better off than previously or, at least, no worse off. It should be responsive to their health needs and priorities in that any product developed is made reasonably available to them, and as far as possible leave the population in a better position to obtain effective health care and protect its own health.

Justice requires also that the research be responsive to the health conditions or needs of vulnerable subjects. The subjects selected should be the least vulnerable necessary to accomplish the purposes of the research. Risk to vulnerable subjects is most easily justified when it arises from interventions or procedures that hold out for them the prospect of direct health-related benefit. Risk that does not hold out such prospect must be justified by the anticipated benefit to the population of which the individual research subject is representative.

PREAMBLE

The term "research" refers to a class of activity designed to develop or contribute to generalizable knowledge. Generalizable knowledge consists of theories, principles or relationships, or the accumulation of information on which they are based, that can be corroborated by accepted scientific methods of observation and inference. In the present context "research" includes both medical and behavioral studies pertaining to human health. Usually "research" is modified by the adjective "biomedical" to indicate its relation to health.

Progress in medical care and disease prevention depends upon an understanding of physiological and pathological processes or epidemiological findings, and requires at some time research involving human subjects. The collection, analysis and interpretation of information obtained from research involving human beings contribute significantly to the improvement of human health. Research involving human subjects includes:

• studies of a physiological, biochemical or pathological process, or of the response to a specific intervention — whether physical, chemical or psychological — in healthy subjects or patients;

• controlled trials of diagnostic, preventive or therapeutic measures in larger groups of persons, designed to demonstrate a specific generalizable response to these measures against a background of individual biological variation;

• studies designed to determine the consequences for individuals and communities of specific preventive or therapeutic measures; and

• studies concerning human health-related behaviour in a variety of circumstances and environments.

Research involving human subjects may employ either observation or physical, chemical or psychological intervention; it may also either generate records or make use of existing records containing biomedical or other information about individuals who may or may not be identifiable from the records or information. The use of such records and the protection of the confidentiality of data obtained from those records are discussed in *International Guidelines for Ethical Review of Epidemiological Studies* (CIOMS, 1991).

The research may be concerned with the social environment, manipulating environmental factors in a way that could affect incidentally exposed individuals. It is defined in broad terms in order to embrace field studies of pathogenic organisms and toxic chemicals under investigation for health-related purposes.

Biomedical research with human subjects is to be distinguished from the practice of medicine, public health and other forms of health care, which is designed to contribute directly to the health of individuals or communities. Prospective subjects may find it confusing when research and practice are to be conducted simultaneously, as when research is designed to obtain new information about the efficacy of a drug or other therapeutic, diagnostic or preventive modality.

As stated in Paragraph 32 of the Declaration of Helsinki, "In the treatment of a patient, where proven prophylactic, diagnostic and therapeutic methods do not exist or have been ineffective, the physician, with informed consent from the patient, must be free to use unproven or new prophylactic, diagnostic and therapeutic measures, if in the physician's judgment it offers hope of saving life, re-establishing health or alleviating suffering. Where possible, these measures should be made the object of research, designed to evaluate their safety and efficacy. In all cases, new information should be recorded and, where appropriate, published. The other relevant guidelines of this Declaration should be followed."

Professionals whose roles combine investigation and treatment have a special obligation to protect the rights and welfare of the patient-subjects. An investigator who agrees to act as physician-investigator undertakes some or all of the legal and eth-ical responsibilities of the subject's primary-care physician. In such a case, if the subject withdraws from the research owing to complications related to the research or in the exercise of the right to withdraw without loss of benefit, the physician has an obligation to continue to provide medical care, or to see that the subject receives the necessary care in the health-care system, or to offer assistance in finding another physician.

Research with human subjects should be carried out only by, or strictly supervised by, suitably qualified and experienced investigators and in accordance with a protocol that clearly states: the aim of the research; the reasons for proposing that it involve human subjects; the nature and degree of any known risks to the subjects; the sources from which it is proposed to recruit subjects; and the means proposed for ensuring that subjects' consent will be adequately informed and voluntary. The protocol should be scientifically and ethically appraised by one or more suitably constituted review bodies, independent of the investigators.

New vaccines and medicinal drugs, before being approved for general use, must be tested on human subjects in clinical trials; such trials constitute a substantial part of all research involving human subjects.

THE GUIDELINES

[The commentaries, which follow each guideline, are omitted.]

Guideline 1: Ethical justification and scientific validity of biomedical research involving human subjects (1993)

The ethical justification of biomedical research involving human subjects is the prospect of discovering new ways of benefiting people's health. Such research can be ethically justifiable only if it is carried out in ways that respect and protect, and are fair to, the subjects of that research and are morally acceptable within the communities in which the research is carried out. Moreover, because scientifically invalid research is unethical in that it exposes research subjects to risks without possible benefit, investigators and sponsors must ensure that proposed studies involving human subjects conform to generally accepted scientific principles and are based on adequate knowledge of the pertinent scientific literature.

Guideline 2: Ethical review committees

All proposals to conduct research involving human subjects must be submitted for review of their scientific merit and ethical acceptability to one or more scientific review and ethical review committees. The review committees must be independent of the research team, and any direct financial or other material benefit they may derive from the research should not be contingent on the outcome of their review. The investigator must obtain their approval or clearance before undertaking the research. The ethical review committee should conduct further reviews as necessary in the course of the research, including monitoring of the progress of the study.

Guideline 3: Ethical review of externally sponsored research

An external sponsoring organization and individual investigators should submit the research protocol for ethical and scientific review in the country of the sponsoring organization, and the ethical standards applied should be no less stringent than they would be for research carried out in that country. The health authorities of the host country, as well as a national or local ethical review committee, should ensure that the proposed research is responsive to the health needs and priorities of the host country and meets the requisite ethical standards.

Guideline 4: Individual informed consent

For all biomedical research involving humans the investigator must obtain the voluntary informed consent of the prospective subject or, in the case of an individual who is not capable of giving informed consent, the permission of a legally authorized representative in accordance with applicable law. Waiver of informed consent is to be regarded as uncommon and exceptional, and must in all cases be approved by an ethical review committee.

Guideline 5: Obtaining informed consent: Essential information for prospective research subjects

Before requesting an individual's consent to participate in research, the investigator must provide the following information, in language or another form of communication that the individual can understand:

1. that the individual is invited to participate in research, the reasons for considering the individual suitable for the research, and that participation is voluntary;

2. that the individual is free to refuse to participate and will be free to withdraw from the research at any time without penalty or loss of benefits to which he or she would otherwise be entitled;

3. the purpose of the research, the procedures to be carried out by the investigator and the subject, and an explanation of how the research differs from routine medical care;

4. for controlled trials, an explanation of features of the research design (e.g., randomization, double-blinding), and that the subject will not be told of the assigned treatment until the study has been completed and the blind has been broken;

5. the expected duration of the individual's participation (including number and duration of visits to the research centre and the total time involved) and the possibility of early termination of the trial or of the individual's participation in it;

6. whether money or other forms of material goods will be provided in return for the individual's participation and, if so, the kind and amount;

7. that, after the completion of the study, subjects will be informed of the findings of the research in general, and individual subjects will be informed of any finding that relates to their particular health status;

8. that subjects have the right of access to their data on demand, even if these data lack immediate clinical utility (unless the ethical review committee has approved temporary or permanent non-disclosure of data, in which case the subject should be informed of, and given, the reasons for such non-disclosure);

9. any foreseeable risks, pain or discomfort, or inconvenience to the individual (or others) associated with participation in the research, including risks to the health or well-being of a subject's spouse or partner;

10. the direct benefits, if any, expected to result to subjects from participating in the research;

11. the expected benefits of the research to the community or to society at large, or contributions to scientific knowledge;

12. whether, when and how any products or interventions proven by the research to be safe and effective will be made available to subjects after they have completed their participation in the research, and whether they will be expected to pay for them;

13. any currently available alternative interventions or courses of treatment;

14. The provisions that will be made to ensure respect for the privacy of subjects and for the confidentiality of records in which subjects are identified;

15. the limits, legal or other, to the investigators' ability to safeguard confidentiality, and the possible consequences of breaches of confidentiality;

16. policy with regard to the use of results of genetic tests and familial genetic information, and the precautions in place to prevent disclosure of the results of a subject's genetic tests to immediate family relatives or to others (e.g., insurance companies or employers) without the consent of the subject;

17. the sponsors of the research, the institutional affiliation of the investigators, and the nature and sources of funding for the research;

18. the possible research uses, direct or secondary, of the subject's medical records and of biological specimens taken in the course of clinical care (See also Guidelines 4 and 18 Commentaries);

19. whether it is planned that biological specimens collected in the research will be destroyed at its conclusion, and, if not, details about their storage (where, how, for how long, and final disposition) and possible future use, and that subjects have the right to decide about such future use, to refuse storage, and to have the material destroyed (See Guideline 4 Commentary);

20. whether commercial products may be developed from biological specimens, and whether the participant will receive monetary or other benefits from the development of such products;

21. whether the investigator is serving only as an investigator or as both investigator and the subject's physician;

22. the extent of the investigator's responsibility to provide medical services to the participant;

23. that treatment will be provided free of charge for specified types of research-related injury or for complications associated with the research, the nature and duration of such care, the name of the organization or individual that will provide the treatment, and whether there is any uncertainty regarding funding of such treatment;

24. in what way, and by what organization, the subject or the subject's family or dependents will be compensated for disability or death resulting from such injury (or, when indicated, that there are no plans to provide such compensation);

25. whether or not, in the country in which the prospective subject is invited to participate in research, the right to compensation is legally guaranteed;

26. that an ethical review committee has approved or cleared the research protocol.

Guideline 6: Obtaining informed consent: Obligations of sponsors and investigators

Sponsors and investigators have a duty to:

• refrain from unjustified deception, undue influence, or intimidation;

• seek consent only after ascertaining that the prospective subject has adequate understanding of the relevant facts and of the consequences of participation and has had sufficient opportunity to consider whether to participate;

• as a general rule, obtain from each prospective subject a signed form as evidence of informed consent — investigators should justify any exceptions to this general rule and obtain the approval of the ethical review committee (See Guideline 4 Commentary, Documentation of consent);

• renew the informed consent of each subject if there are significant changes in the conditions or procedures of the research or if new information becomes available that could affect the willingness of subjects to continue to participate; and,

• renew the informed consent of each subject in long-term studies at pre-determined intervals, even if there are no changes in the design or objectives of the research.

Guideline 7: Inducement to participate

Subjects may be reimbursed for lost earnings, travel costs and other expenses incurred in taking part in a study; they may also receive free medical services. Subjects, particularly those who receive no direct benefit from research, may also be paid or otherwise compensated for inconvenience and time spent. The payments should not be so large, however, or the medical services so extensive as to induce prospective subjects to consent to participate in the research against their better judgment ("undue inducement"). All payments, reimbursements and medical services provided to research subjects must have been approved by an ethical review committee.

Guideline 8: Benefits and risks of study participation

For all biomedical research involving human subjects, the investigator must ensure that potential benefits and risks are reasonably balanced and risks are minimized.

• Interventions or procedures that hold out the prospect of direct diagnostic, therapeutic or preventive benefit for the individual subject must be justified by the expectation that they will be at least as advantageous to the individual subject, in the light of foreseeable risks and benefits, as any available alternative. Risks of such "beneficial" interventions or procedures must be justified in relation to expected benefits to the individual subject.

• Risks of interventions that do not hold out the prospect of direct diagnostic, therapeutic or preventive benefit for the individual must be justified in relation to the expected benefits to society (generalizable knowledge). The risks presented by such interventions must be reasonable in relation to the importance of the knowledge to be gained.

Guideline 9: Special limitations on risk when research involves individuals who are not capable of giving informed consent

When there is ethical and scientific justification to conduct research with individuals incapable of giving informed consent, the risk from research interventions that do not hold out the prospect of direct benefit for the individual subject should be no more likely and not greater than the risk attached to routine medical or psychological examination of such persons. Slight or minor increases above such risk may be permitted when there is an overriding scientific or medical rationale for such increases and when an ethical review committee has approved them.

Guideline 10: Research in populations and communities with limited resources

Before undertaking research in a population or community with limited resources, the sponsor and the investigator must make every effort to ensure that:

• the research is responsive to the health needs and the priorities of the population or community in which it is to be carried out; and

• any intervention or product developed, or knowledge generated, will be made reasonably available for the benefit of that population or community.

Guideline 11: Choice of control in clinical trials

As a general rule, research subjects in the control group of a trial of a diagnostic, therapeutic, or preventive intervention should receive an established effective intervention. In some circumstances it may be ethically acceptable to use an alternative comparator, such as placebo or "no treatment".

Placebo may be used:

• when there is no established effective intervention;

• when withholding an established effective intervention would expose subjects to, at most, temporary discomfort or delay in relief of symptoms;

• when use of an established effective intervention as comparator would not yield scientifically reliable results and use of placebo would not add any risk of serious or irreversible harm to the subjects.

Guideline 12: Equitable distribution of burdens and benefits in the selection of groups of subjects in research

Groups or communities to be invited to be subjects of research should be selected in such a way that the burdens and benefits of the research will be equitably distributed. The exclusion of groups or communities that might benefit from study participation must be justified.

Guideline 13: Research involving vulnerable persons

Special justification is required for inviting vulnerable individuals to serve as research subjects and, if they are selected, the means of protecting their rights and welfare must be strictly applied.

Guideline 14: Research involving children

Before undertaking research involving children, the investigator must ensure that:

• the research might not equally well be carried out with adults;

• the purpose of the research is to obtain knowledge relevant to the health needs of children;

• a parent or legal representative of each child has given permission;

• the agreement (assent) of each child has been obtained to the extent of the child's capabilities; and,

• a child's refusal to participate or continue in the research will be respected.

Guideline 15: Research involving individuals who by reason of mental or behavioral disorders are not capable of giving adequately informed consent

Before undertaking research involving individuals who by reason of mental or behavioral disorders are not capable of giving adequately informed consent, the investigator must ensure that:

• such persons will not be subjects of research that might equally well be carried out on persons whose capacity to give adequately informed consent is not impaired;

• the purpose of the research is to obtain knowledge relevant to the particular health needs of persons with mental or behavioral disorders;

• the consent of each subject has been obtained to the extent of that person's capabilities, and a prospective subject's refusal to participate in research is always respected, unless, in exceptional circumstances, there is no reasonable medical alternative and local law permits overriding the objection; and,

• in cases where prospective subjects lack capacity to consent, permission is obtained from a responsible family member or a legally authorized representative in accordance with applicable law.

Guideline 16: Women as research subjects

Investigators, sponsors or ethical review committees should not exclude women of reproductive age from biomedical research. The potential for becoming pregnant during a study should not, in itself, be used as a reason for precluding or limiting participation. However, a thorough discussion of risks to the pregnant woman and to her fetus is a prerequisite for the woman's ability to make a rational decision to enroll in a clinical study. In this discussion, if participation in the research might be hazardous to a fetus or a woman if she becomes pregnant, the sponsors/investigators should guarantee the prospective subject a pregnancy test and access to effective contraceptive methods before the research commences. Where such access is not possible, for legal or religious reasons, investigators should not recruit for such possibly hazardous research women who might become pregnant.

Guideline 17: Pregnant women as research participants

Pregnant women should be presumed to be eligible for participation in biomedical research. Investigators and ethical review committees should ensure that prospective subjects who are pregnant are adequately informed about the risks and benefits to themselves, their pregnancies, the fetus and their subsequent offspring, and to their fertility.

Research in this population should be performed only if it is relevant to the particular health needs of a pregnant woman or her fetus, or to the health needs of pregnant women in general, and, when appropriate, if it is supported by reliable evidence from animal experiments, particularly as to risks of teratogenicity and mutagenicity.

Guideline 18: Safeguarding confidentiality

The investigator must establish secure safeguards of the confidentiality of subjects' research data. Subjects should be told the limits, legal or other, to the investigators' ability to safeguard confidentiality and the possible consequences of breaches of confidentiality.

Guideline 19: Right of injured subjects to treatment and compensation

Investigators should ensure that research subjects who suffer injury as a result of their participation are entitled to free medical treatment for such injury and to such financial or other assistance as would compensate them equitably for any resultant impairment, disability or handicap. In the case of death as a result of their participation, their dependents are entitled to compensation. Subjects must not be asked to waive the right to compensation.

Guideline 20: Strengthening capacity for ethical and scientific review and biomedical research

Many countries lack the capacity to assess or ensure the scientific quality or ethical acceptability of biomedical research proposed or carried out in their jurisdictions. In externally sponsored collab-

orative research, sponsors and investigators have an ethical obligation to ensure that biomedical research projects for which they are responsible in such countries contribute effectively to national or local capacity to design and conduct biomedical research, and to provide scientific and ethical review and monitoring of such research.

Capacity-building may include, but is not limited to, the following activities:

• establishing and strengthening independent and competent ethical review processes/ committees

• strengthening research capacity

• developing technologies appropriate to health-care and biomedical research

• training of research and health-care staff

• educating the community from which research subjects will be drawn.

(See also Guideline 10: Research in populations and communities with limited resources.)

Guideline 21: Ethical obligation of external sponsors to provide health-care services

External sponsors are ethically obliged to ensure the availability of:

• health-care services that are essential to the safe conduct of the research;

• treatment for subjects who suffer injury as a consequence of research interventions; and,

• services that are a necessary part of the commitment of a sponsor to make a beneficial intervention or product developed as a result of the research reasonably available to the population or community concerned.

[See also International Guidelines for Ethical Review of Epidemiological Studies (Council for International Organizations of Medical Sciences, CIOMS, 1997).]

C. Treatment of Prisoners and Detainees

Note: Other documents relating to torture are located in Part III B.

Standard Minimum Rules for the Treatment of Prisoners and for the Effective Implementation of the Standard Minimum Rules (1955, 1957,1977)

Adopted on 30 August 1955 by the First United Nations Congress on the Prevention of Crime and the Treatment of Offenders. UN Doc. A/CONF/611/annex1, and approved by the Economic and Social Council in Resolution 663C (XXIV) of 31 July 1957 and 2076 (LXII) of 13 May 1977. [Available at http://www.unhcr.ch/html/menu3/b/h_comp34.htm]

PRELIMINARY OBSERVATIONS

1. The following rules are not intended to describe in detail a model system of penal institutions. They seek only, on the basis of the general consensus of contemporary thought and the essential elements of the most adequate systems of today, to set out what is generally accepted as being good principle and practice in the treatment of prisoners and the management of institutions.

2. In view of the great variety of legal, social, economic and geographical conditions of the world, it is evident that not all of the rules are capable of application in all places and at all times. They should, however, serve to stimulate a constant endeavour to overcome practical difficulties in the way of their application, in the knowledge that they represent, as a whole, the minimum conditions which are accepted as suitable by the United Nations.

3. On the other hand, the rules cover a field in which thought is constantly developing. They are not intended to preclude experiment and practices, provided these are in harmony with the principles and seek to further the purposes which derive from the text of the rules as a whole. It will always be justifiable for the central prison administration to authorize departures from the rules in this spirit.

4. (1) Part I of the rules covers the general management of institutions, and is applicable to all categories of prisoners, criminal or civil, untried or convicted, including prisoners subject to "security measures" or corrective measures ordered by the judge.

(2) Part II contains rules applicable only to the special categories dealt with in each section. Nevertheless, the rules under section A, applicable to prisoners under sentence, shall be equally applicable to categories of prisoners dealt with in sections B, C and D, provided they do not conflict with the rules governing those categories and are for their benefit.

5. (1) The rules do not seek to regulate the management of institutions set aside for young persons such as Borstal institutions or correctional schools, but in general part I would be equally applicable in such institutions.

(2) The category of young prisoners should include at least all young persons who come within the jurisdiction of juvenile courts. As a rule, such young persons should not be sentenced to imprisonment.

PART I RULES OF GENERAL APPLICATION

Basic Principle

6. (1) The following rules shall be applied impartially. There shall be no discrimination on grounds of race, colour, sex, language, religion, political or other opinion, national or social origin, property, birth or other status.

(2) On the other hand, it is necessary to respect the religious beliefs and moral precepts of the group to which a prisoner belongs.

* * *

10. All accommodation provided for the use of prisoners and in particular all sleeping accommodation shall meet all requirements of health, due regard being paid to climactic conditions and particularly to cubic content of air, minimum floor space, lighting, heating and ventilation.

11. In all places where prisoners are required to live or work,

(a) The windows shall be large enough to enable the prisoners to read or work by natural light, and shall be so constructed that they can allow the entrance of fresh air whether or not there is artificial ventilation;

(b) Artificial light shall be provided sufficient for the prisoners to read or work without injury to eyesight.

12. The sanitary installations shall be adequate to enable every prisoner to comply with the needs of nature when necessary and in a clean and decent manner.

13. Adequate bathing and shower installations shall be provided so that every prisoner may be enabled and required to have a bath or shower, at a temperature suitable to the climate, as frequently as necessary for general hygiene according to season and geographical region, but at least once a week in a temperate climate.

14. All pans of an institution regularly used by prisoners shall be properly maintained and kept scrupulously clean at all times.

Personal Hygiene

15. Prisoners shall be required to keep their persons clean, and to this end they shall be provided with water and with such toilet articles as are necessary for health and cleanliness.

16. In order that prisoners may maintain a good appearance compatible with their self-respect, facilities shall be provided for the proper care of the hair and beard, and men shall be enabled to shave regularly.

Clothing and Bedding

17. (1) Every prisoner who is not allowed to wear his own clothing shall be provided with an outfit of clothing suitable for the climate and adequate to keep him in good health. Such clothing shall in no manner be degrading or humiliating.

(2) All clothing shall be clean and kept in proper condition. Underclothing shall be changed and washed as often as necessary for the maintenance of hygiene.

(3) In exceptional circumstances, whenever a prisoner is removed outside the institution for an authorized purpose, he shall be allowed to wear his own clothing or other inconspicuous clothing.

18. If prisoners are allowed to wear their own clothing, arrangements shall be made on their admission to the institution to ensure that it shall be clean and fit for use.

19. Every prisoner shall, in accordance with local or national standards, be provided with a separate bed, and with separate and sufficient bedding which shall be clean when issued, kept in good order and changed often enough to ensure its cleanliness.

Food

20. (1) Every prisoner shall be provided by the administration at the usual hours with food of nutritional value adequate for health and strength, of wholesome quality and well prepared and served.

(2) Drinking water shall be available to every prisoner whenever he needs it.

Exercise and Sport

21. (1) Every prisoner who is not employed in outdoor work shall have at least one hour of suitable exercise in the open air daily if the weather permits.

(2) Young prisoners, and others of suitable age and physique, shall receive physical and recreational training during the period of exercise. To this end space, installations and equipment should be provided.

Medical Services

22. (1) At every institution there shall be available the services of at least one qualified medical of-

ficer who should have some knowledge of psychiatry. The medical services should be organized in close relationship to the general health administration of the community or nation. They shall include a psychiatric service for the diagnosis and, in proper cases, the treatment of states of mental abnormality.

(2) Sick prisoners who require specialist treatment shall be transferred to specialized institutions or to civil hospitals. Where hospital facilities are provided in an institution, their equipment, furnishings and pharmaceutical supplies shall be proper for the medical care and treatment of sick prisoners, and there shall be a staff of suitable trained officers.

(3) The services of a qualified dental officer shall be available to every prisoner.

23. (1) In women's institutions there shall be special accommodation for all necessary pre-natal and post-natal care and treatment. Arrangements shall be made wherever practicable for children to be born in a hospital outside the institution. If a child is born in prison, this fact shall not be mentioned in the birth certificate.

(2) Where nursing infants are allowed to remain in the institution with their mothers, provision shall be made for a nursery staffed by qualified persons, where the infants shall be placed when they are not in the care of their mothers.

24. The medical officer shall see and examine every prisoner as soon as possible after his admission and thereafter as necessary, with a view particularly to the discovery of physical or mental illness and the taking of all necessary measures; the segregation of prisoners suspected of infectious or contagious conditions; the noting of physical or mental defects which might hamper rehabilitation, and the determination of the physical capacity of every prisoner for work.

25. (1) The medical officer shall have the care of the physical and mental health of the prisoners and should daily see all sick prisoners, all who complain of illness, and any prisoner to whom his attention is specially directed.

(2) The medical officer shall report to the director whenever he considers that a prisoner's physical or mental health has been or will be injuriously affected by continued imprisonment or by any condition of imprisonment.

26. (1) The medical officer shall regularly inspect and advise the director upon:

(a) The quantity, quality, preparation and service of food;

(b) The hygiene and cleanliness of the institution and the prisoners;

(c) The sanitation, heating, lighting and ventilation of the institution;

(d) The suitability and cleanliness of the prisoners' clothing and bedding;

(e) The observance of the rules concerning physical education and sports, in cases where there is no technical personnel in charge of these activities.

(2) The director shall take into consideration the reports and advice that the medical officer submits according to rules 25 (2) and 26 and, in case he concurs with the recommendations made, shall take immediate steps to give effect to those recommendations; if they are not within his competence or if he does not concur with them, he shall immediately submit his own report and the advice of the medical officer to higher authority.

* * *

32. (1) Punishment by close confinement or reduction of diet shall never be inflicted unless the medical officer has examined the prisoner and certified in writing that he is fit to sustain it.

(2) The same shall apply to any other punishment that may be prejudicial to the physical or mental health of a prisoner. In no case may such punishment be contrary to or depart from the principle stated in rule 31.

(3) The medical officer shall visit daily prisoners undergoing such punishments and shall advise the director if he considers the termination or alteration of the punishment necessary on grounds of physical or mental health.

Instruments of Restraint

33. Instruments of restraint, such as handcuffs, chains, irons and strait-jacket, shall never be applied as a punishment. Furthermore, chains or irons shall not be used as restraints. Other instruments of restraint shall not be used except in the following circumstances:

(a) As a precaution against escape during a transfer, provided that they shall be removed when the prisoner appears before a judicial or administrative authority;

(b) On medical grounds by direction of the medical officer;

(c) By order of the director, if other methods of control fail, in order to prevent a prisoner from injuring himself or others or from damaging property; in such instances the director shall at once consult the medical officer and report to the higher administrative authority.

34. The patterns and manner of use of instruments of restraint shall be decided by the central prison administration. Such instruments must not be applied for any longer time than is strictly necessary.

* * *

Notification of Death, Illness, Transfer, etc.

44. (1) Upon the death or serious illness of, or serious injury to a prisoner, or his removal to an institution for the treatment of mental affections, the director shall at once inform the spouse, if the prisoner is married, or the nearest relative and shall in any event inform any other person previously designated by the prisoner.

(2) A prisoner shall be informed at once of the death or serious illness of any near relative. In case of the critical illness of a near relative, the prisoner should be authorized, whenever circumstances allow, to go to his bedside either under escort or alone.

(3) Every prisoner shall have the right to inform at once his family of his imprisonment or his transfer to another institution.

Removal of Prisoners

45. (1) When the prisoners are being removed to or from an institution, they shall be exposed to public view as little as possible, and proper safeguards shall be adopted to protect them from insult, curiosity and publicity in any form.

(2) The transport of prisoners in conveyances with inadequate ventilation or light, or in any way which would subject them to unnecessary physical hardship, shall be prohibited.

(3) The transport of prisoners shall be carried out at the expense of the administration and equal conditions shall obtain for all of them.

Institutional Personnel

49. (1) So far as possible, the personnel shall include a sufficient number of specialists such as psychiatrists, psychologists, social workers, teachers and trade instructors.

(2) The services of social workers, teachers and trade instructors shall be secured on a permanent basis, without thereby excluding part-time or voluntary workers.

PART II RULES APPLICABLE TO SPECIAL CATEGORIES

A. PRISONERS UNDER SENTENCE

Guiding Principles

56. The guiding principles hereafter are intended to show the spirit in which penal institutions should be administered and the purposes at which they should aim, in accordance with the declaration made under Preliminary Observation 1 of the present text.

57. Imprisonment and other measures which result in cutting off an offender from the outside world are afflictive by the very fact of taking from the person the right of self-determination by depriving him of his liberty. Therefore the prison system shall not, except as incidental to justifiable segregation or the maintenance of discipline, aggravate the suffering inherent in such a situation.

58. The purpose and justification of a sentence of imprisonment or a similar measure deprivative of

liberty is ultimately to protect society against crime. This end can only be achieved if the period of imprisonment is used to ensure, so far as possible, that upon his return to society the offender is not only willing but able to lead a law-abiding and self-supporting life.

59. To this end, the institution should utilize all the remedial, educational, moral, spiritual and other forces and forms of assistance which are appropriate and available, and should seek to apply them according to the individual treatment needs of the prisoners.

60. (1) The regime of the institution should seek to minimize any differences between prison life and life at liberty which tend to lessen the responsibility of the prisoners or the respect due to their dignity as human beings.

(2) Before the completion of the sentence, it is desirable that the necessary steps be taken to ensure for the prisoner a gradual return to life in society. This aim may be achieved, depending on the case, by a pre-release regime organized in the same institution or in another appropriate institution, or by release on trial under some kind of supervision which must not be entrusted to the police but should be combined with effective social aid.

61. The treatment of prisoners should emphasize not their exclusion from the community, but their continuing part in it. Community agencies should, therefore, be enlisted wherever possible to assist the staff of the institution in the task of social rehabilitation of the prisoners. There should be in connection with every institution social workers charged with the duty of maintaining and improving all desirable relations of a prisoner with his family and with valuable social agencies. Steps should be taken to safeguard, to the maximum extent compatible with the law and the sentence, the rights relating to civil interests, social security rights and other social benefits of prisoners.

62. The medical services of the institution shall seek to detect and shall treat any physical or mental illnesses or defects which may hamper a prisoner's rehabilitation. All necessary medical, surgical and psychiatric services shall be provided to that end.

63. (1) The fulfillment of these principles requires individualization of treatment and for this purpose a flexible system of classifying prisoners in groups; it is therefore desirable that such groups should be distributed in separate institutions suitable for the treatment of each group.

(2) These institutions need not provide the same degree of security for every group. It is desirable to provide varying degrees of security according to the needs of different groups. Open institutions, by the very fact that they provide no physical security against escape but rely on the self-discipline of the inmates, provide the conditions most favourable to rehabilitation for carefully selected prisoners.

(3) It is desirable that the number of prisoners in closed institutions should not be so large that the individualization of treatment is hindered. In some countries it is considered that the population of such institutions should not exceed five hundred. In open institutions the population should be as small as possible.

(4) On the other hand, it is undesirable to maintain prisons which are so small that proper facilities cannot be provided.

64. The duty of society does not end with a prisoner's release. There should, therefore, be governmental or private agencies capable of lending the released prisoner efficient after-care directed towards the lessening of prejudice against him and towards his social rehabilitation.

Treatment

65. The treatment of persons sentenced to imprisonment or a similar measure shall have as its purpose, so far as the length of the sentence permits, to establish in them the will to lead law-abiding and self-supporting lives after their release and to fit them to do so. The treatment shall be such as will encourage their self-respect and develop their sense of responsibility.

66. (1) To these ends, all appropriate means shall be used, including religious care in the countries where this is possible, education, vocational guidance and training, social casework, employment counselling, physical development and strengthening of moral character, in accordance with the

individual needs of each prisoner, taking account of his social and criminal history, his physical and mental capacities and aptitudes, his personal temperament, the length of his sentence and his prospects after release.

(2) For every prisoner with a sentence of suitable length, the director shall receive, as soon as possible after his admission, full reports on all the matters referred to in the foregoing paragraph. Such reports shall always include a report by a medical officer, wherever possible qualified in psychiatry, on the physical and mental condition of the prisoner.

(3) The reports and other relevant documents shall be placed in an individual file. This file shall be kept up to date and classified in such a way that it can be consulted by the responsible personnel whenever the need arises.

Work

71. (1) Prison labour must not be of an afflictive nature.

(2) All prisoners under sentence shall be required to work, subject to their physical and mental fitness as determined by the medical officer.

(3) Sufficient work of a useful nature shall be provided to keep prisoners actively employed for a normal working day.

(4) So far as possible the work provided shall be such as will maintain or increase the prisoners, ability to earn an honest living after release.

(5) Vocational training in useful trades shall be provided for prisoners able to profit thereby and especially for young prisoners.

(6) Within the limits compatible with proper vocational selection and with the requirements of institutional administration and discipline, the prisoners shall be able to choose the type of work they wish to perform.

* * *

74. (1) The precautions laid down to protect the safety and health of free workmen shall be equally observed in institutions.

(2) Provision shall be made to indemnify prisoners against industrial injury, including occupational disease, on terms not less favourable than those extended by law to free workmen.

75. (1) The maximum daily and weekly working hours of the prisoners shall be fixed by law or by administrative regulation, taking into account local rules or custom in regard to the employment of free workmen.

(2) The hours so fixed shall leave one rest day a week and sufficient time for education and other activities required as part of the treatment and rehabilitation of the prisoners.

76. (1) There shall be a system of equitable remuneration of the work of prisoners.

(2) Under the system prisoners shall be allowed to spend at least a part of their earnings on approved articles for their own use and to send a part of their earnings to their family.

(3) The system should also provide that a part of the earnings should be set aside by the administration so as to constitute a savings fund to be handed over to the prisoner on his release.

Education and Recreation

77. (1) Provision shall be made for the further education of all prisoners capable of profiting thereby, including religious instruction in the countries where this is possible. The education of illiterates and young prisoners shall be compulsory and special attention shall be paid to it by the administration.

(2) So far as practicable, the education of prisoners shall be integrated with the educational system of the country so that after their release they may continue their education without difficulty.

78. Recreational and cultural activities shall be provided in all institutions for the benefit of the mental and physical health of prisoners.

Social Relations and After-care

79. Special attention shall be paid to the maintenance and improvement of such relations between a prisoner and his family as are desirable in the best interests of both.

80. From the beginning of a prisoner's sentence consideration shall be given to his future after release and he shall be encouraged and assisted to maintain or establish such relations with persons or agencies outside the institution as may promote the best interests of his family and his own social rehabilitation.

81. (1) Services and agencies, governmental or otherwise, which assist released prisoners to re-establish themselves in society shall ensure, so far as is possible and necessary, that released prisoners be provided with appropriate documents and identification papers, have suitable homes and work to go to, are suitably and adequately clothed having regard to the climate and season, and have sufficient means to reach their destination and maintain themselves in the period immediately following their release.

(2) The approved representatives of such agencies shall have all necessary access to the institution and to prisoners and shall be taken into consultation as to the future of a prisoner from the beginning of his sentence.

(3) It is desirable that the activities of such agencies shall be centralized or co-ordinated as far as possible in order to secure the best use of their efforts.

B. INSANE AND MENTALLY ABNORMAL PRISONERS

82. (1) Persons who are found to be insane shall not be detained in prisons and arrangements shall be made to remove them to mental institutions as soon as possible.

(2) Prisoners who suffer from other mental diseases or abnormalities shall be observed and treated in specialized institutions under medical management.

(3) During their stay in a prison, such prisoners shall be placed under the special supervision of a medical officer.

(4) The medical or psychiatric service of the penal institutions shall provide for the psychiatric treatment of all other prisoners who are in need of such treatment.

83. It is desirable that steps should be taken, by arrangement with the appropriate agencies, to ensure if necessary the continuation of psychiatric treatment after release and the provision of social-psychiatric after-care.

C. PRISONERS UNDER ARREST OR AWAITING TRIAL

84. (1) Persons arrested or imprisoned by reason of a criminal charge against them, who are detained either in police custody or in prison custody (jail) but have not yet been tried and sentenced, will be referred to as "untried prisoners,' hereinafter in these rules.

(2) Unconvicted prisoners are presumed to be innocent and shall be treated as such.

(3) Without prejudice to legal rules for the protection of individual liberty or prescribing the procedure to be observed in respect of untried prisoners, these prisoners shall benefit by a special regime which is described in the following rules in its essential requirements only.

85. (1) Untried prisoners shall be kept separate from convicted prisoners.

(2) Young untried prisoners shall be kept separate from adults and shall in principle be detained in separate institutions.

* * *

90. An untried prisoner shall be allowed to procure at his own expense or at the expense of a third party such books, newspapers, writing materials and other means of occupation as are compatible with the interests of the administration of justice and the security and good order of the institution.

91. An untried prisoner shall be allowed to be visited and treated by his own doctor or dentist if there is reasonable ground for his application and he is able to pay any expenses incurred.

92. An untried prisoner shall be allowed to inform immediately his family of his detention and shall be given all reasonable facilities for communicating with his family and friends, and for re-

ceiving visits from them, subject only to restrictions and supervision as are necessary in the interests of the administration of justice and of the security and good order of the institution.

93. For the purposes of his defense, an untried prisoner shall be allowed to apply for free legal aid where such aid is available, and to receive visits from his legal adviser with a view to his defense and to prepare and hand to him confidential instructions. For these purposes, he shall if he so desires be supplied with writing material. Interviews between the prisoner and his legal adviser may be within sight but not within the hearing of a police or institution official.

* * *

Declaration Concerning Support for Medical Doctors Refusing to Participate in, or to Condone, the Use of Torture or Other Forms of Cruel, Inhuman or Degrading Treatment (1997)

World Medical Association, Adopted by the 49th WMA General Assembly Hamburg, Germany, November 1997.
[Available at http://www.wma.net/e/policy/c19.htm]

PREAMBLE

1. On the basis of a number of international ethical declarations and guidelines subscribed to by the medical profession, medical doctors throughout the world are prohibited from countenancing, condoning or participating in the practice of torture or other forms of cruel, inhuman or degrading procedures for any reason.

2. Primary among these declarations are the World Medical Association's International Code of Medical Ethics, Declaration of Geneva, Declaration of Tokyo, and Resolution on Physician Participation in Capital Punishment; the Standing Committee of European Doctors' Statement of Madrid; the Nordic Resolution Concerning Physician Involvement in Capital Punishment; and, the World Psychiatric Association's Declaration of Hawaii.

3. However, none of these declarations or statements addresses explicitly the issue of what protection should be extended to medical doctors if they are pressured, called upon, or ordered to take part in torture or other forms of cruel, inhuman or degrading treatment or punishment. Nor do these declarations or statements express explicit support for, or the obligation to protect, doctors who encounter or become aware of such procedures.

RESOLUTION

4. The World Medical Association (WMA) hereby reiterates and reaffirms the responsibility of the organized medical profession:

i) to encourage doctors to honour their commitment as physicians to serve humanity and to resist any pressure to act contrary to the ethical principles governing their dedication to this task;

ii) to support physicians experiencing difficulties as a result of their resistance to any such pressure or as a result of their attempts to speak out or to act against such inhuman procedures; and,

iii) to extend its support and to encourage other international organisations, as well as the national member associations (NMAs) of the World Medical Association, to support physicians encountering difficulties as a result of their attempts to act in accordance with the highest ethical principles of the profession.

5. Furthermore, in view of the continued employment of such inhumane procedures in many countries throughout the world, and the documented incidents of pressure upon medical doctors to act in contravention to the ethical principles subscribed to by the profession, the WMA finds it necessary:

i) to protest internationally against any involvement of, or any pressure to involve, medical doctors in acts of torture or other forms of cruel, inhuman or degrading treatment or punishment;

ii) to support and protect, and to call upon its NMAs to support and protect, physicians who are resisting involvement in such inhuman procedures or who are working to treat and rehabilitate victims thereof, as well as to secure the right to uphold the highest ethical principles including medical confidentiality;

iii) to publicise information about and to support doctors reporting evidence of torture and to make known proven cases of attempts to involve physicians in such procedures; and,

iv) to encourage national medical associations to ask corresponding academic authorities to teach and investigate in all schools of medicine and hospitals the consequences of torture and its treatment, the rehabilitation of the survivors, the documentation of torture, and the professional protection described in this Declaration.

Nurses' Role in the Care of Prisoners and Detainees (1998)
Adopted in 1998. [Replaces previous ICN Position: "The Nurse's Role in the Care of Detainees and Prisoners."]
[Available at www.icn.ch/psdetainees.htm]

[Footnotes omitted.]

The International Council of Nurses (ICN) endorses the United Nations Universal Declaration of Human Rights, 1948 and the Geneva Convention of 1949 and the additional protocols. ICN therefore asserts that:

• Prisoners and detainees have the right to health care and humane treatment.

• We condemn interrogation procedures harmful to mental and physical health.

• Prisoners and detainees have a right to refuse treatment or diagnostic procedures and to die with dignity and in peaceful manner.

• Nurses have a fundamental responsibility to promote health, to prevent illness, to restore health and to alleviate suffering. Their primary responsibility is to those people who require nursing care. Nurses are often the first health professionals to suspect or detect ill-treatment of detainees and prisoners. It is important that they adhere to ethical principles in caring for detainees and prisoners, and should be guided by the following:

• Nurses who have knowledge of ill-treatment of detainees and prisoners must take appropriate action to safeguard their rights.

• Nurses employed in prison health services do not assume functions of prison security personnel, such as body searches conducted for the purpose of prison security.

• Nurses participate in clinical research on prisoners and detainees only with their informed consent.

• National nurses associations (NNAs) and individual nurses should be protected from abuse related to providing care to detainees and prisoners.

• NNAs should provide access to confidential advice, counsel and support for prison nurses.

D. Patients' Rights

Principles of the Rights of Patients in Europe (1994)

Endorsed by a WHO European Consultation on the Rights of Patients, attended by 60 persons from 36 Member States, meeting in Amsterdam, from 28-30 March 1994, as a set of principles for the promotion and implementation of patients' rights in WHO's European Member States. WHO document ICP/HLE 121 (28 June 1994). Reprinted in International Digest of Health Legislation, vol. 45, p. 411 (1995).
[Available at http://www.who.int/genomics/public/eu_declaration1994.pdf]

* * *

In drafting these Principles of the Rights of Patients in Europe, the following intergovernmental instruments, which together offer a framework and a set of basic concepts which can be applied to the rights of patients, have been taken into account:

• *The Universal Declaration of Human Rights (1948)*

• *The International Covenant on Civil and Political Rights (1966)*

• *The International Covenant on Economic, Social and Cultural Rights (1966)*

• *The European Convention on Human Rights and Fundamental Freedoms (1950)*

• *The European Social Charter (1961)*

THE RIGHTS OF PATIENTS

1. Human Rights and Values in Health Care

The instruments cited in the Introduction should be understood as applying also specifically in the health care setting, and it should therefore be noted that the human values expressed in these instruments shall be reflected in the health care system. It should also be noted that where exceptional limitations are imposed on the rights of patients, these must be in accordance with human rights instruments and have a legal base in the law of the country. It may be further observed that the rights specified below carry a matching responsibility to act with due concern for the health of others and for their same rights.

1.1 Everyone has the right to respect of his or her person as a human being.

1.2 Everyone has the right to self-determination.

1.3 Everyone has the right to physical and mental integrity and to the security of his or her person.

1.4 Everyone has the right to respect for his or her privacy.

1.5 Everyone has the right to have his or her moral and cultural values and religious and philosophical convictions respected.

1.6 Everyone has the right to such protection of health as is afforded by appropriate measures for disease prevention and health care, and to the opportunity to pursue his or her own highest attainable level of health.

2. Information

2.1 Information about health services and how best to use them is to be made available to the public in order to benefit all those concerned.

2.2 Patients have the right to be fully informed about their health status, including the medical facts about their condition; about the proposed medical procedures, together with the potential risks and benefits of each procedure; about alternatives to the proposed procedures, including the effect of non-treatment; and about the diagnosis, prognosis and progress of treatment.

2.3 Information may only be withheld from patients exceptionally when there is good reason to believe that this information would without any expectation of obvious positive effects cause them serious harm.

2.4 Information must be communicated to the patient in a way appropriate to the latter's capacity for understanding, minimizing the use of unfamiliar technical terminology. If the patient does not speak the common language, some form of interpreting should be available.

2.5 Patients have the right not to be informed, at their explicit request.

2.6 Patients have the right to choose who, if any one, should be informed on their behalf.

2.7 Patients should have the possibility of obtaining a second opinion.

2.8 When admitted to a health care establishment, patients should be informed of the identity and professional status of the health care providers taking care of them and of any rules and routines which would bear on their stay and care.

2.9 Patients should be able to request and be given a written summary of their diagnosis, treatment and care on discharge from a health care establishment.

3. Consent

3.1 The informed consent of the patient is a prerequisite for any medical intervention.

3.2 A patient has the right to refuse or to halt a medical intervention. The implications of refusing or halting such an intervention must be carefully explained to the patient

3.3 When a patient is unable to express his or her will and a medical intervention is urgently needed, the consent of the patient may be presumed, unless it is obvious from a previous declared expression of will that consent would be refused in the situation.

3.4 When the consent of a legal representative is required and the proposed intervention is urgently needed, that intervention may be made if it is not possible to obtain, in time, the representative's consent.

3.5 When the consent of a legal representative is required, patients (whether minor or adult) must nevertheless be involved in the decision-making process to the fullest extent which their capacity allows.

3.6 If a legal representative refuses to give consent and the physician or other provider is of the opinion that the intervention is in the interest of the patient, then the decision must be referred to a court or some form of arbitration.

3.7 In all other situations where the patient is unable to give informed consent and where there is no legal representative or representative designated by the patient for this purpose, appropriate measures should be taken to provide for a substitute decision-making process, taking into account what is known and, to the greatest extent possible, what may be presumed about the wishes of the patient.

3.8 The consent of the patient is required for the preservation and use of all substances of the human body. Consent may be presumed when the substances are to be used in the current course of diagnosis, treatment and care of that patient.

3.9 The informed consent of the patient is needed for participation in clinical teaching.

3.10 The informed consent of the patient is a prerequisite for participation in scientific research. All protocols must be submitted to proper ethical review procedures. Such research should not be carried out on those who are unable to express their will, unless the consent of a legal representative has been obtained and the research would likely be in the interest of the patient. As an exception to the requirement of involvement being in the interest of the patient, an incapacitated person may be involved in observational research which is not of direct benefit to his or her health provided that that person offers no objection, that the risk and burden is minimal, that the research is of significant value and that no alternative methods and other research subjects are available.

4. Confidentiality and Privacy

4.1 All information about a patient's health status, medical condition, diagnosis, prognosis and treatment and all other information of a personal kind must be kept confidential, even after death.

4.2 Confidential information can only be disclosed if the patient gives explicit consent or if the law expressly provides for this. Consent may be presumed where disclosure is to other health care providers involved in that patient's treatment.

4.3 All identifiable patient data must be protected. The protection of the data must be appropriate to the manner of their storage. Human substances from which identifiable data can be derived must be likewise protected.

4.4 Patients have the right of access to their medical files and technical records and to any other files and records pertaining to their diagnosis, treatment and care and to receive a copy of their own files and records or parts thereof. Such access excludes data concerning third parties.

4.5 Patients have the right to require the correction, completion, deletion, clarification and/or updating of personal and medical data concerning them which are inaccurate, incomplete, ambiguous or outdated, or which are not relevant to the purposes of diagnosis, treatment and care.

4.6 There can be no intrusion into a patient's private and family life unless and only if, in addition to the patient consenting to it, it can be justified as necessary to the patient's diagnosis, treatment and care.

4.7 Medical interventions may only be carried out when there is proper respect shown for the privacy of the individual. This means that a given intervention may be carried out only in the presence of those persons who are necessary for the intervention unless the patient consents or requests otherwise.

4.8 Patients admitted to health care establishments have the right to expect physical facilities which ensure privacy, particularly when health care providers are offering them personal care or carrying out examinations and treatment.

5. Care and Treatment

5.1 Everyone has the right to receive such health care as is appropriate to his or her health needs, including preventive care and activities aimed at health promotion. Services should be continuously available and accessible to all equitably, without discrimination and according to the financial, human and material resources which can be made available in a given society.

5.2 Patients have a collective right to some form of representation at each level of the health care system in matters pertaining to the planning and evaluation of services, including the range, quality and functioning of the care provided.

5.3 Patients have the right to a quality of care which is marked both by high technical standards and by a humane relationship between the patient and health care providers.

5.4 Patients have the right to continuity of care, including cooperation between all health care providers and/or establishments which may be involved in their diagnosis, treatment and care.

5.5 In circumstances where a choice must be made by providers between potential patients for a particular treatment which is in limited supply, all such patients are entitled to a fair selection procedure for that treatment. That choice must be based on medical criteria and made without discrimination.

5.6 Patients have the right to choose and change their own physician or other health care provider and health care establishment, provided that it is compatible with the functioning of the health care system.

5.7 Patients for whom there are no longer medical grounds for continued stay in a health care establishment are entitled to a full explanation before they can be transferred to another establishment or sent home. Transfer can only take place after another health care establishment has agreed to accept the patient. Where the patient is discharged to home and when his or her condition so requires, community and domiciliary services should be available.

5.8 Patients have the right to be treated with dignity in relation to their diagnosis, treatment and care, which should be rendered with respect for their culture and values.

5.9 Patients have the right to enjoy support from family, relatives and friends during the course of care and treatment and to receive spiritual support and guidance at all times.

5.10 Patients have the right to relief of their suffering according to the current state of knowledge.

5.11 Patients have the right to humane terminal care and to die in dignity.

6. Application

6.1 The exercise of the rights set forth in this document implies that appropriate means are established for this purpose.

6.2 The enjoyment of these rights shall be secured without discrimination.

6.3 In the exercise of these rights, patients shall be subjected only to such limitations as are compatible with human rights instruments and in accordance with a procedure prescribed by law.

6.4 If patients cannot avail themselves of the rights set forth in this document, these rights should be exercised by their legal representative or by a person designated by the patient for that purpose; where neither a legal representative nor a personal surrogate has been appointed, other measures for representation of those patients should be taken.

6.5 Patients must have access to such information and advice as will enable them to exercise the rights set forth in this document. Where patients feel that their rights have not been respected they should be enabled to lodge a complaint. In addition to recourse to the courts, there should be independent mechanisms at institutional and other levels to facilitate the processes of lodging, mediating and adjudicating complaints. These mechanisms would, inter alia, ensure that information relating to complaints procedures was available to patients and that an independent person was available and accessible to them for consultation regarding the most appropriate course of action to take. These mechanisms should further ensure that, where necessary, assistance and advocacy on behalf of the patient would be made available. Patients have the right to have their complaints examined and dealt with in a thorough, just, effective and prompt way and to be informed about their outcome.

7. Definitions

In these Principles of the Rights of Patients in Europe, the following terms have been used with the meanings given:

Patient(s): User(s) of health care services, whether healthy or sick.

Discrimination: Distinction between persons in similar cases on the basis of race, sex, religion, political opinions, national or social origin, associations with a national minority or personal antipathy.

Health Care: Medical, nursing or allied services dispensed by health care providers and health care establishments.

Health Care Providers: Physicians, nurses, dentists or other health professionals.

Medical Intervention: Any examination, treatment or other act having preventive, diagnostic, therapeutic or rehabilitative aims and which is carried out by a physician or other health care provider.

Health Care Establishment: Any health care facility such as a hospital, nursing home or establishment for disabled persons.

Terminal Care: Care given to a patient when it is no longer possible to improve the fatal prognosis of his or her illness/condition with available treatment methods; as well as care at the approach of death.

II. The Right to Health
A. UN Texts

Universal Declaration of Human Rights (1948)

Adopted and proclaimed by General Assembly Resolution 217 A (III)
of 10 December 1948. {Available at http://www.unhchr.ch/udhr/}

---

* * *

Article 25

(1) Everyone has the right to a standard of living adequate for the health and well-being of himself and of his family, including food, clothing, housing and medical care and necessary social services, and the right to security in the event of unemployment, sickness, disability, widowhood, old age or other lack of livelihood in circumstances beyond his control.

(2) Motherhood and childhood are entitled to special care and assistance. All children, whether born in or out of wedlock, shall enjoy the same social protection.

* * *

International Covenant on Economic, Social and Cultural Rights (1966)

Adopted and opened for signature by the United Nations General Assembly
Resolution 2200A (XXI) on 16 December 1966. Entered into force 3 January 1976.
{Available at http://www.unhchr.ch/html/menu3/b/a_cescr.htm}

---

* * *

Article 12

1. The States Parties to the present Covenant recognize the right of everyone to the enjoyment of the highest attainable standard of physical and mental health.

2. The steps to be taken by the States Parties to the present Covenant to achieve the full realization of this right shall include those necessary for:

(a) The provision for the reduction of the still-birth-rate and of infant mortality and for the healthy development of the child;

(b) The improvement of all aspects of environmental and industrial hygiene;

(c) The prevention, treatment and control of epidemic, endemic, occupational and other diseases;

(d) The creation of conditions which would assure to all medical service and medical attention in the event of sickness.

* * *

International Convention on the Elimination of All Forms of Racial Discrimination (1965)

Adopted and opened for signature and ratification by
General Assembly Resolution 2106 (XX) of 21 December 1965.
Entered into force 4 January 1969.
[Available at http://www.unhchr/html/menu3/b/d_icerd.htm]

* * *

Article 5 (e) (iv)

In compliance with the fundamental obligations laid down in article 2 of this Convention, States Parties undertake to prohibit and to eliminate racial discrimination in all its forms and to guarantee the right of everyone, without distinction as to race, colour, or national or ethnic origin, to equality before the law, notably in the enjoyment of the following rights:

(e) Economic, social and cultural rights, in particular:

(iv) The right to public health, medical care, social security and social services;

* * *

Convention on the Elimination of All Forms of Discrimination Against Women (1979)

Adopted and opened for signature, ratification and accession by General Assembly
Resolution 34/180 of 18 December 1979. Entered into force 3 September 1981.
[Available at http://www.unhchr.ch/htm/menu3/b/e1cedaw.htm]

* * *

Article 11

1. States Parties shall take all appropriate measures to eliminate discrimination against women in the field of employment in order to ensure, on a basis of equality of men and women, the same rights, in particular: the right to protection of health and to safety in working conditions, including the safeguarding of the function of reproduction.

* * *

(f) The right to protection of health and to safety in working conditions, including the safeguarding of the function of reproduction.

Article 12

1. States Parties shall take all appropriate measures to eliminate discrimination against women in the field of health care in order to ensure, on a basis of equality of men and women, access to health care services, including those related to family planning.

2. Notwithstanding the provisions of paragraph I of this article, States Parties shall ensure to women appropriate services in connection with pregnancy, confinement and the post-natal period, granting free services where necessary, as well as adequate nutrition during pregnancy and lactation.

* * *

Convention on the Rights of the Child (1989)

Adopted and opened for signature, ratification and accession by General Assembly Resolution 44/25 of 20 November 1989.

* * *

Article 24

1. States Parties recognize the right of the child to the enjoyment of the highest attainable standard of health and to facilities for the treatment of illness and rehabilitation of health. States Parties shall strive to ensure that no child is deprived of his or her right of access to such health care services.

2. States Parties shall pursue full implementation of this right and, in particular, shall take appropriate measures:

(a) To diminish infant and child mortality;

(b) To ensure the provision of necessary medical assistance and health care to all children with emphasis on the development of primary health care;

(c) To combat disease and malnutrition, including within the framework of primary health care, through, inter alia, the application of readily available technology and through the provision of adequate nutritious foods and clean drinking-water, taking into consideration the dangers and risks of environmental pollution;

(d) To ensure appropriate pre-natal and post-natal health care for mothers;

(e) To ensure that all segments of society, in particular parents and children, are informed, have access to education and are supported in the use of basic knowledge of child health and nutrition, the advantages of breast-feeding, hygiene and environmental sanitation and the prevention of accidents;

(f) To develop preventive health care, guidance for parents and family planning education and services.

3. States Parties shall take all effective and appropriate measures with a view to abolishing traditional practices prejudicial to the health of children.

4. States Parties undertake to promote and encourage international co-operation with a view to achieving progressively the full realization of the right recognized in the present article. In this regard, particular account shall be taken of the needs of developing countries.

* * *

General Comment No. 14: The Right to the Highest Attainable Standard of Health (Article 12 of the International Covenant on Economic, Social and Cultural Rights) (2000)

Adopted by the Committee on Economic, Social and Cultural Rights on 11 May 2000.
UN document E/C.12/2000/4, 11 August 2000. [Available at
http://www.unhchr.ch/tbs/doc.nsf/(symbol)/E.C.12.2000.4.En?OpenDocument]

1. Health is a fundamental human right indispensable for the exercise of other human rights. Every human being is entitled to the enjoyment of the highest attainable standard of health conducive to living a life in dignity. The realization of the right to health may be pursued through numerous, complementary approaches, such as the formulation of health policies, or the implementation of health programmes developed by the World Health Organization (WHO), or the adoption of specific legal instruments. Moreover, the right to health includes certain components which are legally enforceable.[1]

2. The human right to health is recognized in numerous international instruments. Article 25.1 of the Universal Declaration of Human Rights affirms: "Everyone has the right to a standard of living adequate for the health of himself and of his family, including food, clothing, housing and medical care and necessary social services". The International Covenant on Economic, Social and Cultural Rights provides the most comprehensive article on the right to health in international human rights law. In accordance with article 12.1 of the Covenant, States parties recognize "the right of everyone to the enjoyment of the highest attainable standard of physical and mental health", while article 12.2 enumerates, by way of illustration, a number of "steps to be taken by the States parties...to achieve the full realization of this right". Additionally, the right to health is recognized, inter alia, in article 5 (e) (iv) of the International Convention on the Elimination of All Forms of Racial Discrimination of 1965, in articles 11.1 (f) and 12 of the Convention on the Elimination of All Forms of Discrimination against Women of 1979 and in article 24 of the Convention on the Rights of the Child of 1989. Several regional human rights instruments also recognize the right to health, such as the European Social Charter of 1961 as revised (art. 11), the African Charter on Human and Peoples' Rights of

1981 (art. 16) and the Additional Protocol to the American Convention on Human Rights in the Area of Economic, Social and Cultural Rights of 1988 (art. 10). Similarly, the right to health has been proclaimed by the Commission on Human Rights,[2] as well as in the Vienna Declaration and Programme of Action of 1993 and other international instruments.[3]

3. The right to health is closely related to and dependent upon the realization of other human rights, as contained in the International Bill of Rights, including the rights to food, housing, work, education, human dignity, life, non-discrimination, equality, the prohibition against torture, privacy, access to information, and the freedoms of association, assembly and movement. These and other rights and freedoms address integral components of the right to health.

4. In drafting article 12 of the Covenant, the Third Committee of the United Nations General Assembly did not adopt the definition of health contained in the preamble to the Constitution of WHO, which conceptualizes health as "a state of complete physical, mental and social well-being and not merely the absence of disease or infirmity". However, the reference in article 12.1 of the Covenant to "the highest attainable standard of physical and mental health" is not confined to the right to health care. On the contrary, the drafting history and the express wording of article 12.2 acknowledge that the right to health embraces a wide range of socio-economic factors that promote conditions in which people can lead a healthy life, and extends to the underlying determinants of health, such as food and nutrition, housing, access to safe and potable water and adequate sanitation, safe and healthy working conditions, and a healthy environment.

5. The Committee is aware that, for millions of people throughout the world, the full enjoyment of

the right to health still remains a distant goal. Moreover, in many cases, especially for those living in poverty, this goal is becoming increasingly remote. The Committee recognizes the formidable structural and other obstacles resulting from international and other factors beyond the control of States that impede the full realization of article 12 in many States parties.

6. With a view to assisting States parties' implementation of the Covenant and the fulfilment of their reporting obligations, this General Comment focuses on the normative content of article 12 (Part I), States parties' obligations (Part II), violations (Part III) and implementation at the national level (Part IV), while the obligations of actors other than States parties are addressed in Part V. The General Comment is based on the Committee's experience in examining States parties' reports over many years.

I. NORMATIVE CONTENT OF ARTICLE 12

7. Article 12.1 provides a definition of the right to health, while article 12.2 enumerates illustrative, non-exhaustive examples of States parties' obligations.

8. The right to health is not to be understood as a right to be healthy. The right to health contains both freedoms and entitlements. The freedoms include the right to control one's health and body, including sexual and reproductive freedom, and the right to be free from interference, such as the right to be free from torture, non-consensual medical treatment and experimentation. By contrast, the entitlements include the right to a system of health protection which provides equality of opportunity for people to enjoy the highest attainable level of health.

9. The notion of "the highest attainable standard of health" in article 12.1 takes into account both the individual's biological and socio-economic preconditions and a State's available resources. There are a number of aspects which cannot be addressed solely within the relationship between States and individuals; in particular, good health cannot be ensured by a State, nor can States provide protection against every possible cause of human ill health. Thus, genetic factors, individual susceptibility to ill health and the adoption of un-

healthy or risky lifestyles may play an important role with respect to an individual's health. Consequently, the right to health must be understood as a right to the enjoyment of a variety of facilities, goods, services and conditions necessary for the realization of the highest attainable standard of health.

10. Since the adoption of the two International Covenants in 1966 the world health situation has changed dramatically and the notion of health has undergone substantial changes and has also widened in scope. More determinants of health are being taken into consideration, such as resource distribution and gender differences. A wider definition of health also takes into account such socially-related concerns as violence and armed conflict.[4] Moreover, formerly unknown diseases, such as Human Immunodeficiency Virus and Acquired Immunodeficiency Syndrome (HIV/AIDS), and others that have become more widespread, such as cancer, as well as the rapid growth of the world population, have created new obstacles for the realization of the right to health which need to be taken into account when interpreting article 12.

11. The Committee interprets the right to health, as defined in article 12.1, as an inclusive right extending not only to timely and appropriate health care but also to the underlying determinants of health, such as access to safe and potable water and adequate sanitation, an adequate supply of safe food, nutrition and housing, healthy occupational and environmental conditions, and access to health-related education and information, including on sexual and reproductive health. A further important aspect is the participation of the population in all health-related decision-making at the community, national and international levels.

12. The right to health in all its forms and at all levels contains the following interrelated and essential elements, the precise application of which will depend on the conditions prevailing in a particular State party:

(a) **Availability**. Functioning public health and health-care facilities, goods and services, as well as programmes, have to be available in sufficient quantity within the State party. The precise nature of the facilities, goods and services will vary depending on numerous factors, including the State party's developmental level. They will include, however, the underlying determinants of health, such as safe and potable drinking water and adequate sanitation facilities, hospitals, clinics and other health-related buildings, trained medical and professional personnel receiving domestically competitive salaries, and essential drugs, as defined by the WHO Action Programme on Essential Drugs.[5]

(b) **Accessibility**. Health facilities, goods and services[6] have to be accessible to everyone without discrimination, within the jurisdiction of the State party. Accessibility has four overlapping dimensions:

Non-discrimination: health facilities, goods and services must be accessible to all, especially the most vulnerable or marginalized sections of the population, in law and in fact, without discrimination on any of the prohibited grounds.[7]

Physical accessibility: health facilities, goods and services must be within safe physical reach for all sections of the population, especially vulnerable or marginalized groups, such as ethnic minorities and indigenous populations, women, children, adolescents, older persons, persons with disabilities and persons with HIV/AIDS. Accessibility also implies that medical services and underlying determinants of health, such as safe and potable water and adequate sanitation facilities, are within safe physical reach, including in rural areas. Accessibility further includes adequate access to buildings for persons with disabilities.

Economic accessibility (affordability): health facilities, goods and services must be affordable for all. Payment for health-care services, as well as services related to the underlying determinants of health, has to be based on the principle of equity, ensuring that these services, whether privately or publicly provided, are affordable for all, including socially disadvantaged groups. Equity demands that poorer households should not be disproportionately burdened with health expenses as compared to richer households.

Information accessibility: accessibility includes the right to seek, receive and impart information and ideas[8] concerning health issues. However, accessibility of information should not impair the right to have personal health data treated with confidentiality.

(c) **Acceptability**. All health facilities, goods and services must be respectful of medical ethics and culturally appropriate, i.e. respectful of the culture of individuals, minorities, peoples and communities, sensitive to gender and life-cycle requirements, as well as being designed to respect confidentiality and improve the health status of those concerned.

(d) **Quality**. As well as being culturally acceptable, health facilities, goods and services must also be scientifically and medically appropriate and of good quality. This requires, inter alia, skilled medical personnel, scientifically approved and unexpired drugs and hospital equipment, safe and potable water, and adequate sanitation.

13. The non-exhaustive catalogue of examples in article 12.2 provides guidance in defining the action to be taken by States. It gives specific generic examples of measures arising from the broad definition of the right to health contained in article 12.1, thereby illustrating the content of that right, as exemplified in the following paragraphs.[9]

Article 12.2 (a)
The Right to Maternal, Child and Reproductive Health

14. "The provision for the reduction of the still-birth rate and of infant mortality and for the healthy development of the child" (art. 12.2 (a))[10] may be understood as requiring measures to improve child and maternal health, sexual and reproductive health services, including access to family planning, pre- and post-natal care,[11] emergency obstetric services and access to information, as well as to resources necessary to act on that information.[12]

Article 12.2 (b)
The Right to Healthy Natural and Workplace Environments

15. "The improvement of all aspects of environmental and industrial hygiene" (art. 12.2 (b)) comprises, inter alia, preventive measures in respect of occupational accidents and diseases; the requirement to ensure an adequate supply of safe and potable water and basic sanitation; the prevention and reduction of the population's exposure to harmful substances such as radiation and harmful chemicals or other detrimental environmental

conditions that directly or indirectly impact upon human health.[13] Furthermore, industrial hygiene refers to the minimization, so far as is reasonably practicable, of the causes of health hazards inherent in the working environment.[14] Article 12.2 (b) also embraces adequate housing and safe and hygienic working conditions, an adequate supply of food and proper nutrition, and discourages the abuse of alcohol, and the use of tobacco, drugs and other harmful substances.

Article 12.2 (c)
The Right to Prevention, Treatment and Control of Diseases

16. "The prevention, treatment and control of epidemic, endemic, occupational and other diseases" (art. 12.2 (c)) requires the establishment of prevention and education programmes for behaviour-related health concerns such as sexually transmitted diseases, in particular HIV/AIDS, and those adversely affecting sexual and reproductive health, and the promotion of social determinants of good health, such as environmental safety, education, economic development and gender equity. The right to treatment includes the creation of a system of urgent medical care in cases of accidents, epidemics and similar health hazards, and the provision of disaster relief and humanitarian assistance in emergency situations. The control of diseases refers to States' individual and joint efforts to, inter alia, make available relevant technologies, using and improving epidemiological surveillance and data collection on a disaggregated basis, the implementation or enhancement of immunization programmes and other strategies of infectious disease control.

Article 12.2 (d)
The Right to Health Facilities, Goods and Services[15]

17. "The creation of conditions which would assure to all medical service and medical attention in the event of sickness" (art. 12.2 (d)), both physical and mental, includes the provision of equal and timely access to basic preventive, curative, rehabilitative health services and health education; regular screening programmes; appropriate treatment of prevalent diseases, illnesses, injuries and disabilities, preferably at community level; the provision of essential drugs; and appropriate mental health treatment and care. A further impor-

tant aspect is the improvement and furtherance of participation of the population in the provision of preventive and curative health services, such as the organization of the health sector, the insurance system and, in particular, participation in political decisions relating to the right to health taken at both the community and national levels.

Article 12
Special Topics of Broad Application

Non-Discrimination and Equal Treatment

18. By virtue of article 2.2 and article 3, the Covenant proscribes any discrimination in access to health care and underlying determinants of health, as well as to means and entitlements for their procurement, on the grounds of race, colour, sex, language, religion, political or other opinion, national or social origin, property, birth, physical or mental disability, health status (including HIV/AIDS), sexual orientation and civil, political, social or other status, which has the intention or effect of nullifying or impairing the equal enjoyment or exercise of the right to health. The Committee stresses that many measures, such as most strategies and programmes designed to eliminate health-related discrimination, can be pursued with minimum resource implications through the adoption, modification or abrogation of legislation or the dissemination of information. The Committee recalls General Comment No. 3, paragraph 12, which states that even in times of severe resource constraints, the vulnerable members of society must be protected by the adoption of relatively low-cost targeted programmes.

19. With respect to the right to health, equality of access to health care and health services has to be emphasized. States have a special obligation to provide those who do not have sufficient means with the necessary health insurance and health-care facilities, and to prevent any discrimination on internationally prohibited grounds in the provision of health care and health services, especially with respect to the core obligations of the right to health.[16] Inappropriate health resource allocation can lead to discrimination that may not be overt. For example, investments should not disproportionately favour expensive curative health services which are often accessible only to a small, privileged fraction of the population, rather than primary and preventive health care benefiting a far larger part of the population.

Gender Perspective

20. The Committee recommends that States integrate a gender perspective in their health-related policies, planning, programmes and research in order to promote better health for both women and men. A gender-based approach recognizes that biological and socio-cultural factors play a significant role in influencing the health of men and women. The disaggregation of health and socioeconomic data according to sex is essential for identifying and remedying inequalities in health.

Women and the Right to Health

21. To eliminate discrimination against women, there is a need to develop and implement a comprehensive national strategy for promoting women's right to health throughout their life span. Such a strategy should include interventions aimed at the prevention and treatment of diseases affecting women, as well as policies to provide access to a full range of high quality and affordable health care, including sexual and reproductive services. A major goal should be reducing women's health risks, particularly lowering rates of maternal mortality and protecting women from domestic violence. The realization of women's right to health requires the removal of all barriers interfering with access to health services, education and information, including in the area of sexual and reproductive health. It is also important to undertake preventive, promotive and remedial action to shield women from the impact of harmful traditional cultural practices and norms that deny them their full reproductive rights.

Children and Adolescents

22. Article 12.2 (a) outlines the need to take measures to reduce infant mortality and promote the healthy development of infants and children. Subsequent international human rights instruments recognize that children and adolescents have the right to the enjoyment of the highest standard of health and access to facilities for the treatment of illness.[17] The Convention on the Rights of the Child directs States to ensure access to essential health services for the child and his or her family, including pre- and post-natal care for mothers. The Convention links these goals with ensuring access to child-friendly information about preventive and health-promoting behaviour and support to families and communities in implementing these practices. Implementation of the principle of non-discrimination requires that girls, as well as boys, have equal access to adequate nutrition, safe environments, and physical as well as mental health services. There is a need to adopt effective and appropriate measures to abolish harmful traditional practices affecting the health of children, particularly girls, including early marriage, female genital mutilation, preferential feeding and care of male children.[18] Children with disabilities should be given the opportunity to enjoy a fulfilling and decent life and to participate within their community.

23. States parties should provide a safe and supportive environment for adolescents, that ensures the opportunity to participate in decisions affecting their health, to build life-skills, to acquire appropriate information, to receive counselling and to negotiate the health-behaviour choices they make. The realization of the right to health of adolescents is dependent on the development of youth-friendly health care, which respects confidentiality and privacy and includes appropriate sexual and reproductive health services.

24. In all policies and programmes aimed at guaranteeing the right to health of children and adolescents their best interests shall be a primary consideration.

Older Persons

25. With regard to the realization of the right to health of older persons, the Committee, in accordance with paragraphs 34 and 35 of General Comment No. 6 (1995), reaffirms the importance of an integrated approach, combining elements of preventive, curative and rehabilitative health treatment. Such measures should be based on periodical check-ups for both sexes; physical as well as psychological rehabilitative measures aimed at maintaining the functionality and autonomy of older persons; and attention and care for chronically and terminally ill persons, sparing them avoidable pain and enabling them to die with dignity.

Persons with Disabilities

26. The Committee reaffirms paragraph 34 of its General Comment No. 5, which addresses the issue of persons with disabilities in the context of the right to physical and mental health. Moreover, the Committee stresses the need to ensure that not only the public health sector but also private

providers of health services and facilities comply with the principle of non-discrimination in relation to persons with disabilities.

Indigenous Peoples

27. In the light of emerging international law and practice and the recent measures taken by States in relation to indigenous peoples,[19] the Committee deems it useful to identify elements that would help to define indigenous peoples' right to health in order better to enable States with indigenous peoples to implement the provisions contained in article 12 of the Covenant. The Committee considers that indigenous peoples have the right to specific measures to improve their access to health services and care. These health services should be culturally appropriate, taking into account traditional preventive care, healing practices and medicines. States should provide resources for indigenous peoples to design, deliver and control such services so that they may enjoy the highest attainable standard of physical and mental health. The vital medicinal plants, animals and minerals necessary to the full enjoyment of health of indigenous peoples should also be protected. The Committee notes that, in indigenous communities, the health of the individual is often linked to the health of the society as a whole and has a collective dimension. In this respect, the Committee considers that development-related activities that lead to the displacement of indigenous peoples against their will from their traditional territories and environment, denying them their sources of nutrition and breaking their symbiotic relationship with their lands, has a deleterious effect on their health.

Limitations

28. Issues of public health are sometimes used by States as grounds for limiting the exercise of other fundamental rights. The Committee wishes to emphasize that the Covenant's limitation clause, article 4, is primarily intended to protect the rights of individuals rather than to permit the imposition of limitations by States. Consequently a State party which, for example, restricts the movement of, or incarcerates, persons with transmissible diseases such as HIV/AIDS, refuses to allow doctors to treat persons believed to be opposed to a government, or fails to provide immunization against the community's major infectious diseases, on grounds such as national security or the preserva-

tion of public order, has the burden of justifying such serious measures in relation to each of the elements identified in article 4. Such restrictions must be in accordance with the law, including international human rights standards, compatible with the nature of the rights protected by the Covenant, in the interest of legitimate aims pursued, and strictly necessary for the promotion of the general welfare in a democratic society.

29. In line with article 5.1, such limitations must be proportional, i.e. the least restrictive alternative must be adopted where several types of limitations are available. Even where such limitations on grounds of protecting public health are basically permitted, they should be of limited duration and subject to review.

II. STATES PARTIES' OBLIGATIONS

General Legal Obligations

30. While the Covenant provides for progressive realization and acknowledges the constraints due to the limits of available resources, it also imposes on States parties various obligations which are of immediate effect. States parties have immediate obligations in relation to the right to health, such as the guarantee that the right will be exercised without discrimination of any kind (art. 2.2) and the obligation to take steps (art. 2.1) towards the full realization of article 12. Such steps must be deliberate, concrete and targeted towards the full realization of the right to health.[20]

31. The progressive realization of the right to health over a period of time should not be interpreted as depriving States parties' obligations of all meaningful content. Rather, progressive realization means that States parties have a specific and continuing obligation to move as expeditiously and effectively as possible towards the full realization of article 12.[21]

32. As with all other rights in the Covenant, there is a strong presumption that retrogressive measures taken in relation to the right to health are not permissible. If any deliberately retrogressive measures are taken, the State party has the burden of proving that they have been introduced after the most careful consideration of all alternatives and that they are duly justified by reference to the totality of the rights provided for in the Covenant in

the context of the full use of the State party's maximum available resources.[22]

33. The right to health, like all human rights, imposes three types or levels of obligations on States parties: the obligations to respect, protect and fulfil. In turn, the obligation to fulfil contains obligations to facilitate, provide and promote.[23] The obligation to respect requires States to refrain from interfering directly or indirectly with the enjoyment of the right to health. The obligation to protect requires States to take measures that prevent third parties from interfering with article 12 guarantees. Finally, the obligation to fulfil requires States to adopt appropriate legislative, administrative, budgetary, judicial, promotional and other measures towards the full realization of the right to health.

Specific Legal Obligations

34. In particular, States are under the obligation to respect the right to health by, inter alia, refraining from denying or limiting equal access for all persons, including prisoners or detainees, minorities, asylum seekers and illegal immigrants, to preventive, curative and palliative health services; abstaining from enforcing discriminatory practices as a State policy; and abstaining from imposing discriminatory practices relating to women's health status and needs. Furthermore, obligations to respect include a State's obligation to refrain from prohibiting or impeding traditional preventive care, healing practices and medicines, from marketing unsafe drugs and from applying coercive medical treatments, unless on an exceptional basis for the treatment of mental illness or the prevention and control of communicable diseases. Such exceptional cases should be subject to specific and restrictive conditions, respecting best practices and applicable international standards, including the Principles for the Protection of Persons with Mental Illness and the Improvement of Mental Health Care.[24]

In addition, States should refrain from limiting access to contraceptives and other means of maintaining sexual and reproductive health, from censoring, withholding or intentionally misrepresenting health-related information, including sexual education and information, as well as from preventing people's participation in health-related matters. States should also refrain from unlaw-fully polluting air, water and soil, e.g. through industrial waste from State-owned facilities, from using or testing nuclear, biological or chemical weapons if such testing results in the release of substances harmful to human health, and from limiting access to health services as a punitive measure, e.g. during armed conflicts in violation of international humanitarian law.

35. Obligations to protect include, inter alia, the duties of States to adopt legislation or to take other measures ensuring equal access to health care and health-related services provided by third parties; to ensure that privatization of the health sector does not constitute a threat to the availability, accessibility, acceptability and quality of health facilities, goods and services; to control the marketing of medical equipment and medicines by third parties; and to ensure that medical practitioners and other health professionals meet appropriate standards of education, skill and ethical codes of conduct. States are also obliged to ensure that harmful social or traditional practices do not interfere with access to pre- and post-natal care and family-planning; to prevent third parties from coercing women to undergo traditional practices, e.g. female genital mutilation; and to take measures to protect all vulnerable or marginalized groups of society, in particular women, children, adolescents and older persons, in the light of gender-based expressions of violence. States should also ensure that third parties do not limit people's access to health-related information and services.

36. The obligation to fulfil requires States parties, inter alia, to give sufficient recognition to the right to health in the national political and legal systems, preferably by way of legislative implementation, and to adopt a national health policy with a detailed plan for realizing the right to health. States must ensure provision of health care, including immunization programmes against the major infectious diseases, and ensure equal access for all to the underlying determinants of health, such as nutritiously safe food and potable drinking water, basic sanitation and adequate housing and living conditions. Public health infrastructures should provide for sexual and reproductive health services, including safe motherhood, particularly in rural areas. States have to ensure the appropriate training of doctors and other medical per-

sonnel, the provision of a sufficient number of hospitals, clinics and other health-related facilities, and the promotion and support of the establishment of institutions providing counselling and mental health services, with due regard to equitable distribution throughout the country. Further obligations include the provision of a public, private or mixed health insurance system which is affordable for all, the promotion of medical research and health education, as well as information campaigns, in particular with respect to HIV/AIDS, sexual and reproductive health, traditional practices, domestic violence, the abuse of alcohol and the use of cigarettes, drugs and other harmful substances. States are also required to adopt measures against environmental and occupational health hazards and against any other threat as demonstrated by epidemiological data. For this purpose they should formulate and implement national policies aimed at reducing and eliminating pollution of air, water and soil, including pollution by heavy metals such as lead from gasoline. Furthermore, States parties are required to formulate, implement and periodically review a coherent national policy to minimize the risk of occupational accidents and diseases, as well as to provide a coherent national policy on occupational safety and health services.[25]

37. The obligation to fulfil (facilitate) requires States inter alia to take positive measures that enable and assist individuals and communities to enjoy the right to health. States parties are also obliged to fulfil (provide) a specific right contained in the Covenant when individuals or a group are unable, for reasons beyond their control, to realize that right themselves by the means at their disposal. The obligation to fulfil (promote) the right to health requires States to undertake actions that create, maintain and restore the health of the population. Such obligations include: (i) fostering recognition of factors favouring positive health results, e.g. research and provision of information; (ii) ensuring that health services are culturally appropriate and that health care staff are trained to recognize and respond to the specific needs of vulnerable or marginalized groups; (iii) ensuring that the State meets its obligations in the dissemination of appropriate information relating to healthy lifestyles and nutrition, harmful traditional practices and the availability of services;

(iv) supporting people in making informed choices about their health.

International Obligations

38. In its General Comment No. 3, the Committee drew attention to the obligation of all States parties to take steps, individually and through international assistance and cooperation, especially economic and technical, towards the full realization of the rights recognized in the Covenant, such as the right to health. In the spirit of article 56 of the Charter of the United Nations, the specific provisions of the Covenant (articles 12, 2.1, 22 and 23) and the Alma-Ata Declaration on primary health care, States parties should recognize the essential role of international cooperation and comply with their commitment to take joint and separate action to achieve the full realization of the right to health. In this regard, States parties are referred to the Alma-Ata Declaration which proclaims that the existing gross inequality in the health status of the people, particularly between developed and developing countries, as well as within countries, is politically, socially and economically unacceptable and is, therefore, of common concern to all countries.[26]

39. To comply with their international obligations in relation to article 12, States parties have to respect the enjoyment of the right to health in other countries, and to prevent third parties from violating the right in other countries, if they are able to influence these third parties by way of legal or political means, in accordance with the Charter of the United Nations and applicable international law. Depending on the availability of resources, States should facilitate access to essential health facilities, goods and services in other countries, wherever possible and provide the necessary aid when required.[27] States parties should ensure that the right to health is given due attention in international agreements and, to that end, should consider the development of further legal instruments. In relation to the conclusion of other international agreements, States parties should take steps to ensure that these instruments do not adversely impact upon the right to health. Similarly, States parties have an obligation to ensure that their actions as members of international organizations take due account of the right to health. Accordingly,

States parties which are members of international financial institutions, notably the International Monetary Fund, the World Bank, and regional development banks, should pay greater attention to the protection of the right to health in influencing the lending policies, credit agreements and international measures of these institutions.

40. States parties have a joint and individual responsibility, in accordance with the Charter of the United Nations and relevant resolutions of the United Nations General Assembly and of the World Health Assembly, to cooperate in providing disaster relief and humanitarian assistance in times of emergency, including assistance to refugees and internally displaced persons. Each State should contribute to this task to the maximum of its capacities. Priority in the provision of international medical aid, distribution and management of resources, such as safe and potable water, food and medical supplies, and financial aid should be given to the most vulnerable or marginalized groups of the population. Moreover, given that some diseases are easily transmissible beyond the frontiers of a State, the international community has a collective responsibility to address this problem. The economically developed States parties have a special responsibility and interest to assist the poorer developing States in this regard.

41. States parties should refrain at all times from imposing embargoes or similar measures restricting the supply of another State with adequate medicines and medical equipment. Restrictions on such goods should never be used as an instrument of political and economic pressure. In this regard, the Committee recalls its position, stated in General Comment No. 8, on the relationship between economic sanctions and respect for economic, social and cultural rights.

42. While only States are parties to the Covenant and thus ultimately accountable for compliance with it, all members of society — individuals, including health professionals, families, local communities, intergovernmental and non-governmental organizations, civil society organizations, as well as the private business sector — have responsibilities regarding the realization of the right to health. State parties should therefore provide an environment which facilitates the discharge of these responsibilities.

Core Obligations

43. In General Comment No. 3, the Committee confirms that States parties have a core obligation to ensure the satisfaction of, at the very least, minimum essential levels of each of the rights enunciated in the Covenant, including essential primary health care. Read in conjunction with more contemporary instruments, such as the Programme of Action of the International Conference on Population and Development,[28] the Alma-Ata Declaration provides compelling guidance on the core obligations arising from article 12. Accordingly, in the Committee's view, these core obligations include at least the following obligations:

(a) To ensure the right of access to health facilities, goods and services on a non-discriminatory basis, especially for vulnerable or marginalized groups;

(b) To ensure access to the minimum essential food which is nutritionally adequate and safe, to ensure freedom from hunger to everyone;

(c) To ensure access to basic shelter, housing and sanitation, and an adequate supply of safe and potable water;

(d) To provide essential drugs, as from time to time defined under the WHO Action Programme on Essential Drugs;

(e) To ensure equitable distribution of all health facilities, goods and services;

(f) To adopt and implement a national public health strategy and plan of action, on the basis of epidemiological evidence, addressing the health concerns of the whole population; the strategy and plan of action shall be devised, and periodically reviewed, on the basis of a participatory and transparent process; they shall include methods, such as right to health indicators and benchmarks, by which progress can be closely monitored; the process by which the strategy and plan of action are devised, as well as their content, shall give particular attention to all vulnerable or marginalized groups.

44. The Committee also confirms that the following are obligations of comparable priority:

(a) To ensure reproductive, maternal (pre-natal as well as post-natal) and child health care;

(b) To provide immunization against the major infectious diseases occurring in the community;

(c) To take measures to prevent, treat and control epidemic and endemic diseases;

(d) To provide education and access to information concerning the main health problems in the community, including methods of preventing and controlling them;

(e) To provide appropriate training for health personnel, including education on health and human rights.

45. For the avoidance of any doubt, the Committee wishes to emphasize that it is particularly incumbent on States parties and other actors in a position to assist, to provide "international assistance and cooperation, especially economic and technical"[29] which enable developing countries to fulfil their core and other obligations indicated in paragraphs 43 and 44 above.

III. VIOLATIONS

46. When the normative content of article 12 (Part I) is applied to the obligations of States parties (Part II), a dynamic process is set in motion which facilitates identification of violations of the right to health. The following paragraphs provide illustrations of violations of article 12.

47. In determining which actions or omissions amount to a violation of the right to health, it is important to distinguish the inability from the unwillingness of a State party to comply with its obligations under article 12. This follows from article 12.1, which speaks of the highest attainable standard of health, as well as from article 2.1 of the Covenant, which obliges each State party to take the necessary steps to the maximum of its available resources. A State which is unwilling to use the maximum of its available resources for the realization of the right to health is in violation of its obligations under article 12. If resource con-

straints render it impossible for a State to comply fully with its Covenant obligations, it has the burden of justifying that every effort has nevertheless been made to use all available resources at its disposal in order to satisfy, as a matter of priority, the obligations outlined above. It should be stressed, however, that a State party cannot, under any circumstances whatsoever, justify its noncompliance with the core obligations set out in paragraph 43 above, which are non-derogable.

48. Violations of the right to health can occur through the direct action of States or other entities insufficiently regulated by States. The adoption of any retrogressive measures incompatible with the core obligations under the right to health, outlined in paragraph 43 above, constitutes a violation of the right to health. Violations through acts of commission include the formal repeal or suspension of legislation necessary for the continued enjoyment of the right to health or the adoption of legislation or policies which are manifestly incompatible with pre-existing domestic or international legal obligations in relation to the right to health.

49. Violations of the right to health can also occur through the omission or failure of States to take necessary measures arising from legal obligations. Violations through acts of omission include the failure to take appropriate steps towards the full realization of everyone's right to the enjoyment of the highest attainable standard of physical and mental health, the failure to have a national policy on occupational safety and health as well as occupational health services, and the failure to enforce relevant laws.

Violations of the Obligation to Respect

50. Violations of the obligation to respect are those State actions, policies or laws that contravene the standards set out in article 12 of the Covenant and are likely to result in bodily harm, unnecessary morbidity and preventable mortality. Examples include the denial of access to health facilities, goods and services to particular individuals or groups as a result of de jure or de facto discrimination; the deliberate withholding or misrepresentation of information vital to health protection or treatment; the suspension of legislation or the adoption of laws or policies that interfere with the enjoyment of any of the components of the

right to health; and the failure of the State to take into account its legal obligations regarding the right to health when entering into bilateral or multilateral agreements with other States, international organizations and other entities, such as multinational corporations.

Violations of the Obligation to Protect

51. Violations of the obligation to protect follow from the failure of a State to take all necessary measures to safeguard persons within their jurisdiction from infringements of the right to health by third parties. This category includes such omissions as the failure to regulate the activities of individuals, groups or corporations so as to prevent them from violating the right to health of others; the failure to protect consumers and workers from practices detrimental to health, e.g. by employers and manufacturers of medicines or food; the failure to discourage production, marketing and consumption of tobacco, narcotics and other harmful substances; the failure to protect women against violence or to prosecute perpetrators; the failure to discourage the continued observance of harmful traditional medical or cultural practices; and the failure to enact or enforce laws to prevent the pollution of water, air and soil by extractive and manufacturing industries.

Violations of the Obligation to Fulfil

52. Violations of the obligation to fulfil occur through the failure of States parties to take all necessary steps to ensure the realization of the right to health. Examples include the failure to adopt or implement a national health policy designed to ensure the right to health for everyone; insufficient expenditure or misallocation of public resources which results in the non-enjoyment of the right to health by individuals or groups, particularly the vulnerable or marginalized; the failure to monitor the realization of the right to health at the national level, for example by identifying right to health indicators and benchmarks; the failure to take measures to reduce the inequitable distribution of health facilities, goods and services; the failure to adopt a gender-sensitive approach to health; and the failure to reduce infant and maternal mortality rates.

IV. IMPLEMENTATION AT THE NATIONAL LEVEL

Framework Legislation

53. The most appropriate feasible measures to implement the right to health will vary significantly from one State to another. Every State has a margin of discretion in assessing which measures are most suitable to meet its specific circumstances. The Covenant, however, clearly imposes a duty on each State to take whatever steps are necessary to ensure that everyone has access to health facilities, goods and services so that they can enjoy, as soon as possible, the highest attainable standard of physical and mental health. This requires the adoption of a national strategy to ensure to all the enjoyment of the right to health, based on human rights principles which define the objectives of that strategy, and the formulation of policies and corresponding right to health indicators and benchmarks. The national health strategy should also identify the resources available to attain defined objectives, as well as the most cost-effective way of using those resources.

54. The formulation and implementation of national health strategies and plans of action should respect, inter alia, the principles of non-discrimination and people's participation. In particular, the right of individuals and groups to participate in decision-making processes, which may affect their development, must be an integral component of any policy, programme or strategy developed to discharge governmental obligations under article 12. Promoting health must involve effective community action in setting priorities, making decisions, planning, implementing and evaluating strategies to achieve better health. Effective provision of health services can only be assured if people's participation is secured by States.

55. The national health strategy and plan of action should also be based on the principles of accountability, transparency and independence of the judiciary, since good governance is essential to the effective implementation of all human rights, including the realization of the right to health. In order to create a favourable climate for the realization of the right, States parties should take appropriate steps to ensure that the private business

sector and civil society are aware of, and consider the importance of, the right to health in pursuing their activities.

56. States should consider adopting a framework law to operationalize their right to health national strategy. The framework law should establish national mechanisms for monitoring the implementation of national health strategies and plans of action. It should include provisions on the targets to be achieved and the time-frame for their achievement; the means by which right to health benchmarks could be achieved; the intended collaboration with civil society, including health experts, the private sector and international organizations; institutional responsibility for the implementation of the right to health national strategy and plan of action; and possible recourse procedures. In monitoring progress towards the realization of the right to health, States parties should identify the factors and difficulties affecting implementation of their obligations.

Right to Health Indicators and Benchmarks

57. National health strategies should identify appropriate right to health indicators and benchmarks. The indicators should be designed to monitor, at the national and international levels, the State party's obligations under article 12. States may obtain guidance on appropriate right to health indicators, which should address different aspects of the right to health, from the ongoing work of WHO and the United Nations Children's Fund (UNICEF) in this field. Right to health indicators require disaggregation on the prohibited grounds of discrimination.

58. Having identified appropriate right to health indicators, States parties are invited to set appropriate national benchmarks in relation to each indicator. During the periodic reporting procedure the Committee will engage in a process of scoping with the State party. Scoping involves the joint consideration by the State party and the Committee of the indicators and national benchmarks which will then provide the targets to be achieved during the next reporting period. In the following five years, the State party will use these national benchmarks to help monitor its implementation of article 12. Thereafter, in the subsequent reporting process, the State party and the Committee will consider whether or not the benchmarks have been achieved, and the reasons for any difficulties that may have been encountered.

Remedies and Accountability

59. Any person or group victim of a violation of the right to health should have access to effective judicial or other appropriate remedies at both national and international levels.[30] All victims of such violations should be entitled to adequate reparation, which may take the form of restitution, compensation, satisfaction or guarantees of nonrepetition. National ombudsmen, human rights commissions, consumer forums, patients' rights associations or similar institutions should address violations of the right to health.

60. The incorporation in the domestic legal order of international instruments recognizing the right to health can significantly enhance the scope and effectiveness of remedial measures and should be encouraged in all cases.[31] Incorporation enables courts to adjudicate violations of the right to health, or at least its core obligations, by direct reference to the Covenant.

61. Judges and members of the legal profession should be encouraged by States parties to pay greater attention to violations of the right to health in the exercise of their functions.

62. States parties should respect, protect, facilitate and promote the work of human rights advocates and other members of civil society with a view to assisting vulnerable or marginalized groups in the realization of their right to health.

V. OBLIGATIONS OF ACTORS OTHER THAN STATES PARTIES

63. The role of the United Nations agencies and programmes, and in particular the key function assigned to WHO in realizing the right to health at the international, regional and country levels, is of particular importance, as is the function of UNICEF in relation to the right to health of chil-

dren. When formulating and implementing their right to health national strategies, States parties should avail themselves of technical assistance and cooperation of WHO. Further, when preparing their reports, States parties should utilize the extensive information and advisory services of WHO with regard to data collection, disaggregation, and the development of right to health indicators and benchmarks.

64. Moreover, coordinated efforts for the realization of the right to health should be maintained to enhance the interaction among all the actors concerned, including the various components of civil society. In conformity with articles 22 and 23 of the Covenant, WHO, The International Labour Organization, the United Nations Development Programme, UNICEF, the United Nations Population Fund, the World Bank, regional development banks, the International Monetary Fund, the World Trade Organization and other relevant bodies within the United Nations system, should cooperate effectively with States parties, building on their respective expertise, in relation to the implementation of the right to health at the national level, with due respect to their individual mandates. In particular, the international financial institutions, notably the World Bank and the International Monetary Fund, should pay greater attention to the protection of the right to health in their lending policies, credit agreements and structural adjustment programmes. When examining the reports of States parties and their ability to meet the obligations under article 12, the Committee will consider the effects of the assistance provided by all other actors. The adoption of a human rights-based approach by United Nations specialized agencies, programmes and bodies will greatly facilitate implementation of the right to health. In the course of its examination of States parties' reports, the Committee will also consider the role of health professional associations and other non-governmental organizations in relation to the States' obligations under article 12.

65. The role of WHO, the Office of the United Nations High Commissioner for Refugees, the International Committee of the Red Cross/Red Crescent and UNICEF, as well as non governmental organizations and national medical associations, is of particular importance in relation to disaster relief and humanitarian assistance in times of emergencies, including assistance to refugees and internally displaced persons. Priority in the provision of international medical aid, distribution and management of resources, such as safe and potable water, food and medical supplies, and financial aid should be given to the most vulnerable or marginalized groups of the population.

Notes

1. For example, the principle of non-discrimination in relation to health facilities, goods and services is legally enforceable in numerous national jurisdictions.

2. In its resolution 1989/11.

3. The Principles for the Protection of Persons with Mental Illness and for the Improvement of Mental Health Care adopted by the United Nations General Assembly in 1991 (resolution 46/119) and the Committee's General Comment No. 5 on persons with disabilities apply to persons with mental illness; the Programme of Action of the International Conference on Population and Development held at Cairo in 1994, as well as the Declaration and Programme for Action of the Fourth World Conference on Women held in Beijing in 1995 contain definitions of reproductive health and women's health, respectively.

4. Common article 3 of the Geneva Conventions for the protection of war victims (1949); Additional Protocol I (1977) relating to the Protection of Victims of International Armed Conflicts, art. 75 (2) (a); Additional Protocol II (1977) relating to the Protection of Victims of Non-International Armed Conflicts, art. 4 (a).

5. See WHO Model List of Essential Drugs, revised December 1999, WHO Drug Information, vol. 13, No. 4, 1999.

6. Unless expressly provided otherwise, any reference in this General Comment to health facilities, goods and services includes the underlying determinants of health outlined in paras. 11 and 12 (a) of this General Comment.

7. See paras. 18 and 19 of this General Comment.

8. See article 19.2 of the International Covenant on Civil and Political Rights. This General Comment gives particular emphasis to access to information because of the special importance of this issue in relation to health.

9. In the literature and practice concerning the right to health, three levels of health care are frequently referred to: primary health care typically deals with common and relatively minor illnesses

and is provided by health professionals and/or generally trained doctors working within the community at relatively low cost; secondary health care is provided in centres, usually hospitals, and typically deals with relatively common minor or serious illnesses that cannot be managed at community level, using specialty-trained health professionals and doctors, special equipment and sometimes in-patient care at comparatively higher cost; tertiary health care is provided in relatively few centres, typically deals with small numbers of minor or serious illnesses requiring specialty-trained health professionals and doctors and special equipment, and is often relatively expensive. Since forms of primary, secondary and tertiary health care frequently overlap and often interact, the use of this typology does not always provide sufficient distinguishing criteria to be helpful for assessing which levels of health care States parties must provide, and is therefore of limited assistance in relation to the normative understanding of article 12.

10. According to WHO, the stillbirth rate is no longer commonly used, infant and under-five mortality rates being measured instead.

11. Prenatal denotes existing or occurring before birth; perinatal refers to the period shortly before and after birth (in medical statistics the period begins with the completion of 28 weeks of gestation and is variously defined as ending one to four weeks after birth); neonatal, by contrast, covers the period pertaining to the first four weeks after birth; while post-natal denotes occurrence after birth. In this General Comment, the more generic terms pre- and post-natal are exclusively employed.

12. Reproductive health means that women and men have the freedom to decide if and when to reproduce and the right to be informed and to have access to safe, effective, affordable and acceptable methods of family planning of their choice as well as the right of access to appropriate health-care services that will, for example, enable women to go safely through pregnancy and childbirth.

13. The Committee takes note, in this regard, of Principle 1 of the Stockholm Declaration of 1972 which states: "Man has the fundamental right to freedom, equality and adequate conditions of life, in an environment of a quality that permits a life of dignity and well-being", as well as of recent developments in international law, including General Assembly resolution 45/94 on the need to ensure a healthy environment for the well-being

of individuals; Principle 1 of the Rio Declaration; and regional human rights instruments such as article 10 of the San Salvador Protocol to the American Convention on Human Rights.

14. ILO Convention No. 155, art. 4.2.

15. See para. 12 (b) and note 8 above.

16. For the core obligations, see paras. 43 and 44 of the present General Comments.

17. Article 24.1 of the Convention on the Rights of the Child.

18. See World Health Assembly resolution WHA47.10, 1994, entitled "Maternal and child health and family planning: traditional practices harmful to the health of women and children".

19. Recent emerging international norms relevant to indigenous peoples include the ILO Convention No. 169 concerning Indigenous and Tribal Peoples in Independent Countries (1989); articles 29 (c) and (d) and 30 of the Convention on the Rights of the Child (1989); article 8 (j) of the Convention on Biological Diversity (1992), recommending that States respect, preserve and maintain knowledge, innovation and practices of indigenous communities; Agenda 21 of the United Nations Conference on Environment and Development (1992), in particular chapter 26; and Part I, paragraph 20, of the Vienna Declaration and Programme of Action (1993), stating that States should take concerted positive steps to ensure respect for all human rights of indigenous people, on the basis of non-discrimination. See also the preamble and article 3 of the United Nations Framework Convention on Climate Change (1992); and article 10 (2) (e) of the United Nations Convention to Combat Desertification in Countries Experiencing Serious Drought and/or Desertification, Particularly in Africa (1994). During recent years an increasing number of States have changed their constitutions and introduced legislation recognizing specific rights of indigenous peoples.

20. See General Comment No. 13, para. 43.

21. See General Comment No. 3, para. 9; General Comment No. 13, para. 44.

22. See General Comment No. 3, para. 9; General Comment No. 13, para. 45.

23. According to General Comments Nos. 12 and 13, the obligation to fulfil incorporates an obligation to facilitate and an obligation to provide. In the present General Comment, the obligation to fulfil also incorporates an obligation to promote because of the critical importance of health pro-

motion in the work of WHO and elsewhere.

24. General Assembly resolution 46/119 (1991).

25. Elements of such a policy are the identification, determination, authorization and control of dangerous materials, equipment, substances, agents and work processes; the provision of health information to workers and the provision, if needed, of adequate protective clothing and equipment; the enforcement of laws and regulations through adequate inspection; the requirement of notification of occupational accidents and diseases, the conduct of inquiries into serious accidents and diseases, and the production of annual statistics; the protection of workers and their representatives from disciplinary measures for actions properly taken by them in conformity with such a policy; and the provision of occupational health services with essentially preventive functions. See ILO Occupational Safety and Health Convention, 1981 (No. 155) and Occupational Health Services Convention, 1985 (No. 161).

26. Article II, Alma-Ata Declaration, Report of the International Conference on Primary Health Care, Alma-Ata, 6-12 September 1978, in: World Health Organization, "Health for All" Series, No. 1, WHO, Geneva, 1978.

27. See para. 45 of this General Comment.

28. Report of the International Conference on Population and Development, Cairo, 5-13 September 1994 (United Nations publication, Sales No. E.95.XIII.18), chap. I, resolution 1, annex, chaps. VII and VIII.

29. Covenant, art. 2.1.

30. Regardless of whether groups as such can seek remedies as distinct holders of rights, States parties are bound by both the collective and individual dimensions of article 12. Collective rights are critical in the field of health; modern public health policy relies heavily on prevention and promotion which are approaches directed primarily to groups.

31. See General Comment No. 2, para. 9.

B. Regional Texts

European Social Charter (1961 as Revised in 1996) (1996)
[Available at http://conventions.coe.int/treaty/en/Treaties/Html/163.htm]

* * *

Article 11: The Right to Protection of Health

With a view to ensuring the effective exercise of the right to protection of health, the Parties undertake, either directly or in cooperation with public or private organisations, to take appropriate measures designed inter alia:

1. To remove as far as possible the causes of ill-health;

2. to provide advisory and educational facilities for the promotion of health and the encouragement of individual responsibility in matters of health;

3. To prevent as far as possible epidemic, endemic and other diseases, as well as accidents.

* * *

African Charter on Human and Peoples' Rights (1981)
[Available at http://www1.umn.edu/humanrts/instree/z1afchar.htm]

* * *

Article 16

1. Every individual shall have the right to enjoy the best attainable state of physical and mental health.

2. States Parties to the present Charter shall take the necessary measures to protect the health of their people and to ensure that they receive medical attention when they are sick.

* * *

Additional Protocol to the American Convention on Human Rights in the Area of Economic, Social and Cultural Rights (1988)
[Available at http://www.oas.org/juridico/english/Treaties/a-52.html]

* * *

Article 10
Right to Health

1. Everyone shall have the right to health, understood to mean the enjoyment of the highest level of physical, mental and social well-being.

2. In order to ensure the exercise of the right to health, the States Parties agree to recognize health as a public good and, particularly, to adopt the following measures to ensure that right:

a. Primary health care, that is, essential health care made available to all individuals and families in the community;

b. Extension of the benefits of health services to all individuals subject to the State's jurisdiction;

c. Universal immunization against the principal infectious diseases;

d. Prevention and treatment of endemic, occupational and other diseases;

e. Education of the population on the prevention and treatment of health problems, and

f. Satisfaction of the health needs of the highest risk groups and of those whose poverty makes them the most vulnerable.

* * *

C. Other General Texts on Health and Human Rights

Declaration of Alma-Ata (1978)
Adopted by the International Conference on Primary Health Care,
Alma-Ata, USSR, 6-12 September 1978.
[Available at: http://www.who.int/hpr/NPH/docs/declaration_almaata.pdf]

The International Conference on Primary Health Care, meeting in Alma-Ata this twelfth day of September in the year Nineteen hundred and seventy-eight, expressing the need for urgent action by all governments, all health and development workers, and the world community to protect and promote the health of all the people of the world, hereby makes the following Declaration:

I

The Conference strongly reaffirms that health, which is a state of complete physical, mental and social wellbeing, and not merely the absence of disease or infirmity, is a fundamental human right and that the attainment of the highest possible level of health is a most important world-wide social goal whose realization requires the action of many other social and economic sectors in addition to the health sector.

II

The existing gross inequality in the health status of the people particularly between developed and developing countries as well as within countries is politically, socially and economically unacceptable and is, therefore, of common concern to all countries.

III

Economic and social development, based on a New International Economic Order, is of basic importance to the fullest attainment of health for all and to the reduction of the gap between the health status of the developing and developed countries. The promotion and protection of the health of the people is essential to sustained economic and social development and contributes to a better quality of life and to world peace.

IV

The people have the right and duty to participate individually and collectively in the planning and implementation of their health care.

V

Governments have a responsibility for the health of their people which can be fulfilled only by the provision of adequate health and social measures. A main social target of governments, international organizations and the whole world community in the coming decades should be the attainment by all peoples of the world by the year 2000 of a level of health that will permit them to lead a socially and economically productive life. Primary health care is the key to attaining this target as part of development in the spirit of social justice.

VI

Primary health care is essential health care based on practical, scientifically sound and socially acceptable methods and technology made universally accessible to individuals and families in the community through their full participation and at a cost that the community and country can afford to maintain at every stage of their development in the spirit of self-reliance and self-determination. It forms an integral part both of the country's health system, of which it is the central function and main focus, and of the overall social and economic development of the community. It is the first level of contact of individuals, the family and community with the national health system bringing health care as close as possible to where people live and work, and constitutes the first element of a continuing health care process.

VII

Primary Health Care:

reflects and evolves from the economic conditions and sociocultural and political characteristics of the country and its communities and is based on the application of the relevant results of social, biomedical and health services research and public health experience;

addresses the main health problems in the community, providing promotive, preventive, curative and rehabilitative services accordingly;

includes at least: education concerning prevailing health problems and the methods of preventing and controlling them; promotion of food supply and proper nutrition; an adequate supply of safe water and basic sanitation; maternal and child health care, including family planning; immunization against the major infectious diseases; prevention and control of locally endemic diseases; appropriate treatment of common diseases and injuries; and provision of essential drugs;

involves, in addition to the health sector, all related sectors and aspects of national and community development, in particular agriculture, animal husbandry, food, industry, education, housing, public works, communications and other sectors; and demands the coordinated efforts of all those sectors;

requires and promotes maximum community and individual self-reliance and participation in the planning, organization, operation and control of primary health care, making fullest use of local, national and other available resources; and to this end develops through appropriate education the ability of communities to participate;

should be sustained by integrated, functional and mutually supportive referral systems, leading to the progressive improvement of comprehensive health care for all, and giving priority to those most in need;

relies, at local and referral levels, on health workers, including physicians, nurses, midwives, auxiliaries and community workers as applicable, as well as traditional practitioners as needed, suitably trained socially and technically to work as a health team and to respond to the expressed health needs of the community.

VIII

All governments should formulate national policies, strategies and plans of action to launch and sustain primary health care as part of a comprehensive national health system and in coordination with other sectors. To this end, it will be necessary to exercise political will, to mobilize the country's resources and to use available external resources rationally.

IX

All countries should cooperate in a spirit of partnership and service to ensure primary health care for all people since the attainment of health by people in any one country directly concerns and benefits every other country. In this context the joint WHO/UNICEF report on primary health care constitutes a solid basis for the further development and operation of primary health care throughout the world.

X

An acceptable level of health for all the people of the world by the year 2000 can be attained through a fuller and better use of the world's resources, a considerable part of which is now spent on armaments and military conflicts. A genuine policy of independence, peace, détente and disarmament could and should release additional resources that could well be devoted to peaceful aims and in particular to the acceleration of social and economic development of which primary health care, as an essential part, should be allotted its proper share.

The International Conference on Primary Health Care calls for urgent and effective national and international action to develop and implement primary health care throughout the world and particularly in developing countries in a spirit of technical cooperation and in keeping with a New International Economic Order. It urges governments, WHO and UNICEF, and other international organizations, as well as multilateral and bilateral agencies, non-governmental organizations, funding agencies, all health workers and the whole world community to support national and international commitment to primary health care and to channel increased technical and financial support to it, particularly in developing countries. The Conference calls on all the aforementioned to collaborate in introducing, developing and maintaining primary health care in accordance with the spirit and content of this Declaration.

Peoples' Charter for Health (2000)

Adopted on 8 December 2000 by the People's Health Assembly (PHA), a meeting of more than 1,400 people from over 90 countries in Savar, Bangladesh, from 4-8 December 2000. [Available at: http://phmovement.org/pdf/charter/phm-pch-english.pdf]

PREAMBLE

Health is a social, economic and political issue and above all a fundamental human right. Inequality, poverty, exploitation, violence and injustice are at the root of ill-health and the deaths of poor and marginalised people. Health for all means that powerful interests have to be challenged, that globalisation has to be opposed, and that political and economic priorities have to be drastically changed.

This Charter builds on perspectives of people whose voices have rarely been heard before, if at all. It encourages people to develop their own solutions and to hold accountable local authorities, national governments, international organisations and corporations.

VISION

Equity, ecologically-sustainable development and peace are at the heart of our vision of a better world — a world in which a healthy life for all is a reality; a world that respects, appreciates and celebrates all life and diversity; a world that enables the flowering of people's talents and abilities to enrich each other; a world in which people's voices guide the decisions that shape our lives. There are more than enough resources to achieve this vision.

THE HEALTH CRISIS

"Illness and death every day anger us. Not because there are people who get sick or because there are people who die. We are angry because many illnesses and deaths have their roots in the economic and social policies that are imposed on us."

(A voice from Central America)

In recent decades, economic changes world-wide have profoundly affected people's health and their access to health care and other social services.

Despite unprecedented levels of wealth in the world, poverty and hunger are increasing. The gap between rich and poor nations has widened, as have inequalities within countries, between social classes, between men and women and between young and old.

A large proportion of the world's population still lacks access to food, education, safe drinking water, sanitation, shelter, land and its resources, employment and health care services. Discrimination continues to prevail. It affects both the occurrence of disease and access to health care.

The planet's natural resources are being depleted at an alarming rate. The resulting degradation of the environment threatens everyone's health, especially the health of the poor. There has been an upsurge of new conflicts while weapons of mass destruction still pose a grave threat.

The world's resources are increasingly concentrated in the hands of a few who strive to maximise their private profit. Neoliberal political and economic policies are made by a small group of powerful governments, and by international institutions such as the World Bank, the International Monetary Fund and the World Trade Organisation. These policies, together with the unregulated activities of transnational corporations, have had severe effects on the lives and livelihoods, health and well-being of people in both North and South.

Public services are not fulfilling people's needs, not least because they have deteriorated as a result of cuts in governments' social budgets. Health services have become less accessible, more unevenly distributed and more inappropriate.

Privatisation threatens to undermine access to health care still further and to compromise the essential principle of equity. The persistence of preventable ill health, the resurgence of diseases such as tuberculosis and malaria, and the emergence and spread of new diseases such as HIV/AIDS are a stark reminder of our world's lack of commitment to principles of equity and justice.

PRINCIPLES OF THE PEOPLE'S CHARTER FOR HEALTH

• The attainment of the highest possible level of health and well-being is a fundamental human right, regardless of a person's colour, ethnic background, religion, gender, age, abilities, sexual orientation or class.

• The principles of universal, comprehensive Primary Health Care (PHC), envisioned in the 1978 Alma Ata Declaration, should be the basis for formulating policies related to health. Now more than ever an equitable, participatory and intersectoral approach to health and health care is needed.

• Governments have a fundamental responsibility to ensure universal access to quality health care, education and other social services according to people's needs, not according to their ability to pay.

• The participation of people and people's organisations is essential to the formulation, implementation and evaluation of all health and social policies and programmes.

• Health is primarily determined by the political, economic, social and physical environment and should, along with equity and sustainable development, be a top priority in local, national and international policy-making.

A CALL FOR ACTION

To combat the global health crisis, we need to take action at all levels — individual, community, national, regional and global — and in all sectors. The demands presented below provide a basis for action.

HEALTH AS A HUMAN RIGHT

Health is a reflection of a society's commitment to equity and justice. Health and human rights should prevail over economic and political concerns.

This Charter calls on people of the world to:

• Support all attempts to implement the right to health.

• Demand that governments and international organisations reformulate, implement and enforce policies and practices which respect the right to health.

• Build broad-based popular movements to pressure governments to incorporate health and human rights into national constitutions and legislation.

• Fight the exploitation of people's health needs for purposes of profit.

TACKLING THE BROADER DETERMINANTS OF HEALTH
Economic Challenges

The economy has a profound influence on people's health. Economic policies that prioritise equity, health and social well-being can improve the health of the people as well as the economy.

Political, financial, agricultural and industrial policies which respond primarily to capitalist needs, imposed by national governments and international organisations, alienate people from their lives and livelihoods. The processes of economic globalisation and liberalisation have increased inequalities between and within nations.

Many countries of the world and especially the most powerful ones are using their resources, including economic sanctions and military interventions, to consolidate and expand their positions, with devastating effects on people's lives.

This Charter calls on people of the world to:

• Demand transformation of the World Trade Organisation and the global trading system so that it ceases to violate social, environmental, economic and health rights of people and begins to discriminate positively in favour of countries of the South. In order to protect public health, such transformation must include intellectual property regimes such as patents and the Trade Related aspects of Intellectual Property Rights (TRIPS) agreement.

• Demand the cancellation of Third World debt.

• Demand radical transformation of the World Bank and International Monetary Fund so that these institutions reflect and actively promote the rights and interests of developing countries.

• Demand effective regulation to ensure that TNCs do not have negative effects on people's health, exploit their workforce, degrade the environment or impinge on national sovereignty.

• Ensure that governments implement agricultural policies attuned to people's needs and not to the demands of the market, thereby guaranteeing food security and equitable access to food.

• Demand that national governments act to protect public health rights in intellectual property laws.

• Demand the control and taxation of speculative international capital flows.

• Insist that all economic policies be subject to health, equity, gender and environmental impact assessments and include enforceable regulatory measures to ensure compliance.

• Challenge growth-centred economic theories and replace them with alternatives that create humane and sustainable societies. Economic theories should recognise environmental constraints, the fundamental importance of equity and health, and the contribution of unpaid labour, especially the unrecognised work of women.

Social and Political Challenges

Comprehensive social policies have positive effects on people's lives and livelihoods. Economic globalisation and privatisation have profoundly disrupted communities, families and cultures. Women are essential to sustaining the social fabric of societies everywhere, yet their basic needs are often ignored or denied, and their rights and persons violated.

Public institutions have been undermined and weakened. Many of their responsibilities have been transferred to the private sector, particularly corporations, or to other national and international institutions, which are rarely accountable to the people. Furthermore, the power of political parties and trade unions has been severely curtailed, while conservative and fundamentalist forces are on the rise. Participatory democracy in political organisations and civic structures should thrive. There is an urgent need to foster and ensure transparency and accountability.

This Charter calls on people of the world to:

• Demand and support the development and implementation of comprehensive social policies with full participation of people.

• Ensure that all women and all men have equal rights to work, livelihoods, to freedom of expression, to political participation, to exercise religious choice, to education and to freedom from violence.

• Pressure governments to introduce and enforce legislation to protect and promote the physical, mental and spiritual health and human rights of marginalised groups.

• Demand that education and health are placed at the top of the political agenda. This calls for free and compulsory quality education for all children and adults, particularly girl children and women, and for quality early childhood education and care.

• Demand that the activities of public institutions, such as child care services, food distribution systems, and housing provisions, benefit the health of individuals and communities.

• Condemn and seek the reversal of any policies, which result in the forced displacement of people from their lands, homes or jobs.

• Oppose fundamentalist forces that threaten the rights and liberties of individuals, particularly the lives of women, children and minorities.

• Oppose sex tourism and the global traffic of women and children.

Environmental Challenges

Water and air pollution, rapid climate change, ozone layer depletion, nuclear energy and waste, toxic chemicals and pesticides, loss of biodiversity, deforestation and soil erosion have far-reaching effects on people's health. The root causes of this destruction include the unsustainable exploitation of natural resources, the absence of a long-term holistic vision, the spread of individualistic and profit-maximising behaviours, and over-consumption by the rich. This destruction must be confronted and reversed immediately and effectively.

This Charter calls on people of the world to:

• Hold transnational and national corporations, public institutions and the military accountable for their destructive and hazardous activities that impact on the environment and people's health.

• Demand that all development projects be evaluated against health and environmental criteria and that caution and restraint be applied whenever technologies or policies pose potential threats to health and the environment (the precautionary principle).

• Demand that governments rapidly commit themselves to reductions of greenhouse gases from their own territories far stricter than those set out in the international climate change agreement, without resorting to hazardous or inappropriate technologies and practices.

• Oppose the shifting of hazardous industries and toxic and radioactive waste to poorer countries and marginalised communities and encourage solutions that minimise waste production.

• Reduce over-consumption and non-sustainable lifestyles — both in the North and the South. Pressure wealthy industrialised countries to reduce their consumption and pollution by 90 percent.

• Demand measures to ensure occupational health and safety, including worker-centred monitoring of working conditions.

• Demand measures to prevent accidents and injuries in the workplace, the community and in homes.

• Reject patents on life and oppose bio-piracy of traditional and indigenous knowledge and resources.

• Develop people-centred, community-based indicators of environmental and social progress, and to press for the development and adoption of regular audits that measure environmental degradation and the health status of the population.

War, Violence, Conflict and Natural Disasters

War, violence, conflict and natural disasters devastate communities and destroy human dignity. They have a severe impact on the physical and mental health of their members, especially women and children. Increased arms procurement and an aggressive and corrupt international arms trade undermine social, political and economic stability and the allocation of resources to the social sector.

This Charter calls on people of the world to:

• Support campaigns and movements for peace and disarmament.

• Support campaigns against aggression, and the research, production, testing and use of weapons of mass destruction and other arms, including all types of landmines.

• Support people's initiatives to achieve a just and lasting peace, especially in countries with experiences of civil war and genocide.

• Condemn the use of child soldiers, and the abuse and rape, torture and killing of women and children.

• Demand the end of occupation as one of the most destructive tools to human dignity.

• Oppose the militarisation of humanitarian relief interventions.

• Demand the radical transformation of the UN Security Council so that it functions democratically.

• Demand that the United Nations and individual states end all kinds of sanctions used as an instrument of aggression which can damage the health of civilian populations.

• Encourage independent, people-based initiatives to declare neighbourhoods, communities and cities areas of peace and zones free of weapons.

• Support actions and campaigns for the prevention and reduction of aggressive and violent behaviour, especially in men, and the fostering of peaceful coexistence.

• Support actions and campaigns for the prevention of natural disasters and the reduction of subsequent human suffering.

A PEOPLE-CENTERED HEALTH SECTOR

This Charter calls for the provision of universal and comprehensive primary health care, irrespective of people's ability to pay. Health services must be democratic and accountable with sufficient resources to achieve this.

This Charter calls on people of the world to:

• Oppose international and national policies that privatise health care and turn it into a commodity.

• Demand that governments promote, finance and provide comprehensive Primary Health Care as the most effective way of addressing health problems and organising public health services so as to ensure free and universal access.

• Pressure governments to adopt, implement and enforce national health and drugs policies.

• Demand that governments oppose the privatisation of public health services and ensure effective regulation of the private medical sector, including charitable and NGO medical services.

• Demand a radical transformation of the World Health Organization (WHO) so that it responds to health challenges in a manner which benefits the poor, avoids vertical approaches, ensures intersectoral work, involves people's organisations in the World Health Assembly, and ensures independence from corporate interests.

• Promote, support and engage in actions that encourage people's power and control in decision-making in health at all levels, including patient and consumer rights.

• Support, recognise and promote traditional and holistic healing systems and practitioners and their integration into Primary Health Care.

• Demand changes in the training of health personnel so that they become more problem-oriented and practice-based, understand better the impact of global issues in their communities, and are encouraged to work with and respect the community and its diversities.

• Demystify medical and health technologies (including medicines) and demand that they be subordinated to the health needs of the people.

• Demand that research in health, including genetic research and the development of medicines and reproductive technologies, is carried out in a participatory, needs-based manner by accountable institutions. It should be people- and public health-oriented, respecting universal ethical principles.

• Support people's rights to reproductive and sexual self-determination and oppose all coercive measures in population and family planning policies. This support includes the right to the full range of safe and effective methods of fertility regulation.

PEOPLE'S PARTICIPATION FOR A HEALTHY WORLD

Strong people's organisations and movements are fundamental to more democratic, transparent and accountable decision-making processes. It is essential that people's civil, political, economic, social and cultural rights are ensured. While governments have the primary responsibility for promoting a more equitable approach to health and human rights, a wide range of civil society groups and movements, and the media have an important role to play in ensuring people's power and control in policy development and in the monitoring of its implementation.

This Charter calls on people of the world to:

• Build and strengthen people's organisations to create a basis for analysis and action.

• Promote, support and engage in actions that encourage people's involvement in decision-making in public services at all levels.

• Demand that people's organisations be represented in local, national and international fora that are relevant to health.

• Support local initiatives towards participatory democracy through the establishment of people-centred solidarity networks across the world.

III. Protection of Existence and Physical Integrity

A. The Right to Life

Universal Declaration of Human Rights (1948)

Adopted and proclaimed by General Assembly Resolution 217 A (III)
of 10 December 1948.

---

* * *

Article 3

Everyone has the right to life, liberty and security of person.

* * *

International Covenant on Civil and Political Rights (1966)

Adopted and opened for signature, ratification and accession by General Assembly
Resolution 2200A (XXI) of 16 December 1966. Entered into force on 23 March 1976.
[Available at http://www.unhchr.ch/html/menu3/b/a_ccpr.htm]

---

* * *

Article 6

1. Every human being has the inherent right to life. This right shall be protected by law. No one shall be arbitrarily deprived of his life.

2. In countries which have not abolished the death penalty, sentence of death may be imposed only for the most serious crimes in accordance with the law in force at the time of the commission of the crime and not contrary to the provisions of the present Covenant and to the Convention on the Prevention and Punishment of the Crime of Genocide. This penalty can only be carried out pursuant to a final judgement rendered by a competent court.

3. When deprivation of life constitutes the crime of genocide, it is understood that nothing in this article shall authorize any State Party to the present Covenant to derogate in any way from any obligation assumed under the provisions of the Convention on the Prevention and Punishment of the Crime of Genocide.

4. Anyone sentenced to death shall have the right to seek pardon or commutation of the sentence. Amnesty, pardon or commutation of the sentence of death may be granted in all cases.

5. Sentence of death shall not be imposed for crimes committed by persons below eighteen years of age and shall not be carried out on pregnant women.

6. Nothing in this article shall be invoked to delay or to prevent the abolition of capital punishment by any State Party to the present Covenant.

* * *

Second Optional Protocol to the International Covenant on Civil and Political Rights, Aiming at the Abolition of the Death Penalty (1989)

Adopted and General Assembly Resolution 44/128, annex, 44 U.N. GAOR Supp. (No. 49) at 207, U.N. Doc. A/44/49 (1989), entered into force 11 July 1991.
[Available at http://www1.umn.edu/humanrts/instree/b5ccprp2.htm]

The States Parties to the Present Protocol,

Believing that abolition of the death penalty contributes to enhancement of human dignity and progressive development of human rights,

Recalling article 3 of the Universal Declaration of Human Rights, adopted on 10 December 1948, and article 6 of the International Covenant on Civil and Political Rights, adopted on 16 December 1966,

Noting that article 6 of the International Covenant on Civil and Political Rights refers to abolition of the death penalty in terms that strongly suggest that abolition is desirable,

Convinced that all measures of abolition of the death penalty should be considered as progress in the enjoyment of the right to life,

Desirous to undertake hereby an international commitment to abolish the death penalty,

Have agreed as follows:

Article 1

1. No one within the jurisdiction of a State Party to the present Protocol shall be executed.

2. Each State Party shall take all necessary measures to abolish the death penalty within its jurisdiction.

Article 2

1. No reservation is admissible to the present Protocol, except for a reservation made at the time of ratification or accession that provides for the application of the death penalty in time of war pursuant to a conviction for a most serious crime of a military nature committed during wartime.

2. The State Party making such a reservation shall at the time of ratification or accession communicate to the Secretary-General of the United Nations the relevant provisions of its national legislation applicable during wartime.

3. The State Party having made such a reservation shall notify the Secretary-General of the United Nations of any beginning or ending of a state of war applicable to its territory.

Article 3

The States Parties to the present Protocol shall include in the reports they submit to the Human Rights Committee, in accordance with article 40 of the Covenant, information on the measures that they have adopted to give effect to the present Protocol.

Article 4

With respect to the States Parties to the Covenant that have made a declaration under article 41, the competence of the Human Rights Committee to receive and consider communications when a State Party claims that another State Party is not fulfilling its obligations shall extend to the provisions of the present Protocol, unless the State Party concerned has made a statement to the contrary at the moment of ratification or accession.

Article 5

With respect to the States Parties to the first Optional Protocol to the International Covenant on Civil and Political Rights adopted on 16 December 1966, the competence of the Human Rights Committee to receive and consider communications from individuals subject to its jurisdiction shall extend to the provisions of the present Protocol, unless the State Party concerned has made a statement to the contrary at the moment of ratification or accession.

Article 6

1. The provisions of the present Protocol shall apply as additional provisions to the Covenant.

2. Without prejudice to the possibility of a reservation under article 2 of the present Protocol, the right guaranteed in article 1, paragraph 1, of the present Protocol shall not be subject to any derogation under article 4 of the Covenant.

Article 7

1. The present Protocol is open for signature by any State that has signed the Covenant.

2. The present Protocol is subject to ratification by any State that has ratified the Covenant or acceded to it. Instruments of ratification shall be deposited with the Secretary-General of the United Nations.

3. The present Protocol shall be open to accession by any State that has ratified the Covenant or acceded to it.

4. Accession shall be effected by the deposit of an instrument of accession with the Secretary-General of the United Nations.

5. The Secretary-General of the United Nations shall inform all States that have signed the present Protocol or acceded to it of the deposit of each instrument of ratification or accession.

Article 8

1. The present Protocol shall enter into force three months after the date of the deposit with the Secretary-General of the United Nations of the tenth instrument of ratification or accession.

2. For each State ratifying the present Protocol or acceding to it after the deposit of the tenth instrument of ratification or accession, the present Protocol shall enter into force three months after the date of the deposit of its own instrument of ratification or accession.

Article 9

The provisions of the present Protocol shall extend to all parts of federal States without any limitations or exceptions.

Article 10

The Secretary-General of the United Nations shall inform all States referred to in article 48, paragraph 1, of the Covenant of the following particulars:

(a) Reservations, communications and notifications under article 2 of the present Protocol;

(b) Statements made under articles 4 or 5 of the present Protocol;

(c) Signatures, ratifications and accessions under article 7 of the present Protocol:

(d) The date of the entry into force of the present Protocol under article 8 thereof.

Article 11

1. The present Protocol, of which the Arabic, Chinese, English, French, Russian and Spanish texts are equally authentic, shall be deposited in the archives of the United Nations.

2. The Secretary-General of the United Nations shall transmit certified copies of the present Protocol to all States referred to in article 48 of the Covenant.

World Medical Association Resolution on Physician Participation in Capital Punishment (1981)

Adopted by the 34th World Medical Assembly Lisbon, Portugal, September 28-October 2, 1981 and amended by the 52nd WMA General Assembly in Edinburgh, Scotland, during October 2000.
[Available at http://www.wma.net/e/policy/c1.htm]

RESOLVED, that it is unethical for physicians to participate in capital punishment, in any way, or during any step of the execution process.

Torture, Death Penalty and Participation by Nurses in Executions (1998)

Adopted by the International Council of Nurses in 1998. Replaces previous ICN Positions "Nurses and Torture", adopted 1989 and "Death penalty and participation by nurses in execution" adopted 1989. [Available at http://www.icn.ch/pstorture.htm]

[Footnotes omitted.]

The International Council of Nurses (ICN) supports the United Nations Universal Declaration of Human Rights. Furthermore we declare:

The nurse's primary responsibility is to those people who require nursing care.

Nurses have the duty to provide the highest possible level of care to victims of cruel, degrading and inhumane treatment.

The nurse shall not voluntarily participate in any deliberate infliction of physical or mental suffering.

The nurse's responsibility to a prisoner sentenced to death continues until execution.

ICN considers the death penalty to be the ultimate form of inhumanity.

Participation by nurses, either directly or indirectly, in the preparation for and the implementation of executions is a violation of nursing's ethical code.

ICN advocates that its member national nurses' associations (NNAs) lobby for abolition of the death penalty. ICN further advocates that NNAs develop mechanisms to ensure nurses have access to confidential advice and support in caring for prisoners sentenced to death or subjected to torture.

ICN advocates that all levels of nursing education curricula include the following: recognition of human rights issues and violations, such as torture and death penalty; awareness of the use of medical technology for executions; and recognition of the nurse's right to refuse participation in executions.

Declaration on the Participation of Psychiatrists in the Death Penalty (1989)

Adopted by the General Assembly of the World Psychiatric Association at its World Congress in Athens, October 1989.
[Available at http://www.wpanet.org/generalinfo/ethic7.html]

Psychiatrists are physicians and adhere to the Hippocratic Oath "to practice for the good of their patients and never to do harm."

The World Psychiatric Association is an international association with 77 Member Societies.

Considering that the United Nations' Principles of Medical Ethics enjoins physicians — and thus psychiatrists — to refuse to enter into any relationship with a prisoner, other than one directed at evaluation, protecting or improving their physical and mental health, and further, considering that the Declaration of Hawaii of the WPA resolves that the psychiatrist shall serve the best interests of the patient and treat every patient with the solicitude and respect due to the dignity of all human beings and that the psychiatrist must refuse to cooperate if some third party demands actions contrary to ethical principles.

Conscious that psychiatrists may be called on to participate in any action connected to executions

Declares that the participation of psychiatrists in any such action is a violation of professional ethics.

B. Freedom from Torture

Universal Declaration of Human Rights (1948)
Adopted and proclaimed by General Assembly
Resolution 217 A (III) of 10 December 1948.

* * *

Article 5

No one shall be subjected to torture or to cruel,
inhuman or degrading treatment or punishment.

* * *

International Covenant on Civil and Political Rights (1966)
Adopted and opened for signature, ratification and accession by General Assembly
Resolution 2200A (XXI) of 16 December 1966.
Entered into force 23 March 1976.
[Available at http://www.unhchr.ch/html/menu3/b/a_ccpr.htm]

* * *

Article 7

No one shall be subjected to torture or to cruel, inhuman or degrading treatment or punishment. In
particular, no one shall be subjected without his free
consent to medical or scientific experimentation.

* * *

Convention Against Torture and Other Cruel, Inhuman or Degrading Treatment or Punishment (1984)
Adopted and opened for signature, ratification and accession by UN General Assembly
Resolution 39/46 of 10 December 1984. Entered into force on 26 June 1987.
[Available at http://www.hrweb.org/legal/cat.html]

* * *

PART I

Article 1

1. For the purposes of this Convention, torture
means any act by which severe pain or suffering,
whether physical or mental, is intentionally inflicted on a person for such purposes as obtaining
from him or a third person information or a confession, punishing him for an act he or a third
person has committed or is suspected of having
committed, or intimidating or coercing him or a
third person, or for any reason based on discrimination of any kind, when such pain or suffering is
inflicted by or at the instigation of or with the consent or acquiescence of a public official or other
person acting in an official capacity. It does not in-

clude pain or suffering arising only from, inherent in or incidental to lawful sanctions.

2. This article is without prejudice to any international instrument or national legislation which does or may contain provisions of wider application.

Article 2

1. Each State Party shall take effective legislative, administrative, judicial or other measures to prevent acts of torture in any territory under its jurisdiction.

2. No exceptional circumstances whatsoever, whether a state of war or a threat or war, internal political instability or any other public emergency, may be invoked as a justification of torture.

3. An order from a superior officer or a public authority may not be invoked as a justification of torture.

Article 3

1. No State Party shall expel, return ("refouler") or extradite a person to another State where there are substantial grounds for believing that he would be in danger of being subjected to torture.

2. For the purpose of determining whether there are such grounds, the competent authorities shall take into account all relevant considerations including, where applicable, the existence in the State concerned of a consistent pattern of gross, flagrant or mass violations of human rights.

Article 4

1. Each State Party shall ensure that all acts of torture are offences under its criminal law. The same shall apply to an attempt to commit torture and to an act by any person which constitutes complicity or participation in torture.

2. Each State Party shall make these offences punishable by appropriate penalties which take into account their grave nature.

* * *

Declaration of Tokyo: Guidelines for Medical Doctors Concerning Torture and Other Cruel, Inhuman or Degrading Treatment or Punishment in Relation to Detention and Imprisonment (1975)
Adopted by the 29th World Medical Assembly Tokyo, Japan, October 1975.
[Available at http://www.wma.net/e/policy/c18.htm]

PREAMBLE

It is the privilege of the medical doctor to practise medicine in the service of humanity, to preserve and restore bodily and mental health without distinction as to persons, to comfort and to ease the suffering of his or her patients. The utmost respect for human life is to be maintained even under threat, and no use made of any medical knowledge contrary to the laws of humanity.

For the purpose of this Declaration, torture is defined as the deliberate, systematic or wanton infliction of physical or mental suffering by one or more persons acting alone or on the orders of any authority, to force another person to yield information, to make a confession, or for any other reason.

DECLARATION

1. The doctor shall not countenance, condone or participate in the practice of torture or other forms of cruel, inhuman or degrading procedures, whatever the offense of which the victim of such procedures is suspected, accused or guilty, and whatever the victim's beliefs or motives, and in all situations, including armed conflict and civil strife.

2. The doctor shall not provide any premises, instruments, substances or knowledge to facilitate the practice of torture or other forms of cruel, inhuman or degrading treatment or to diminish the ability of the victim to resist such treatment.

3. The doctor shall not be present during any procedure during which torture or other forms of

cruel, inhuman or degrading treatment is used or threatened.

4. A doctor must have complete clinical independence in deciding upon the care of a person for whom he or she is medically responsible. The doctor's fundamental role is to alleviate the distress of his or her fellow men, and no motive whether personal, collective or political shall prevail against this higher purpose.

5. Where a prisoner refuses nourishment and is considered by the doctor as capable of forming an unimpaired and rational judgment concerning the consequences of such a voluntary refusal of nour-ishment, he or she shall not be fed artificially. The decision should be confirmed by at least one other independent doctor. The consequences of the refusal of nourishment shall be explained by the doctor to the prisoner.

6. The World Medical Association will support, and should encourage the international community, the national medical associations and fellow doctors to support the doctor and his or her family in the face of threats or reprisals resulting from a refusal to condone the use of torture or other forms of cruel, inhuman or degrading treatment.

Principles of Medical Ethics Relevant to the Role of Health Personnel, Particularly Physicians, in the Protection of Prisoners and Detainees Against Torture and Other Cruel, Inhuman or Degrading Treatment or Punishment (1982)

General Assembly Resolution of 18 December 1982.
[Available at http://www.unhchr.ch/html/menu3/b/h_comp40.htm]

[Footnotes omitted.]

Principle 1

Health personnel, particularly physicians, charged with the medical care of prisoners and detainees have a duty to provide them with protection of their physical and mental health and treatment of disease of the same quality and standard as is afforded to those who are not imprisoned or detained.

Principle 2

It is a gross contravention of medical ethics, as well as an offence under applicable international instruments, for health personnel, particularly physicians, to engage, actively or passively, in acts which constitute participation in, complicity in, incitement to or attempts to commit torture or other cruel, inhuman or degrading treatment or punishment.

Principle 3

It is a contravention of medical ethics for health personnel, particularly physicians, to be involved in any professional relationship with prisoners or detainees the purpose of which is not solely to evaluate, protect or improve their physical and mental health.

Principle 4

It is a contravention of medical ethics for health personnel, particularly physicians:

(a) To apply their knowledge and skills in order to assist in the interrogation of prisoners and detainees in a manner that may adversely affect the physical or mental health or condition of such prisoners or detainees and which is not in accordance with the relevant international instruments;

(b) To certify, or to participate in the certification of, the fitness of prisoners or detainees for any form of treatment or punishment that may adversely affect their physical or mental health and which is not in accordance with the relevant international instruments, or to participate in any way in the infliction of any such treatment or punishment which is not in accordance with the relevant international instruments.

Principle 5

It is a contravention of medical ethics for health personnel, particularly physicians, to participate in any procedure for restraining a prisoner or detainee unless such a procedure is determined in accordance with purely medical criteria as being necessary for the protection of the physical or mental health or the safety of the prisoner or detainee himself, of his fellow prisoners or detainees, or of his guardians, and presents no hazard to his physical or mental health.

Principle 6

There may be no derogation from the foregoing principles on any ground whatsoever, including public emergency.

Torture, Death Penalty and Participation by Nurses in Executions (1998)

[See text on page 68.]

Manual on the Effective Investigation and Documentation of Torture and Other Cruel, Inhuman or Degrading Treatment or Punishment (Istanbul Protocol) (1999)
Submitted to the United Nations High Commissioner for Human Rights 9 August 1999.
[United Nations Publication Sales No. E.01.XIV.1
Available at http:// www.unhchr.ch/pdf/8istprot.pdf]

[Footnotes omitted.]

From the Introduction: *The Manual on the Effective Investigation and Documentation of Torture and Other Cruel, Inhuman or Degrading Treatment or Punishment* (the Istanbul Protocol) is intended to serve as international guidelines for the assessment of persons who allege torture and ill-treatment, for investigating cases of alleged torture and for reporting findings to the judiciary or any other investigative body. … These principles outline minimum standards for States in order to ensure the effective documentation of torture. The guidelines contained in this manual are not presented as a fixed protocol. Rather, they represent minimum standards based on the principles and should be used taking into account available resources.

CHAPTER I

RELEVANT INTERNATIONAL LEGAL STANDARDS
* * *

CHAPTER II
RELEVANT ETHICAL CODES

* * *

CHAPTER III

LEGAL INVESTIGATION OF TORTURE

73. States are required under international law to investigate reported incidents of torture promptly and impartially. Where evidence warrants it, a State in whose territory a person alleged to have committed or participated in torture is present, must either extradite the alleged perpetrator to another State that has competent jurisdiction or submit the case to its own competent authorities for the purpose of prosecution under national or local criminal laws. The fundamental principles of any viable investigation into incidents of torture are competence, impartiality, independence, promptness and thoroughness. These elements can be adapted to any legal system and should guide all investigations of alleged torture.

74. Where investigative procedures are inadequate because of a lack of resources or expertise, the appearance of bias, the apparent existence of a pattern of abuse or other substantial reasons, States shall pursue investigations through an independent

commission of inquiry or similar procedure. Members of that commission must be chosen for their recognized impartiality, competence and independence as individuals. In particular, they must be independent of any institution, agency or person that may be the subject of the inquiry.

75. Section A describes the broad purpose of an investigation into torture. Section B sets forth basic principles on the effective investigation and documentation of torture and other cruel, inhuman or degrading treatment or punishment. Section C sets forth suggested procedures for conducting an investigation into alleged torture, first considering the decision regarding the appropriate investigative authority, then offering guidelines regarding collection of oral testimony from the reported victim and other witnesses and collection of physical evidence. Section D provides guidelines for establishing a special independent commission of inquiry. These guidelines are based on the experiences of several countries that have established independent commissions to investigate alleged human rights abuses, including extrajudicial killing, torture and disappearances.

A. Purposes of an Investigation into Torture

76. The broad purpose of the investigation is to establish the facts relating to alleged incidents of torture, with a view to identifying those responsible for the incidents and facilitating their prosecution, or for use in the context of other procedures designed to obtain redress for victims. The issues addressed here may also be relevant for other types of investigations of torture. To fulfill this purpose, those carrying out the investigation must, at a minimum, seek to obtain statements from the victims of alleged torture; to recover and preserve evidence, including medical evidence, related to the alleged torture to aid in any potential prosecution of those responsible; to identify possible witnesses and obtain statements from them concerning the alleged torture; and to determine how, when and where the alleged incidents of torture occurred as well as any pattern or practice that may have brought about the torture.

B. Principles for the Effective Investigation and Documentation of Torture and Other Cruel, Inhuman or Degrading Treatment or Punishment

* * *

C. Procedures of a Torture Investigation
* * *

D. Commission of Inquiry
* * *

CHAPTER IV

GENERAL CONSIDERATIONS FOR INTERVIEWS

119. When a person who has allegedly been tortured is interviewed, there are a number of issues and practical factors that have to be taken into consideration. These considerations apply to all persons carrying out interviews, whether they are lawyers, medical doctors, psychologists, psychiatrists, human rights monitors or members of any other profession. The following section takes up this "common ground" and attempts to put it into contexts that may be encountered when investigating torture and interviewing victims of torture.

A. Purpose of Inquiry, Examination and Documentation
* * *

B. Procedural Safeguards with Respect to Detainees
* * *

C. Official Visits to Detention Centres
* * *

D. Techniques of Questioning
* * *

E. Documenting the Background
1. Psychosocial History and Pre-Arrest
* * *
2. Summary of Detention and Abuse
* * *
3. Circumstances of Detention
* * *
4. Place and Conditions of Detention
* * *
5. Methods of Torture and Ill-Treatment
* * *

F. Assessment of the Background
* * *

G. Review of Torture Methods
* * *

H. Risk of Re-Traumatization of the Interviewee
* * *

I. Use of Interpreters
* * *

CHAPTER V

PHYSICAL EVIDENCE OF TORTURE

160. Witness and survivor testimony are necessary components in the documentation of torture. To the extent that physical evidence of torture exists, it provides important confirmatory evidence that a person was tortured. However, the absence of such physical evidence should not be construed to suggest that torture did not occur, since such acts of violence against persons frequently leave no marks or permanent scars.

161. A medical evaluation for legal purposes should be conducted with objectivity and impartiality. The evaluation should be based on the physician's clinical expertise and professional experience. The ethical obligation of beneficence demands uncompromising accuracy and impartiality in order to establish and maintain professional credibility. When possible, clinicians who conduct evaluations of detainees should have specific essential training in forensic documentation of torture and other forms of physical and psychological abuse. They should have knowledge of prison conditions and torture methods used in the particular region where the patient was imprisoned and the common after-effects of torture. The medical report should be factual and carefully worded. Jargon should be avoided. All medical terminology should be defined so that it is understandable to lay persons. The physician should not assume that the official requesting a medical-legal evaluation has related all the material facts. It is the physician's responsibility to discover and report upon any material findings that he or she considers relevant, even if they may be considered irrelevant or adverse to the case of the party requesting the medical examination. Findings that are consistent with torture or other forms of ill-treatment must not be excluded from a medical-legal report under any circumstance.

CHAPTER VI
PSYCHOLOGICAL EVIDENCE
OF TORTURE

A. General Considerations

1. The Central Role of the Psychological Evaluation

233. It is a widely held view that torture is an extraordinary life experience capable of causing a wide range of physical and psychological suffering. Most clinicians and researchers agree that the extreme nature of the torture event is powerful enough on its own to produce mental and emotional consequences, regardless of the individual's pre-torture psychological status. The psychological consequences of torture, however, occur in the context of personal attribution of meaning, personality development and social, political and cultural factors. For this reason, it cannot be assumed that all forms of torture have the same outcome. For example, the psychological consequences of a mock execution are not the same as those due to a sexual assault, and solitary confine-

ment and isolation are not likely to produce the same effects as physical acts of torture. Likewise, one cannot assume that the effects of detention and torture on an adult will be the same as those on a child. Nevertheless, there are clusters of symptoms and psychological reactions that have been observed and documented in torture survivors with some regularity.

234. Perpetrators often attempt to justify their acts of torture and ill-treatment by the need to gather information. Such conceptualizations obscure the purpose of torture and its intended consequences. One of the central aims of torture is to reduce an individual to a position of extreme helplessness and distress that can lead to a deterioration of cognitive, emotional and behavioural functions. Thus, torture is a means of attacking an individual's fundamental modes of psychological and social functioning. Under such circumstances, the torturer strives not only to incapacitate physically a victim but also to disintegrate the individual's personality. The torturer attempts to destroy a victim's sense of being grounded in a family and society as a human being with dreams, hopes and aspirations for the future. By dehumanizing and breaking the will of their victims, torturers set horrific examples for those who later come in contact with the victim. In this way, torture can break or damage the will and coherence of entire communities. In addition, torture can profoundly damage intimate relationships between spouses, parents, children, other family members and relationships between the victims and their communities.

235. It is important to recognize that not everyone who has been tortured develops a diagnosable mental illness. However, many victims experience profound emotional reactions and psychological symptoms. The main psychiatric disorders associated with torture are post-traumatic stress disorder (PTSD) and major depression. While these disorders are present in the general population, their prevalence is much higher among traumatized populations. The unique cultural, social and polit-

ical implications that torture has for each individual influence his or her ability to describe and speak about it. These are important factors that contribute to the impact that torture inflicts psychologically and socially and that must be considered when performing an evaluation of an individual from another culture. Cross-cultural research reveals that phenomenological or descriptive methods are the most rational approaches to use when attempting to evaluate psychological or psychiatric disorders. What is considered disordered behaviour or a disease in one culture may not be viewed as pathological in another. Since the Second World War, progress has been made towards understanding the psychological consequences of violence. Certain psychological symptoms and clusters of symptoms have been observed and documented among survivors of torture and other types of violence.

236. In recent years, the diagnosis of post-traumatic stress disorder has been applied to an increasingly broad array of individuals suffering from the impact of widely varying types of violence. However, the utility of this diagnosis in non-western cultures has not been established. Nevertheless, evidence suggests that there are high rates of post-traumatic stress disorder and depression symptoms among traumatized refugee populations from many different ethnic and cultural backgrounds. The World Health Organization's cross-cultural study of depression provides helpful information. While some symptoms may be present across different cultures, they may not be the symptoms that concern the individual the most.

2. The Context of the Psychological Evaluation

* * *

B. Psychological Consequences of Torture
* * *

C. The Psychological/Psychiatric Evaluation
* * *

Principles on the Effective Investigation and Documentation of Torture and Other Cruel, Inhuman or Degrading Treatment or Punishment (2000)

Adopted by General Assembly Resolution 55/89 Annex, 4 December 2000.
[Available at http://www.unhchr/html/menu3/b/h_comp51.htm]

1. The purposes of effective investigation and documentation of torture and other cruel, inhuman or degrading treatment or punishment (hereinafter "torture or other ill-treatment") include the following:

(a) Clarification of the facts and establishment and acknowledgement of individual and State responsibility for victims and their families;

(b) Identification of measures needed to prevent recurrence;

(c) Facilitation of prosecution and/or, as appropriate, disciplinary sanctions for those indicated by the investigation as being responsible and demonstration of the need for full reparation and redress from the State, including fair and adequate financial compensation and provision of the means for medical care and rehabilitation.

2. States shall ensure that complaints and reports of torture or ill-treatment are promptly and effectively investigated. Even in the absence of an express complaint, an investigation shall be undertaken if there are other indications that torture or ill-treatment might have occurred. The investigators, who shall be independent of the suspected perpetrators and the agency they serve, shall be competent and impartial. They shall have access to, or be empowered to commission investigations by, impartial medical or other experts. The methods used to carry out such investigations shall meet the highest professional standards and the findings shall be made public.

3. (a) The investigative authority shall have the power and obligation to obtain all the information necessary to the inquiry. The persons conducting the investigation shall have at their disposal all the necessary budgetary and technical resources for effective investigation. They shall also have the authority to oblige all those acting in an official capacity allegedly involved in torture or ill-treatment to appear and testify. The same shall apply to any witness. To this end, the investigative authority shall be entitled to issue summonses to witnesses, including any officials allegedly involved, and to demand the production of evidence.

(b) Alleged victims of torture or ill-treatment, witnesses, those conducting the investigation and their families shall be protected from violence, threats of violence or any other form of intimidation that may arise pursuant to the investigation. Those potentially implicated in torture or ill-treatment shall be removed from any position of control or power, whether direct or indirect, over complainants, witnesses and their families, as well as those conducting the investigation.

4. Alleged victims of torture or ill-treatment and their legal representatives shall be informed of, and have access to, any hearing, as well as to all information relevant to the investigation, and shall be entitled to present other evidence.

5. (a) In cases in which the established investigative procedures are inadequate because of insufficient expertise or suspected bias, or because of the apparent existence of a pattern of abuse or for other substantial reasons, States shall ensure that investigations are undertaken through an independent commission of inquiry or similar procedure. Members of such a commission shall be chosen for their recognized impartiality, competence and independence as individuals. In particular, they shall be independent of any suspected perpetrators and the institutions or agencies they may serve. The commission shall have the authority to obtain all information necessary to the inquiry and shall conduct the inquiry as provided for under these Principles.

(b) A written report, made within a reasonable time, shall include the scope of the inquiry, procedures and methods used to evaluate evidence as well as conclusions and recommendations based on findings of fact and on applicable law. Upon completion, the report shall be made public. It shall also describe in detail specific events that were found to have occurred and the evidence upon which such findings were based and list the names of witnesses who testified, with the exception of those whose identities have been withheld for their own protection. The State shall, within a reasonable period of time, reply to the report of the investigation and, as appropriate, indicate steps to be taken in response.

6. (a) Medical experts involved in the investigation of torture or ill-treatment shall behave at all times in conformity with the highest ethical standards and, in particular, shall obtain informed consent before any examination is undertaken. The examination must conform to established standards of medical practice. In particular, examinations shall be conducted in private under the control of the medical expert and outside the presence of security agents and other government officials.

(b) The medical expert shall promptly prepare an accurate written report, which shall include at least the following:

(i) Circumstances of the interview: name of the subject and name and affiliation of those present at the examination; exact time and date; location, nature and address of the institution (including, where appropriate, the room) where the examination is being conducted (e.g., detention centre, clinic or house); circumstances of the subject at the time of the examination (e.g., nature of any restraints on arrival or during the examination, presence of security forces during the examination, demeanour of those accompanying the prisoner or threatening statements to the examiner); and any other relevant factors;

(ii) History: detailed record of the subject's story as given during the interview, including alleged methods of torture or ill-treatment, times when torture or ill-treatment is alleged to have occurred and all complaints of physical and psychological symptoms;

(iii) Physical and psychological examination: record of all physical and psychological findings on clinical examination, including appropriate diagnostic tests and, where possible, colour photographs of all injuries;

(iv) Opinion: interpretation as to the probable relationship of the physical and psychological findings to possible torture or ill-treatment. A recommendation for any necessary medical and psychological treatment and/or further examination shall be given;

(v) Authorship: the report shall clearly identify those carrying out the examination and shall be signed.

(c) The report shall be confidential and communicated to the subject or his or her nominated representative. The views of the subject and his or her representative about the examination process shall be solicited and recorded in the report. It shall also be provided in writing, where appropriate, to the authority responsible for investigating the allegation of torture or ill-treatment. It is the responsibility of the State to ensure that it is delivered securely to these persons. The report shall not be made available to any other person, except with the consent of the subject or on the authorization of a court empowered to enforce such a transfer.

C. Disappearances and Summary and Extra-Judicial Execution

Declaration on the Protection of All Persons from Enforced Disappearances (1992)

General Assembly Resolution 47/133. Adopted 18 December 1992.
[Available at: http://www.unhchr.ch/huridocda/huridoca.nsf/
(Symbol)/A.RES.47.133.En?OpenDocument]

The General Assembly,

Considering that, in accordance with the principles proclaimed in the Charter of the United Nations and other international instruments, recognition of the inherent dignity and of the equal and inalienable rights of all members of the human family is the foundation of freedom, justice and peace in the world,

Bearing in mind the obligation of States under the Charter, in particular Article 55, to promote universal respect for, and observance of, human rights and fundamental freedoms,

Deeply concerned that in many countries, often in a persistent manner, enforced disappearances occur, in the sense that persons are arrested, detained or abducted against their will or otherwise deprived of their liberty by officials of different branches or levels of Government, or by organized groups or private individuals acting on behalf of, or with the support, direct or indirect, consent or acquiescence of the Government, followed by a refusal to disclose the fate or whereabouts of the persons concerned or a refusal to acknowledge the deprivation of their liberty, which places such persons outside the protection of the law,

Considering that enforced disappearance undermines the deepest values of any society committed to respect for the rule of law, human rights and fundamental freedoms, and that the systematic practice of such acts is of the nature of a crime against humanity,

Recalling its resolution 33/173 of 20 December 1978, in which it expressed concern about the reports from various parts of the world relating to enforced or involuntary disappearances, as well as

about the anguish and sorrow caused by those disappearances, and called upon Governments to hold law enforcement and security forces legally responsible for excesses which might lead to enforced or involuntary disappearances of persons,

Recalling also the protection afforded to victims of armed conflicts by the Geneva Conventions of 12 August 1949 and the Additional Protocols thereto, of 1977,

Having regard in particular to the relevant articles of the Universal Declaration of Human Rights and the International Covenant on Civil and Political Rights, which protect the right to life, the right to liberty and security of the person, the right not to be subjected to torture and the right to recognition as a person before the law,

Having regard also to the Convention against Torture and Other Cruel, Inhuman or Degrading Treatment or Punishment, which provides that States parties shall take effective measures to prevent and punish acts of torture,

Bearing in mind the Code of Conduct for Law Enforcement Officials, the Basic Principles on the Use of Force and Firearms by Law Enforcement officials, the Declaration of Basic Principles of Justice for Victims of Crime and Abuse of Power and the Standard Minimum Rules for the Treatment of Prisoners,

Affirming that, in order to prevent enforced disappearances, it is necessary to ensure strict compliance with the Body of Principles for the Protection of All Persons under any form of Detention or Imprisonment contained in the annex to its resolution 43/173 of 9 December 1988, and with the Principles on the Effective Prevention and

Investigation of Extra-legal, Arbitrary and Summary Executions, set forth in the annex to Economic and Social Council resolution 1989/65 of 24 May 1989 and endorsed by the General Assembly in its resolution 44/162 of 15 December 1989,

Bearing in mind that, while the acts which comprise enforced disappearance constitute a violation of the prohibition found in the aforementioned international instruments, it is none the less important to devise an instrument which characterizes all acts of enforced disappearance of persons as very serious offences and sets forth standards designed to punish and prevent their commission,

1. Proclaims the present Declaration on the Protection of all Persons from Enforced Disappearance, as a body of principles for all States;

2. Urges that all efforts be made so that the Declaration becomes generally known and respected;

Article 1

1. Any act of enforced disappearance is an offence to human dignity. It is condemned as a denial of the purposes of the Charter of the United Nations and as a grave and flagrant violation of the human rights and fundamental freedoms proclaimed in the Universal Declaration of Human Rights and reaffirmed and developed in international instruments in this field.

2. Any act of enforced disappearance places the persons subjected thereto outside the protection of the law and inflicts severe suffering on them and their families. It constitutes a violation of the rules of international law guaranteeing, inter alia, the right to recognition as a person before the law, the right to liberty and security of the person and the right not to be subjected to torture and other cruel, inhuman or degrading treatment or punishment. It also violates or constitutes a grave threat to the right to life.

Article 2

1. No State shall practise, permit or tolerate enforced disappearances.

2. States shall act at the national and regional levels and in cooperation with the United Nations to contribute by all means to the prevention and eradication of enforced disappearance.

Article 3

Each State shall take effective legislative, administrative, judicial or other measures to prevent and terminate acts of enforced disappearance in any territory under its jurisdiction.

Article 4

1. All acts of enforced disappearance shall be offences under criminal law punishable by appropriate penalties which shall take into account their extreme seriousness.

2. Mitigating circumstances may be established in national legislation for persons who, having participated in enforced disappearances, are instrumental in bringing the victims forward alive or in providing voluntarily information which would contribute to clarifying cases of enforced disappearance.

Article 5

In addition to such criminal penalties as are applicable, enforced disappearances render their perpetrators and the State or State authorities which organize, acquiesce in or tolerate such disappearances liable under civil law, without prejudice to the international responsibility of the State concerned in accordance with the principles of international law.

Article 6

1. No order or instruction of any public authority, civilian, military or other, may be invoked to justify an enforced disappearance. Any person receiving such an order or instruction shall have the right and duty not to obey it.

2. Each State shall ensure that orders or instructions directing, authorizing or encouraging any enforced disappearance are prohibited.

3. Training of law enforcement officials shall emphasize the provisions in paragraphs 1 and 2 of the present article.

Article 7

No circumstances whatsoever, whether a threat of war, a state of war, internal political instability or any other public emergency, may be invoked to justify enforced disappearances.

Article 8

1. No State shall expel, return (refouler) or extradite a person to another State where there are substantial grounds to believe that he would be in danger of enforced disappearance.

2. For the purpose of determining whether there are such grounds, the competent authorities shall take into account all relevant considerations including, where applicable, the existence in the State concerned of a consistent pattern of gross, flagrant or mass violations of human rights.

Article 9

1. The right to a prompt and effective judicial remedy as a means of determining the whereabouts or state of health of persons deprived of their liberty and/or identifying the authority ordering or carrying out the deprivation of liberty is required to prevent enforced disappearances under all circumstances, including those referred to in article 7 above.

2. In such proceedings, competent national authorities shall have access to all places where persons deprived of their liberty are being held and to each part of those places, as well as to any place in which there are grounds to believe that such persons may be found.

3. Any other competent authority entitled under the law of the State or by any international legal instrument to which the State is a party may also have access to such places.

Article 10

1. Any person deprived of liberty shall be held in an officially recognized place of detention and, in conformity with national law. be brought before a judicial authority promptly after detention.

2. Accurate information on the detention of such persons and their place or places of detention, including transfers, shall be made promptly avail-able to their family members, their counsel or to any other persons having a legitimate interest in the information unless a wish to the contrary has been manifested by the persons concerned.

3. An official up-to-date register of all persons deprived of their liberty shall be maintained in every place of detention. Additionally, each State shall take steps to maintain similar centralized registers. The information contained in these registers shall be made available to the persons mentioned in the preceding paragraph, to any judicial or other competent and independent national authority and to any other competent authority entitled under the law of the State concerned or any international legal instrument to which a State concerned is a party, seeking to trace the whereabouts of a detained person.

Article 11

All persons deprived of liberty must be released in a manner permitting reliable verification that they have actually been released and, further, have been released in conditions in which their physical integrity and ability fully to exercise their rights are assured.

Article 12

1. Each State shall establish rules under its national law indicating those officials authorized to order deprivation of liberty, establishing the conditions under which such orders may be given, and stipulating penalties for officials who, without legal justification, refuse to provide information on any detention.

2. Each State shall likewise ensure strict supervision, including a clear chain of command, of all law enforcement officials responsible for apprehensions, arrests, detentions, custody, transfers and imprisonment, and of other officials authorized by law to use force and firearms.

Article 13

1. Each State shall ensure that any person having knowledge or a legitimate interest who alleges that a person has been subjected to enforced disappearance has the right to complain to a competent and independent State authority and to have that complaint promptly, thoroughly and impartially investigated by that authority. Whenever

there are reasonable grounds to believe that an enforced disappearance has been committed, the State shall promptly refer the matter to that authority for such an investigation, even if there has been no formal complaint. No measure shall be taken to curtail or impede the investigation.

2. Each State shall ensure that the competent authority shall have the necessary powers and resources to conduct the investigation effectively, including powers to compel attendance of witnesses and production of relevant documents and to make immediate on-site visits.

3. Steps shall be taken to ensure that all involved in the investigation, including the complainant, counsel, witnesses and those conducting the investigation, are protected against ill-treatment, intimidation or reprisal.

4. The findings of such an investigation shall be made available upon request to all persons concerned, unless doing so would jeopardize an ongoing criminal investigation.

5. Steps shall be taken to ensure that any ill-treatment, intimidation or reprisal or any other form of interference on the occasion of the lodging of a complaint or during the investigation procedure is appropriately punished.

6. An investigation, in accordance with the procedures described above, should be able to be conducted for as long as the fate of the victim of enforced disappearance remains unclarified.

Article 14

Any person alleged to have perpetrated an act of enforced disappearance in a particular State shall, when the facts disclosed by an official investigation so warrant, be brought before the competent civil authorities of that State for the purpose of prosecution and trial unless he has been extradited to another State wishing to exercise jurisdiction in accordance with the relevant international agreements in force. All States should take any lawful and appropriate action available to them to bring to justice all persons presumed responsible for an act of enforced disappearance, who are found to be within their jurisdiction or under their control.

Article 15

The fact that there are grounds to believe that a person has participated in acts of an extremely serious nature such as those referred to in article 4, paragraph 1, above, regardless of the motives, shall be taken into account when the competent authorities of the State decide whether or not to grant asylum.

Article 16

1. Persons alleged to have committed any of the acts referred to in article 4, paragraph 1, above, shall be suspended from any official duties during the investigation referred to in article 13 above.

2. They shall be tried only by the competent ordinary courts in each State, and not by any other special tribunal, in particular military courts.

3. No privileges, immunities or special exemptions shall be admitted in such trials, without prejudice to the provisions contained in the Vienna Convention on Diplomatic Relations.

4. The persons presumed responsible for such acts shall be guaranteed fair treatment in accordance with the relevant provisions of the Universal Declaration of Human Rights and other relevant international agreements in force at all stages of the investigation and eventual prosecution and trial.

Article 17

1. Acts constituting enforced disappearance shall be considered a continuing offence as long as the perpetrators continue to conceal the fate and the whereabouts of persons who have disappeared and these facts remain unclarified.

2. When the remedies provided for in article 2 of the International Covenant on Civil and Political Rights are no longer effective, the statute of limitations relating to acts of enforced disappearance shall be suspended until these remedies are re-established.

3. Statutes of limitations, where they exist, relating to acts of enforced disappearance shall be substantial and commensurate with the extreme seriousness of the offence.

Article 18

1. Persons who have or are alleged to have committed offences referred to in article 4, paragraph 1, above, shall not benefit from any special amnesty law or similar measures that might have the effect of exempting them from any criminal proceedings or sanction.

2. In the exercise of the right of pardon, the extreme seriousness of acts of enforced disappearance shall be taken into account.

Article 19

The victims of acts of enforced disappearance and their family shall obtain redress and shall have the right to adequate compensation, including the means for as complete a rehabilitation as possible. In the event of the death of the victim as a result of an act of enforced disappearance, their dependants shall also be entitled to compensation.

Article 20

1. States shall prevent and suppress the abduction of children of parents subjected to enforced disappearance and of children born during their mother's enforced disappearance, and shall devote their efforts to the search for and identification of such children and to the restitution of the children to their families of origin.

2. Considering the need to protect the best interests of children referred to in the preceding paragraph, there shall be an opportunity, in States which recognize a system of adoption, for a review of the adoption of such children and, in particular, for annulment of any adoption which originated in enforced disappearance. Such adoption should, however, continue to be in force if consent is given, at the time of the review, by the child's closest relatives.

3. The abduction of children of parents subjected to enforced disappearance or of children born during their mother's enforced disappearance, and the act of altering or suppressing documents attesting to their true identity, shall constitute an extremely serious offence, which shall be punished as such.

4. For these purposes, States shall, where appropriate, conclude bilateral and multilateral agreements.

Article 21

The provisions of the present Declaration are without prejudice to the provisions enunciated in the Universal Declaration of Human Rights or in any other international instrument, and shall not be construed as restricting or derogating from any of those provisions.

Inter-American Convention on Forced Disappearance of Persons (1994)

Adopted by the 24th regular session of the General Assembly of the Organization of American States on 9 June 1994. Entered into force 28 March 1996.
[Available at: http://www.oas.org/juridico/english/Treaties/a-60.html]

PREAMBLE

The member states of the Organization of American States signatory to the present Convention,

Disturbed by the persistence of the forced disappearance of persons;

Reaffirming that the true meaning of American solidarity and good neighborliness can be none other than that of consolidating in this Hemisphere, in the framework of democratic institutions, a system of individual freedom and social justice based on respect for essential human rights;

Considering that the forced disappearance of persons is an affront to the conscience of the Hemisphere and a grave and abominable offense against the inherent dignity of the human being, and one that contradicts the principles and purposes enshrined in the Charter of the Organization of American States;

Considering that the forced disappearance of persons violates numerous non-derogable and essential human rights enshrined in the American Convention on Human Rights, in the American Declaration of the Rights and Duties of Man, and in the Universal Declaration of Human Rights;

Recalling that the international protection of human rights is in the form of a convention reinforcing or complementing the protection provided by domestic law and is based upon the attributes of the human personality;

Reaffirming that the systematic practice of the forced disappearance of persons constitutes a crime against humanity;

Hoping that this Convention may help to prevent, punish, and eliminate the forced disappearance of persons in the Hemisphere and make a decisive contribution to the protection of human rights and the rule of law,

Resolve to adopt the following Inter-American Convention on Forced Disappearance of Persons:

Article I

The States Parties to this Convention undertake:

a. Not to practice, permit, or tolerate the forced disappearance of persons, even in states of emergency or suspension of individual guarantees;

b. To punish within their jurisdictions, those persons who commit or attempt to commit the crime of forced disappearance of persons and their accomplices and accessories;

c. To cooperate with one another in helping to prevent, punish, and eliminate the forced disappearance of persons;

d. To take legislative, administrative, judicial, and any other measures necessary to comply with the commitments undertaken in this Convention.

Article II

For the purposes of this Convention, forced disappearance is considered to be the act of depriving a person or persons of his or their freedom, in whatever way, perpetrated by agents of the state or by persons or groups of persons acting with the authorization, support, or acquiescence of the state, followed by an absence of information or a refusal to acknowledge that deprivation of freedom or to give information on the whereabouts of that person, thereby impeding his or her recourse to the applicable legal remedies and procedural guarantees.

Article III

The States Parties undertake to adopt, in accordance with their constitutional procedures, the legislative measures that may be needed to define the forced disappearance of persons as an offense and to impose an appropriate punishment commensurate with its extreme gravity. This offense shall be deemed continuous or permanent as long as the fate or whereabouts of the victim has not been determined.

The States Parties may establish mitigating circumstances for persons who have participated in acts constituting forced disappearance when they help to cause the victim to reappear alive or provide information that sheds light on the forced disappearance of a person.

Article IV

The acts constituting the forced disappearance of persons shall be considered offenses in every State Party. Consequently, each State Party shall take measures to establish its jurisdiction over such cases in the following instances:

a. When the forced disappearance of persons or any act constituting such offense was committed within its jurisdiction;

b. When the accused is a national of that state;

c. When the victim is a national of that state and that state sees fit to do so.

Every State Party shall, moreover, take the necessary measures to establish its jurisdiction over the crime described in this Convention when the alleged criminal is within its territory and it does not proceed to extradite him.

This Convention does not authorize any State Party to undertake, in the territory of another State Party, the exercise of jurisdiction or the performance of functions that are placed within the exclusive purview of the authorities of that other Party by its domestic law.

Article V

The forced disappearance of persons shall not be considered a political offense for purposes of extradition.

The forced disappearance of persons shall be deemed to be included among the extraditable offenses in every extradition treaty entered into between States Parties.

The States Parties undertake to include the offense of forced disappearance as one which is extra-ditable in every extradition treaty to be concluded between them in the future.

Every State Party that makes extradition conditional on the existence of a treaty and receives a request for extradition from another State Party with which it has no extradition treaty may consider this Convention as the necessary legal basis for extradition with respect to the offense of forced disappearance.

States Parties which do not make extradition conditional on the existence of a treaty shall recognize such offense as extraditable, subject to the conditions imposed by the law of the requested state.

Extradition shall be subject to the provisions set forth in the constitution and other laws of the request state.

Article VI

When a State Party does not grant the extradition, the case shall be submitted to its competent authorities as if the offense had been committed within its jurisdiction, for the purposes of investigation and when appropriate, for criminal action, in accordance with its national law. Any decision adopted by these authorities shall be communicated to the state that has requested the extradition.

Article VII

Criminal prosecution for the forced disappearance of persons and the penalty judicially imposed on its perpetrator shall not be subject to statutes of limitations.

However, if there should be a norm of a fundamental character preventing application of the stipulation contained in the previous paragraph, the period of limitation shall be equal to that which applies to the gravest crime in the domestic laws of the corresponding State Party.

Article VIII

The defense of due obedience to superior orders or instructions that stipulate, authorize, or encourage forced disappearance shall not be admitted. All persons who receive such orders have the right and duty not to obey them.

The States Parties shall ensure that the training of public law-enforcement personnel or officials includes the necessary education on the offense of forced disappearance of persons.

Article IX

Persons alleged to be responsible for the acts constituting the offense of forced disappearance of persons may be tried only in the competent jurisdictions of ordinary law in each state, to the exclusion of all other special jurisdictions, particularly military jurisdictions.

The acts constituting forced disappearance shall not be deemed to have been committed in the course of military duties.

Privileges, immunities, or special dispensations shall not be admitted in such trials, without prejudice to the provisions set forth in the Vienna Convention on Diplomatic Relations.

Article X

In no case may exceptional circumstances such as a state of war, the threat of war, internal political instability, or any other public emergency be invoked to justify the forced disappearance of persons. In such cases, the right to expeditious and effective judicial procedures and recourse shall be retained as a means of determining the whereabouts or state of health of a person who has been deprived of freedom, or of identifying the official who ordered or carried out such deprivation of freedom.

In pursuing such procedures or recourse, and in keeping with applicable domestic law, the competent judicial authorities shall have free and immediate access to all detention centers and to each of their units, and to all places where there is reason to believe the disappeared person might be found including places that are subject to military jurisdiction.

Article XI

Every person deprived of liberty shall be held in an officially recognized place of detention and be brought before a competent judicial authority without delay, in accordance with applicable domestic law.

The States Parties shall establish and maintain official up-to-date registries of their detainees and, in accordance with their domestic law, shall make them available to relatives, judges, attorneys, any other person having a legitimate interest, and other authorities.

Article XII

The States Parties shall give each other mutual assistance in the search for, identification, location, and return of minors who have been removed to another state or detained therein as a consequence of the forced disappearance of their parents or guardians.

Article XIII

For the purposes of this Convention, the processing of petitions or communications presented to the Inter-American Commission on Human Rights alleging the forced disappearance of persons shall be subject to the procedures established in the American Convention on Human Rights and to the Statute and Regulations of the Inter-American Commission on Human Rights and to the Statute and Rules of Procedure of the Inter-American Court of Human Rights, including the provisions on precautionary measures.

Article XIV

Without prejudice to the provisions of the preceding article, when the Inter-American Commission on Human Rights receives a petition or communication regarding an alleged forced disappearance, its Executive Secretariat shall urgently and confidentially address the respective government, and shall request that government to provide as soon as possible information as to the whereabouts of the allegedly disappeared person together with any other information it considers pertinent, and such request shall be without prejudice as to the admissibility of the petition.

Article XV

None of the provisions of this Convention shall be interpreted as limiting other bilateral or multilateral treaties or other agreements signed by the Parties.

This Convention shall not apply to the international armed conflicts governed by the 1949 Geneva Conventions and their Protocols, concerning protection of wounded, sick, and ship-wrecked members of the armed forces; and prisoners of war and civilians in time of war.

Article XVI

This Convention is open for signature by the member states of the Organization of American States.

Article XVII

This Convention is subject to ratification. The instruments of ratification shall be deposited with the General Secretariat of the Organization of American States.

Article XVIII

This Convention shall be open to accession by any other state. The instruments of accession shall be deposited with the General Secretariat of the Organization of American States.

Article XIX

The states may express reservations with respect to this Convention when adopting, signing, ratifying or acceding to it, unless such reservations are incompatible with the object and purpose of the Convention and as long as they refer to one or more specific provisions.

Article XX

This Convention shall enter into force for the ratifying states on the thirtieth day from the date of deposit of the second instrument of ratification.

For each state ratifying or acceding to the Convention after the second instrument of ratification has been deposited, the Convention shall enter into force on the thirtieth day from the date on which that state deposited its instrument of ratification or accession.

Article XXI

This Convention shall remain in force indefinitely, but may be denounced by any State Party. The instrument of denunciation shall be deposited with the General Secretariat of the Organization of American States. The Convention shall cease to be in effect for the denouncing state and shall remain in force for the other States Parties one year from the date of deposit of the instrument of denunciation.

Article XXII

The original instrument of this Convention, the Spanish, English, Portuguese, and French texts of which are equally authentic, shall be deposited with the General Secretariat of the Organization of American States, which shall forward certified copies thereof to the United Nations Secretariat, for registration and publication, in accordance with Article 102 of the Charter of the United Nations. The General Secretariat of the Organization of American States shall notify member states of the Organization and states acceding to the Convention of the signatures and deposit of instruments of ratification, accession or denunciation, as well as of any reservations that may be expressed.

Principles on the Effective Prevention and Investigation of Extra-Legal, Arbitrary and Summary Executions (1989)

*Recommended by Economic and Social Council Resolution 1989/65 of 24 May 1989
to be taken into account and respected by Governments within
the framework of their national legislation and practices.
[Available at http://www.unhchr.ch/html/menu3/b/54.htm#top]*

1. Governments shall prohibit by law all extra-legal, arbitrary and summary executions and shall ensure that any such executions are recognized as offences under their criminal laws, and are punishable by appropriate penalties which take into account the seriousness of such offences. Exceptional circumstances including a state of war or threat of war, internal political instability or any other public emergency may not be invoked as a justification of such executions.

Such executions shall not be carried out under any circumstances including, but not limited to, situations of internal armed conflict, excessive or illegal use of force by a public official or other person acting in an official capacity or by a person acting at the instigation, or with the consent or acquiescence of such person, and situations in which deaths occur in custody. This prohibition shall prevail over decrees issued by governmental authority.

2. In order to prevent extra-legal, arbitrary and summary executions, Governments shall ensure strict control, including a clear chain of command over all officials responsible for apprehension, arrest, detention, custody and imprisonment, as well as those officials authorized by law to use force and firearms.

3. Governments shall prohibit orders from superior officers or public authorities authorizing or inciting other persons to carry out any such extralegal, arbitrary or summary executions. All persons shall have the right and the duty to defy such orders. Training of law enforcement officials shall emphasize the above provisions.

4. Effective protection through judicial or other means shall be guaranteed to individuals and groups who are in danger of extra-legal, arbitrary or summary executions, including those who receive death threats.

5. No one shall be involuntarily returned or extradited to a country where there are substantial grounds for believing that he or she may become a victim of extra-legal, arbitrary or summary execution in that country.

6. Governments shall ensure that persons deprived of their liberty are held in officially recognized places of custody, and that accurate information on their custody and whereabouts, including transfers, is made promptly available to their relatives and lawyer or other persons of confidence.

7. Qualified inspectors, including medical personnel, or an equivalent independent authority, shall conduct inspections in places of custody on a regular basis, and be empowered to undertake unannounced inspections on their own initiative, with full guarantees of independence in the exercise of this function. The inspectors shall have unrestricted access to all persons in such places of custody, as well as to all their records.

8. Governments shall make every effort to prevent extra-legal, arbitrary and summary executions through measures such as diplomatic intercession, improved access of complainants to intergovernmental and judicial bodies, and public denunciation. Intergovernmental mechanisms shall be used to investigate reports of any such executions and to take effective action against such practices. Governments, including those of countries where extra-legal, arbitrary and summary executions are reasonably suspected to occur, shall cooperate fully in international investigations on the subject.

Investigation

9. There shall be thorough, prompt and impartial investigation of all suspected cases of extra-legal, arbitrary and summary executions, including cases where complaints by relatives or other reliable reports suggest unnatural death in the above circumstances. Governments shall maintain inves-

tigative offices and procedures to undertake such inquiries. The purpose of the investigation shall be to determine the cause, manner and time of death, the person responsible, and any pattern or practice which may have brought about that death. It shall include an adequate autopsy, collection and analysis of all physical and documentary evidence and statements from witnesses. The investigation shall distinguish between natural death, accidental death, suicide and homicide.

10. The investigative authority shall have the power to obtain all the information necessary to the inquiry. Those persons conducting the investigation shall have at their disposal all the necessary budgetary and technical resources for effective investigation. They shall also have the authority to oblige officials allegedly involved in any such executions to appear and testify. The same shall apply to any witness. To this end, they shall be entitled to issue summonses to witnesses, including the officials allegedly involved and to demand the production of evidence.

11. In cases in which the established investigative procedures are inadequate because of lack of expertise or impartiality, because of the importance of the matter or because of the apparent existence of a pattern of abuse, and in cases where there are complaints from the family of the victim about these inadequacies or other substantial reasons, Governments shall pursue investigations through an independent commission of inquiry or similar procedure. Members of such a commission shall be chosen for their recognized impartiality, competence and independence as individuals. In particular, they shall be independent of any institution, agency or person that may be the subject of the inquiry. The commission shall have the authority to obtain all information necessary to the inquiry and shall conduct the inquiry as provided for under these Principles.

12. The body of the deceased person shall not be disposed of until an adequate autopsy is conducted by a physician, who shall, if possible, be an expert in forensic pathology. Those conducting the autopsy shall have the right of access to all investigative data, to the place where the body was discovered, and to the place where the death is thought to have occurred. If the body has been buried and it later appears that an investigation is

required, the body shall be promptly and competently exhumed for an autopsy. If skeletal remains are discovered, they should be carefully exhumed and studied according to systematic anthropological techniques.

13. The body of the deceased shall be available to those conducting the autopsy for a sufficient amount of time to enable a thorough investigation to be carried out. The autopsy shall, at a minimum, attempt to establish the identity of the deceased and the cause and manner of death. The time and place of death shall also be determined to the extent possible. Detailed colour photographs of the deceased shall be included in the autopsy report in order to document and support the findings of the investigation. The autopsy report must describe any and all injuries to the deceased including any evidence of torture.

14. In order to ensure objective results, those conducting the autopsy must be able to function impartially and independently of any potentially implicated persons or organizations or entities.

15. Complainants, witnesses, those conducting the investigation and their families shall be protected from violence, threats of violence or any other form of intimidation. Those potentially implicated in extra-legal, arbitrary or summary executions shall be removed from any position of control or power, whether direct or indirect, over complainants, witnesses and their families, as well as over those conducting investigations.

16. Families of the deceased and their legal representatives shall be informed of, and have access to, any hearing as well as to all information relevant to the investigation, and shall be entitled to present other evidence. The family of the deceased shall have the right to insist that a medical or other qualified representative be present at the autopsy. When the identity of a deceased person has been determined, a notification of death shall be posted, and the family or relatives of the deceased shall be informed immediately. The body of the deceased shall be returned to them upon completion of the investigation.

17. A written report shall be made within a reasonable period of time on the methods and findings of such investigaptions. The report shall be made

public immediately and shall include the scope of the inquiry, procedures and methods used to evaluate evidence as well as conclusions and recommendations based on findings of fact and on applicable law. The report shall also describe in detail specific events that were found to have occurred and the evidence upon which such findings were based, and list the names of witnesses who testified, with the exception of those whose identities have been withheld for their own protection. The Government shall, within a reasonable period of time, either reply to the report of the investigation, or indicate the steps to be taken in response to it.

Legal Proceedings

18. Governments shall ensure that persons identified by the investigation as having participated in extra-legal, arbitrary or summary executions in any territory under their jurisdiction are brought to justice. Governments shall either bring such persons to justice or cooperate to extradite any such persons to other countries wishing to exercise jurisdiction. This principle shall apply irrespective of who and where the perpetrators or the victims are, their nationalities or where the offence was committed.

19. Without prejudice to principle 3 above, an order from a superior officer or a public authority may not be invoked as a justification for extra-legal, arbitrary or summary executions. Superiors, officers or other public officials may be held responsible for acts committed by officials under their authority if they had a reasonable opportunity to prevent such acts. In no circumstances, including a state of war, siege or other public emergency, shall blanket immunity from prosecution be granted to any person allegedly involved in extra-legal, arbitrary or summary executions.

20. The families and dependents of victims of extra-legal, arbitrary or summary executions shall be entitled to fair and adequate compensation within a reasonable period of time.

D. War Crimes, Crimes Against Humanity, Genocide

Common Article 3 of the Geneva Conventions (1949)

Adopted on 12 August 1949 by the Diplomatic Conference for the Establishment of International Conventions for the Protection of Victims of War, held in Geneva from April 21 to August 1, 1949. Entered into force 21 October 1950.
[Available at http://www.icrc.org/Web/Eng/siteeng0.nsf/html/genevaconventions]

* * *

Article 3

In the case of armed conflict not of an international character occurring in the territory of one of the High Contracting Parties, each party to the conflict shall be bound to apply, as a minimum, the following provisions:

1. Persons taking no active part in the hostilities, including members of armed forces who have laid down their arms and those placed hors de combat by sickness, wounds, detention, or any other cause, shall in all circumstances be treated humanely, without any adverse distinction founded on race, colour, religion or faith, sex, birth or wealth, or any other similar criteria.

To this end the following acts are and shall remain prohibited at any time and in any place whatsoever with respect to the above-mentioned persons:

a. Violence to life and person, in particular murder of all kinds, mutilation, cruel treatment and torture;

b. Taking of hostages;

c. Outrages upon personal dignity, in particular, humiliating and degrading treatment;

d. The passing of sentences and the carrying out of executions without previous judgment pronounced by a regularly constituted court affording all the judicial guarantees which are recognized as indispensable by civilized peoples.

2. The wounded and sick shall be collected and cared for.

An impartial humanitarian body, such as the International Committee of the Red Cross, may offer its services to the Parties to the conflict.

The Parties to the conflict should further endeavour to bring into force, by means of special agreements, all or part of the other provisions of the present Convention.

The application of the preceding provisions shall not affect the legal status of the Parties to the conflict.

* * *

Convention on the Prevention and Punishment of the Crime of Genocide (1948)

Approved and proposed for signature and ratification or accession by General Assembly Resolution 260 A (III) of 9 December 1948. Entered into force 12 January 1951.
[Available at http://www.unchcr.ch/html/menu3/b/p_genoci.htm]

The Contracting Parties,

Having considered the declaration made by the General Assembly of the United Nations in its resolution 96 (I) dated 11 December 1946 that genocide is a crime under international law, contrary to the spirit and aims of the United Nations and condemned by the civilized world,

Recognizing that at all periods of history genocide has inflicted great losses on humanity, and

Being convinced that, in order to liberate mankind from such an odious scourge, international co-operation is required,

Hereby agree as hereinafter provided:

Article 1

The Contracting Parties confirm that genocide, whether committed in time of peace or in time of war, is a crime under international law which they undertake to prevent and to punish.

Article 2

In the present Convention, genocide means any of the following acts committed with intent to destroy, in whole or in part, a national, ethnical, racial or religious group, as such:

(a) Killing members of the group;

(b) Causing serious bodily or mental harm to members of the group;

(c) Deliberately inflicting on the group conditions of life calculated to bring about its physical destruction in whole or in part;

(d) Imposing measures intended to prevent births within the group;

(e) Forcibly transferring children of the group to another group.

Article 3

The following acts shall be punishable:

(a) Genocide;

(b) Conspiracy to commit genocide;

(c) Direct and public incitement to commit genocide;

(d) Attempt to commit genocide;

(e) Complicity in genocide.

Article 4

Persons committing genocide or any of the other acts enumerated in article III shall be punished, whether they are constitutionally responsible rulers, public officials or private individuals.

Article 5

The Contracting Parties undertake to enact, in accordance with their respective Constitutions, the necessary legislation to give effect to the provisions of the present Convention, and, in particular, to provide effective penalties for persons guilty of genocide or any of the other acts enumerated in article III.

Article 6

Persons charged with genocide or any of the other acts enumerated in article III shall be tried by a competent tribunal of the State in the territory of which the act was committed, or by such international penal tribunal as may have jurisdiction with respect to those Contracting Parties which shall have accepted its jurisdiction.

Article 7

Genocide and the other acts enumerated in article III shall not be considered as political crimes for the purpose of extradition.

The Contracting Parties pledge themselves in such cases to grant extradition in accordance with their laws and treaties in force.

Article 8

Any Contracting Party may call upon the competent organs of the United Nations to take such action under the Charter of the United Nations as they consider appropriate for the prevention and suppression of acts of genocide or any of the other acts enumerated in article III.

Article 9

Disputes between the Contracting Parties relating to the interpretation, application or fulfillment of the present Convention, including those relating to the responsibility of a State for genocide or for any of the other acts enumerated in article III, shall be submitted to the International Court of Justice at the request of any of the parties to the dispute.

Article 10

The present Convention, of which the Chinese, English, French, Russian and Spanish texts are equally authentic, shall bear the date of 9 December 1948.

Article 11

The present Convention shall be open until 31 December 1949 for signature on behalf of any Member of the United Nations and of any non-member State to which an invitation to sign has been addressed by the General Assembly.

The present Convention shall be ratified, and the instruments of ratification shall be deposited with the Secretary-General of the United Nations.

After 1 January 1950, the present Convention may be acceded to on behalf of any Member of the United Nations and of any non-member State which has received an invitation as aforesaid. Instruments of accession shall be deposited with the Secretary-General of the United Nations.

Article 12

Any Contracting Party may at any time, by notification addressed to the Secretary-General of the United Nations, extend the application of the present Convention to all or any of the territories for the conduct of whose foreign relations that Contracting Party is responsible.

Article 13

On the day when the first twenty instruments of ratification or accession have been deposited, the Secretary-General shall draw up a process-verbal and transmit a copy thereof to each Member of the United Nations and to each of the non-member States contemplated in article 11.

The present Convention shall come into force on the ninetieth day following the date of deposit of the twentieth instrument of ratification or accession.

Any ratification or accession effected, subsequent to the latter date shall become effective on the ninetieth day following the deposit of the instrument of ratification or accession.

Article 14

The present Convention shall remain in effect for a period of ten years as from the date of its coming into force.

It shall thereafter remain in force for successive periods of five years for such Contracting Parties as have not denounced it at least six months before the expiration of the current period.

Denunciation shall be effected by a written notification addressed to the Secretary-General of the United Nations.

Article 15

If, as a result of denunciations, the number of Parties to the present Convention should become less than sixteen, the Convention shall cease to be in force as from the date on which the last of these denunciations shall become effective.

Article 16

A request for the revision of the present Convention may be made at any time by any Contracting Party by means of a notification in writing addressed to the Secretary-General.

The General Assembly shall decide upon the steps, if any, to be taken in respect of such request.

Article 17

The Secretary-General of the United Nations shall notify all Members of the United Nations and the non-member States contemplated in article XI of the following:

(a) Signatures, ratifications and accessions received in accordance with article 11;

(b) Notifications received in accordance with article 12;

(c) The date upon which the present Convention comes into force in accordance with article 13;

(d) Denunciations received in accordance with article 14;

(e) The abrogation of the Convention in accordance with article 15;

(f) Notifications received in accordance with article 16.

Article 18

The original of the present Convention shall be deposited in the archives of the United Nations.

A certified copy of the Convention shall be transmitted to each Member of the United Nations and to each of the non-member States contemplated in article XI.

Article 19

The present Convention shall be registered by the Secretary-General of the United Nations on the date of its coming into force.

Protocol Additional to the Geneva Conventions of 12 August 1949, and Relating to the Protection of Victims of International Armed Conflicts (Protocol I): Grave Breaches (1977)

Adopted on 8 June 1977 by the Diplomatic Conference on the Reaffirmation and Development of International Humanitarian Law Applicable in Armed Conflicts. Entered into force on 7 December 1978.
[Available at: http://www.icrc.org/ihl.nsf/WebCONVFULL?OpenView]

* * *

Article 11
Protection of Persons

1. The physical or mental health and integrity of persons who are in the power of the adverse Party or who are interned, detained or otherwise deprived of liberty as a result of a situation referred to in Article 1 shall not be endangered by any unjustified act or omission. Accordingly, it is prohibited to subject the persons described in this Article to any medical procedure which is not indicated by the state of health of the person concerned and which is not consistent with generally accepted medical standards which would be applied under similar medical circumstances to persons who are nationals of the Party conducting the procedure and who are in no way deprived of liberty.

2. It is, in particular, prohibited to carry out on such persons, even with their consent:

(a) physical mutilations;

(b) medical or scientific experiments;

(c) removal of tissue or organs for transplantation, except where these acts are justified in conformity with the conditions provided for in paragraph 1.

3. Exceptions to the prohibition in paragraph 2 (c) may be made only in the case of donations of blood for transfusion or of skin for grafting, provided that they are given voluntarily and without any coercion or inducement, and then only for therapeutic purposes, under conditions consistent with generally accepted medical standards and controls designed for the benefit of both the donor and the recipient.

4. Any wilful act or omission which seriously endangers the physical or mental health or integrity of any person who is in the power of a Party other than the one on which he depends and which either violates any of the prohibitions in paragraphs 1 and 2 or fails to comply with the requirements of paragraph 3 shall be a grave breach of this Protocol.

5. The persons described in paragraph 1 have the right to refuse any surgical operation. In case of refusal, medical personnel shall endeavour to obtain a written statement to that effect, signed or acknowledged by the patient.

6. Each Party to the conflict shall keep a medical record for every donation of blood for transfusion or skin for grafting by persons referred to in paragraph 1, if that donation is made under the responsibility of that Party. In addition, each Party to the conflict shall endeavour to keep a record of all medical procedures undertaken with respect to any person who is interned, detained or otherwise deprived of liberty as a result of a situation referred to in Article 1. These records shall be available at all times for inspection by the Protecting Power.

* * *

Article 85
Repression of Breaches
of This Protocol

* * *

3. In addition to the grave breaches defined in Article 11, the following acts shall be regarded as grave breaches of this Protocol, when committed wilfully, in violation of the relevant provisions of this Protocol, and causing death or serious injury to body or health:

(a) making the civilian population or individual civilians the object of attack;

(b) launching an indiscriminate attack affecting the civilian population or civilian objects in the knowledge that such attack will cause excessive loss of life, injury to civilians or damage to civilian objects, as defined in Article 57, paragraph 2 (a)(iii);

(c) launching an attack against works or installations containing dangerous forces in the knowledge that such attack will cause excessive loss of life, injury to civilians or damage to civilian objects, as defined in Article 57, paragraph 2. (a)(iii);

(d) making non-defended localities and demilitarized zones the object of attack;

(e) making a person the object of attack in the knowledge that he is hors de combat;

(f) the perfidious use, in violation of Article 37, of the distinctive emblem of the red cross, red crescent or red lion and sun or of other protective signs recognized by the Conventions or this Protocol.

Protocol Additional to the Geneva Conventions of 12 August 1949, and Relating to the Protection of Victims of Non-International Armed Conflicts (Protocol II) (1977)

Adopted on 8 June 1977 by the Diplomatic Conference on the Reaffirmation and Development of International Humanitarian Law Applicable in Armed Conflicts Entered into force 7 December 1978.
[Available at http://www.icrc.org/ihl.nsf/7c4d08d9b287a42141256739003e636b/ d67c3971bcff1c10c125641e0052b545?OpenDocument]

PREAMBLE

The High Contracting Parties, Recalling that the humanitarian principles enshrined in Article 3 common to the Geneva Conventions of 12 August 1949, constitute the foundation of respect for the human person in cases of armed conflict not of an international character,

Recalling furthermore that international instruments relating to human rights offer a basic protection to the human person,

Emphasizing the need to ensure a better protection for the victims of those armed conflicts,

Recalling that, in cases not covered by the law in force, the human person remains under the protection of the principles of humanity and the dictates or the public conscience,

Have agreed on the following:

PART I.
SCOPE OF THIS PROTOCOL

Article 1
Material Field of Application

1. This Protocol, which develops and supplements Article 3 common to the Geneva Conventions of 12 August 1949 without modifying its existing conditions or application, shall apply to all armed conflicts which are not covered by Article 1 of the Protocol Additional to the Geneva Conventions of 12 August 1949, and relating to the Protection of Victims of International Armed Conflicts (Protocol I) and which take place in the territory of a High Contracting Party between its armed forces and dissident armed forces or other organized armed groups which, under responsible command, exercise such control over a part of its territory as to enable them to carry out sustained and concerted military operations and to implement this Protocol.

2. This Protocol shall not apply to situations of internal disturbances and tensions, such as riots, isolated and sporadic acts of violence and other acts of a similar nature, as not being armed conflicts.

Article 2
Personal Field of Application

1. This Protocol shall be applied without any adverse distinction founded on race, colour, sex, language, religion or belief, political or other opinion, national or social origin, wealth, birth or other status, or on any other similar criteria (hereinafter referred to as "adverse distinction") to all persons affected by an armed conflict as defined in Article 1.

2. At the end of the armed conflict, all the persons who have been deprived of their liberty or whose liberty has been restricted for reasons related to such conflict, as well as those deprived of their liberty or whose liberty is restricted after the conflict for the same reasons, shall enjoy the protection of Articles 5 and 6 until the end of such deprivation or restriction of liberty.

Article 3
Non-Intervention

1. Nothing in this Protocol shall be invoked for the purpose of affecting the sovereignty of a State or the responsibility of the government, by all legitimate means, to maintain or re-establish law and order in the State or to defend the national unity and territorial integrity of the State.

2. Nothing in this Protocol shall be invoked as a justification for intervening, directly or indirectly, for any reason whatever, in the armed conflict or in the internal or external affairs of the High Contracting Party in the territory of which that conflict occurs.

PART II.
HUMANE TREATMENT

Article 4
Fundamental Guarantees

1. All persons who do not take a direct part or who have ceased to take part in hostilities, whether or not their liberty has been restricted, are entitled to respect for their person, honour and convictions and religious practices. They shall in all circumstances be treated humanely, without any adverse distinction. It is prohibited to order that there shall be no survivors.

2. Without prejudice to the generality of the foregoing, the following acts against the persons referred to in paragraph I are and shall remain prohibited at any time and in any place whatsoever:

(a) violence to the life, health and physical or mental well-being of persons, in particular murder as well as cruel treatment such as torture, mutilation or any form of corporal punishment;

(b) collective punishments;

(c) taking of hostages;

(d) acts of terrorism;

(e) outrages upon personal dignity, in particular humiliating and degrading treatment, rape, enforced prostitution and any form or indecent assault;

(f) slavery and the slave trade in all their forms;

(g) pillage;

(h) threats to commit any or the foregoing acts.

3. Children shall be provided with the care and aid they require, and in particular:

(a) they shall receive an education, including religious and moral education, in keeping with the wishes of their parents, or in the absence of parents, of those responsible for their care;

(b) all appropriate steps shall be taken to facilitate the reunion of families temporarily separated;

(c) children who have not attained the age of fifteen years shall neither be recruited in the armed forces or groups nor allowed to take part in hostilities;

(d) the special protection provided by this Article to children who have not attained the age of fifteen years shall remain applicable to them if they take a direct part in hostilities despite the provisions of subparagraph (c) and are captured;

(e) measures shall be taken, if necessary, and whenever possible with the consent of their parents or persons who by law or custom are primarily responsible for their care, to remove children temporarily from the area in which hostilities are taking place to a safer area within the country and ensure that they are accompanied by persons responsible for their safety and well-being.

Article 5
Persons Whose Liberty Has Been Restricted

1. In addition to the provisions of Article 4 the following provisions shall be respected as a minimum with regard to persons deprived of their liberty for reasons related to the armed conflict, whether they are interned or detained;

(a) the wounded and the sick shall be treated in accordance with Article 7;

(b) the persons referred to in this paragraph shall, to the same extent as the local civilian population, be provided with food and drinking water and be afforded safeguards as regards health and hygiene and protection against the rigours of the climate and the dangers of the armed conflict;

(c) they shall be allowed to receive individual or collective relief;

(d) they shall be allowed to practise their religion and, if requested and appropriate, to receive spiritual assistance from persons, such as chaplains, performing religious functions;

(e) they shall, if made to work, have the benefit of working conditions and safeguards similar to those enjoyed by the local civilian population.

2. Those who are responsible for the internment or detention of the persons referred to in paragraph 1 shall also, within the limits of their capabilities, respect the following provisions relating to such persons:

(a) except when men and women of a family are accommodated together, women shall be held in quarters separated from those of men and shall be under the immediate supervision of women;

(b) they shall be allowed to send and receive letters and cards, the number of which may be limited by competent authority if it deems necessary;

(c) places of internment and detention shall not be located close to the combat zone. The persons referred to in paragraph 1 shall be evacuated when the places where they are interned or detained become particularly exposed to danger arising out of the armed conflict, if their evacuation can be carried out under adequate conditions of safety;

(d) they shall have the benefit of medical examinations;

(e) their physical or mental health and integrity shall not be endangered by any unjustified act or omission. Accordingly, it is prohibited to subject the persons described in this Article to any medical procedure which is not indicated by the state of health of the person concerned, and which is not consistent with the generally accepted medical standards applied to free persons under similar medical circumstances.

3. Persons who are not covered by paragraph 1 but whose liberty has been restricted in any way whatsoever for reasons related to the armed conflict shall be treated humanely in accordance with Article 4 and with paragraphs 1 (a), (c) and (d), and 2 (b) of this Article.

4. If it is decided to release persons deprived of their liberty, necessary measures to ensure their safety shall be taken by those so deciding.

Article 6
Penal Prosecutions

1. This Article applies to the prosecution and punishment of criminal offenses related to the armed conflict.

2. No sentence shall be passed and no penalty shall be executed on a person found guilty of an offense except pursuant to a conviction pronounced by a court offering the essential guarantees of independence and impartiality.
In particular:

(a) the procedure shall provide for an accused to be informed without delay of the particulars of the offense alleged against him and shall afford the accused before and during his trial all necessary rights and means of defence;

(b) no one shall be convicted of an offense except on the basis of individual penal responsibility;

PROTECTION OF EXISTENCE AND PHYSICAL INTEGRITY

(c) no one shall be held guilty of any criminal offense on account of any act or omission which did not constitute a criminal offense, under the law, at the time when it was committed; nor shall a heavier penalty be imposed than that which was applicable at the time when the criminal offense was committed; if, after the commission of the offense, provision is made by law for the imposition of a lighter penalty, the offender shall benefit thereby;

(d) anyone charged with an offense is presumed innocent until proved guilty according to law;

(e) anyone charged with an offense shall have the right to be tried in his presence;

(f) no one shall be compelled to testify against himself or to confess guilt.

3. A convicted person shall be advised on conviction of his judicial and other remedies and of the time-limits within which they may be exercised.

4. The death penalty shall not be pronounced on persons who were under the age of eighteen years at the time of the offense and shall not be carried out on pregnant women or mothers of young children.

5. At the end of hostilities, the authorities in power shall endeavour to grant the broadest possible amnesty to persons who have participated in the armed conflict, or those deprived of their liberty for reasons related to the armed conflict, whether they are interned or detained.

PART III.
WOUNDED, SICK AND
SHIPWRECKED

Article 7
Protection and Care

1. All the wounded, sick and shipwrecked, whether or not they have taken part in the armed conflict, shall be respected and protected.

2. In all circumstances they shall be treated humanely and shall receive to the fullest extent practicable and with the least possible delay, the medical care and attention required by their condition. There shall be no distinction among them founded on any grounds other than medical ones.

Article 8
Search

Whenever circumstances permit and particularly after an engagement, all possible measures shall be taken, without delay, to search for and collect the wounded, sick and shipwrecked, to protect them against pillage and ill-treatment, to ensure their adequate care, and to search for the dead, prevent their being despoiled, and decently dispose of them.

Article 9
Protection of Medical and
Religious Personnel

1. Medical and religious personnel shall be respected and protected and shall be granted all available help for the performance of their duties. They shall not be compelled to carry out tasks which are not compatible with their humanitarian mission.

2. In the performance of their duties medical personnel may not be required to give priority to any person except on medical grounds.

Article 10
General Protection of Medical Duties

1. Under no circumstances shall any person be punished for having carried out medical activities compatible with medical ethics, regardless of the person benefiting therefrom.

2. Persons engaged in medical activities shall neither be compelled to perform acts or to carry out work contrary to, nor be compelled to refrain from acts required by, the rules of medical ethics or other rules designed for the benefit of the wounded and sick, or this Protocol.

3. The professional obligations of persons engaged in medical activities regarding information which they may acquire concerning the wounded and sick under their care shall, subject to national law, be respected.

4. Subject to national law, no person engaged in medical activities may be penalized in any way for refusing or failing to give information concerning the wounded and sick who are, or who have been, under his care.

Article 11
Protection of Medical Units
and Transports

1. Medical units and transports shall be respected and protected at all times and shall not be the object of attack.

2. The protection to which medical units and transports are entitled shall not cease unless they are used to commit hostile acts, outside their humanitarian function. Protection may, however, cease only after a warning has been given, setting, whenever appropriate, a reasonable time-limit, and after such warning has remained unheeded.

Article 12
The Distinctive Emblem

Under the direction of the competent authority concerned, the distinctive emblem of the red cross, red crescent or red lion and sun on a white ground shall be displayed by medical and religious personnel and medical units, and on medical transports. It shall be respected in all circumstances. It shall not be used improperly.

PART IV.
CIVILIAN POPULATION

Article 13
Protection of the Civilian Population

1. The civilian population and individual civilians shall enjoy general protection against the dangers arising from military operations. To give effect to this protection, the following rules shall be observed in all circumstances.

2. The civilian population as such, as well as individual civilians, shall not be the object of attack. Acts or threats of violence the primary purpose of which is to spread terror among the civilian population are prohibited.

3. Civilians shall enjoy the protection afforded by this part, unless and for such time as they take a direct part in hostilities.

Article 14
Protection of Objects Indispensable to
the Survival of the Civilian Population

Starvation of civilians as a method of combat is prohibited. It is therefore prohibited to attack, destroy, remove or render useless for that purpose, objects indispensable to the survival of the civilian population such as food-stuffs, agricultural areas for the production of food-stuffs, crops, livestock, drinking water installations and supplies and irrigation works.

Article 15
Protection of Works and Installations
Containing Dangerous Forces

Works or installations containing dangerous forces, namely dams, dykes and nuclear electrical generating stations, shall not be made the object of attack, even where these objects are military objectives, if such attack may cause the release of dangerous forces and consequent severe losses among the civilian population.

Article 16
Protection of Cultural Objects
and of Places of Worship

Without prejudice to the provisions of the Hague Convention for the Protection of Cultural Property in the Event of Armed Conflict of 14 May 1954, it is prohibited to commit any acts of hostility directed against historic monuments, works of art or places of worship which constitute the cultural or spiritual heritage of peoples, and to use them in support of the military effort.

Article 17
Prohibition of Forced Movement
of Civilians

1. The displacement of the civilian population shall not be ordered for reasons related to the conflict unless the security of the civilians involved or imperative military reasons so demand. Should such displacements have to be carried out, all possible measures shall be taken in order that the civilian population may be received under satisfactory conditions of shelter, hygiene, health, safety and nutrition.

2. Civilians shall not be compelled to leave their own territory for reasons connected with the conflict.

Article 18
Relief Societies and Relief Actions

1. Relief societies located in the territory of the High Contracting Party, such as Red Cross (Red Crescent, Red Lion and Sun) organizations may offer their services for the performance of their traditional functions in relation to the victims of the armed conflict. The civilian population may, even on its own initiative, offer to collect and care for the wounded, sick and shipwrecked.

2. If the civilian population is suffering undue hardship owing to a lack of the supplies essential for its survival, such as food-stuffs and medical supplies, relief actions for the civilian population which are of an exclusively humanitarian and impartial nature and which are conducted without any adverse distinction shall be undertaken subject to the consent of the High Contracting Party concerned.

PART V.
FINAL PROVISIONS

* * *

Statute of the International Criminal Court (1998)

Text of the Rome Statute circulated as document A/CONF.183/9 of 17 July 1998 and corrected by procès-verbaux of 10 November 1998, 12 July 1999, 30 November 1999, 8 May 2000, 17 January 2001 and 16 January 2002. The Statute entered into force on 1 July 2002. [Available at http://www.icc-cpi.int/library/basicdocuments/rome_statute(e).pdf]

PREAMBLE

The States Parties to this Statute,

Conscious that all peoples are united by common bonds, their cultures pieced together in a shared heritage, and concerned that this delicate mosaic may be shattered at any time,

Mindful that during this century millions of children, women and men have been victims of unimaginable atrocities that deeply shock the conscience of humanity,

Recognizing that such grave crimes threaten the peace, security and well-being of the world,

Affirming that the most serious crimes of concern to the international community as a whole must not go unpunished and that their effective prosecution must be ensured by taking measures at the national level and by enhancing international cooperation,

Determined to put an end to impunity for the perpetrators of these crimes and thus to contribute to the prevention of such crimes,

Recalling that it is the duty of every State to exercise its criminal jurisdiction over those responsible for international crimes,

Reaffirming the Purposes and Principles of the Charter of the United Nations, and in particular that all States shall refrain from the threat or use of force against the territorial integrity or political independence of any State, or in any other manner inconsistent with the Purposes of the United Nations,

Emphasizing in this connection that nothing in this Statute shall be taken as authorizing any State Party to intervene in an armed conflict or in the internal affairs of any State,

Determined to these ends and for the sake of present and future generations, to establish an independent permanent International Criminal Court in relationship with the United Nations system, with jurisdiction over the most serious crimes of concern to the international community as a whole,

Emphasizing that the International Criminal Court established under this Statute shall be complementary to national criminal jurisdictions,

Resolved to guarantee lasting respect for and the enforcement of international justice,

Have agreed as follows:

PART 1.
ESTABLISHMENT OF THE COURT
Article 1
The Court

An International Criminal Court ("the Court") is hereby established. It shall be a permanent institution and shall have the power to exercise its jurisdiction over persons for the most serious crimes of international concern, as referred to in this Statute, and shall be complementary to national criminal jurisdictions. The jurisdiction and functioning of the Court shall be governed by the provisions of this Statute.

Article 2
Relationship of the
Court with the United Nations

The Court shall be brought into relationship with the United Nations through an agreement to be approved by the Assembly of States Parties to this Statute and thereafter concluded by the President of the Court on its behalf.

Article 3
Seat of the Court

1. The seat of the Court shall be established at The Hague in the Netherlands ("the host State").

2. The Court shall enter into a headquarters agreement with the host State, to be approved by the Assembly of States Parties and thereafter concluded by the President of the Court on its behalf.

3. The Court may sit elsewhere, whenever it considers it desirable, as provided in this Statute.

Article 4
Legal Status and Powers of the Court

1. The Court shall have international legal personality. It shall also have such legal capacity as may be necessary for the exercise of its functions and the fulfillment of its purposes.

2. The Court may exercise its functions and powers, as provided in this Statute, on the territory of any State Party and, by special agreement, on the territory of any other State.

PART 2.
JURISDICTION, ADMISSIBILITY
AND APPLICABLE LAW
Article 5
Crimes Within the Jurisdiction
of the Court

1. The jurisdiction of the Court shall be limited to the most serious crimes of concern to the international community as a whole. The Court has jurisdiction in accordance with this Statute with respect to the following crimes:

(a) The crime of genocide;

(b) Crimes against humanity;

(c) War crimes;

(d) The crime of aggression.

2. The Court shall exercise jurisdiction over the crime of aggression once a provision is adopted in accordance with articles 121 and 123 defining the crime and setting out the conditions under which the Court shall exercise jurisdiction with respect to this crime. Such a provision shall be consistent with the relevant provisions of the Charter of the United Nations.

Article 6
Genocide

For the purpose of this Statute, "genocide" means any of the following acts committed with intent to destroy, in whole or in part, a national, ethnical, racial or religious group, as such:

(a) Killing members of the group;

(b) Causing serious bodily or mental harm to members of the group;

(c) Deliberately inflicting on the group conditions of life calculated to bring about its physical destruction in whole or in part;

(d) Imposing measures intended to prevent births within the group;

(e) Forcibly transferring children of the group to another group.

Article 7
Crimes Against Humanity

1. For the purpose of this Statute, "crime against humanity" means any of the following acts when committed as part of a widespread or systematic attack directed against any civilian population, with knowledge of the attack:

(a) Murder;

(b) Extermination;

(c) Enslavement;

(d) Deportation or forcible transfer of population;

(e) Imprisonment or other severe deprivation of physical liberty in violation of fundamental rules of international law;

(f) Torture;

(g) Rape, sexual slavery, enforced prostitution, forced pregnancy, enforced sterilization, or any other form of sexual violence of comparable gravity;

(h) Persecution against any identifiable group or collectivity on political, racial, national, ethnic, cultural, religious, gender as defined in paragraph 3, or other grounds that are universally recognized as impermissible under international law, in connection with any act referred to in this paragraph or any crime within the jurisdiction of the Court;

(i) Enforced disappearance of persons;

(j) The crime of apartheid;

(k) Other inhumane acts of a similar character intentionally causing great suffering, or serious injury to body or to mental or physical health.

2. For the purpose of paragraph 1:

(a) "Attack directed against any civilian popula-

tion" means a course of conduct involving the multiple commission of acts referred to in paragraph 1 against any civilian population, pursuant to or in furtherance of a State or organizational policy to commit such attack;

(b) "Extermination" includes the intentional infliction of conditions of life, inter alia the deprivation of access to food and medicine, calculated to bring about the destruction of part of a population;

(c) "Enslavement" means the exercise of any or all of the powers attaching to the right of ownership over a person and includes the exercise of such power in the course of trafficking in persons, in particular women and children;

(d) "Deportation or forcible transfer of population" means forced displacement of the persons concerned by expulsion or other coercive acts from the area in which they are lawfully present, without grounds permitted under international law;

(e) "Torture" means the intentional infliction of severe pain or suffering, whether physical or mental, upon a person in the custody or under the control of the accused; except that torture shall not include pain or suffering arising only from, inherent in or incidental to, lawful sanctions;

(f) "Forced pregnancy" means the unlawful confinement of a woman forcibly made pregnant, with the intent of affecting the ethnic composition of any population or carrying out other grave violations of international law. This definition shall not in any way be interpreted as affecting national laws relating to pregnancy;

(g) "Persecution" means the intentional and severe deprivation of fundamental rights contrary to international law by reason of the identity of the group or collectivity;

(h) "The crime of apartheid" means inhumane acts of a character similar to those referred to in paragraph 1, committed in the context of an institutionalized regime of systematic oppression and domination by one racial group over any other racial group or groups and committed with the intention of maintaining that regime;

(i) "Enforced disappearance of persons" means the arrest, detention or abduction of persons by, or with the authorization, support or acquiescence of, a State or a political organization, followed by a refusal to acknowledge that deprivation of freedom or to give information on the fate or whereabouts of those persons, with the intention of removing them from the protection of the law for a prolonged period of time.

3. For the purpose of this Statute, it is understood that the term "gender" refers to the two sexes, male and female, within the context of society. The term "gender" does not indicate any meaning different from the above.

Article 8
War Crimes

1. The Court shall have jurisdiction in respect of war crimes in particular when committed as part of a plan or policy or as part of a large-scale commission of such crimes.

2. For the purpose of this Statute, "war crimes" means:

(a) Grave breaches of the Geneva Conventions of 12 August 1949, namely, any of the following acts against persons or property protected under the provisions of the relevant Geneva Convention:

(i) Wilful killing;

(ii) Torture or inhuman treatment, including biological experiments;

(iii) Wilfully causing great suffering, or serious injury to body or health;

(iv) Extensive destruction and appropriation of property, not justified by military necessity and carried out unlawfully and wantonly;

(v) Compelling a prisoner of war or other protected person to serve in the forces of a hostile Power;

(vi) Wilfully depriving a prisoner of war or other protected person of the rights of fair and regular trial;

(vii) Unlawful deportation or transfer or unlawful confinement;

(viii) Taking of hostages.

(b) Other serious violations of the laws and customs applicable in international armed conflict, within the established framework of international law, namely, any of the following acts:

(i) Intentionally directing attacks against the civilian population as such or against individual civilians not taking direct part in hostilities;

(ii) Intentionally directing attacks against civilian objects, that is, objects which are not military objectives;

(iii) Intentionally directing attacks against personnel, installations, material, units or vehicles involved in a humanitarian assistance or peacekeeping mission in accordance with the Charter of the United Nations, as long as they are entitled to the protection given to civilians or civilian objects under the international law of armed conflict;

(iv) Intentionally launching an attack in the knowledge that such attack will cause incidental loss of life or injury to civilians or damage to civilian objects or widespread, long-term and severe damage to the natural environment which would be clearly excessive in relation to the concrete and direct overall military advantage anticipated;

(v) Attacking or bombarding, by whatever means, towns, villages, dwellings or buildings which are undefended and which are not military objectives;

(vi) Killing or wounding a combatant who, having laid down his arms or having no longer means of defence, has surrendered at discretion;

(vii) Making improper use of a flag of truce, of the flag or of the military insignia and uniform of the enemy or of the United Nations, as well as of the distinctive emblems of the Geneva Conventions, resulting in death or serious personal injury;

(viii) The transfer, directly or indirectly, by the Occupying Power of parts of its own civilian population into the territory it occupies, or the deportation or transfer of all or parts of the population of the occupied territory within or outside this territory;

(ix) Intentionally directing attacks against buildings dedicated to religion, education, art, science or charitable purposes, historic monuments, hospitals and places where the sick and wounded are collected, provided they are not military objectives;

(x) Subjecting persons who are in the power of an adverse party to physical mutilation or to medical or scientific experiments of any kind which are neither justified by the medical, dental or hospital treatment of the person concerned nor carried out in his or her interest, and which cause death to or seriously endanger the health of such person or persons;

(xi) Killing or wounding treacherously individuals belonging to the hostile nation or army;

(xii) Declaring that no quarter will be given;

(xiii) Destroying or seizing the enemy's property unless such destruction or seizure be imperatively demanded by the necessities of war;

(xiv) Declaring abolished, suspended or inadmissible in a court of law the rights and actions of the nationals of the hostile party;

(xv) Compelling the nationals of the hostile party to take part in the operations of war directed against their own country, even if they were in the belligerent's service before the commencement of the war;

(xvi) Pillaging a town or place, even when taken by assault;

(xvii) Employing poison or poisoned weapons;

(xviii) Employing asphyxiating, poisonous or other gases, and all analogous liquids, materials or devices;

(xix) Employing bullets which expand or flatten easily in the human body, such as bullets with a hard envelope which does not entirely cover the core or is pierced with incisions;

(xx) Employing weapons, projectiles and material and methods of warfare which are of a nature to cause superfluous injury or unnecessary suffering or which are inherently indiscriminate in violation of the international law of armed conflict, provided that such weapons, projectiles and material and methods of warfare are the subject of a comprehensive prohibition and are included in an annex to this Statute, by an amendment in accordance with the relevant provisions set forth in articles 121 and 123;

(xxi) Committing outrages upon personal dignity, in particular humiliating and degrading treatment;

(xxii) Committing rape, sexual slavery, enforced prostitution, forced pregnancy, as defined in article 7, paragraph 2 (f), enforced sterilization, or any other form of sexual violence also constituting a grave breach of the Geneva Conventions;

(xxiii) Utilizing the presence of a civilian or other protected person to render certain points, areas or military forces immune from military operations;

(xxiv) Intentionally directing attacks against buildings, material, medical units and transport, and personnel using the distinctive emblems of the Geneva Conventions in conformity with international law;

(xxv) Intentionally using starvation of civilians as a method of warfare by depriving them of objects indispensable to their survival, including wilfully impeding relief supplies as provided for under the Geneva Conventions;

(xxvi) Conscripting or enlisting children under the age of fifteen years into the national armed forces or using them to participate actively in hostilities.

(c) In the case of an armed conflict not of an international character, serious violations of article 3 common to the four Geneva Conventions of 12 August 1949, namely, any of the following acts committed against persons taking no active part in the hostilities, including members of armed forces who have laid down their arms and those placed hors de combat by sickness, wounds, detention or any other cause:

(i) Violence to life and person, in particular murder of all kinds, mutilation, cruel treatment and torture;

(ii) Committing outrages upon personal dignity, in particular humiliating and degrading treatment;

(iii) Taking of hostages;

(iv) The passing of sentences and the carrying out of executions without previous judgement pronounced by a regularly constituted court, affording all judicial guarantees which are generally recognized as indispensable.

(d) Paragraph 2 (c) applies to armed conflicts not of an international character and thus does not apply to situations of internal disturbances and tensions, such as riots, isolated and sporadic acts of violence or other acts of a similar nature.

(e) Other serious violations of the laws and customs applicable in armed conflicts not of an international character, within the established framework of international law, namely, any of the following acts:

(i) Intentionally directing attacks against the civilian population as such or against individual civilians not taking direct part in hostilities;

(ii) Intentionally directing attacks against buildings, material, medical units and transport, and personnel using the distinctive emblems of the Geneva Conventions in conformity with international law;

(iii) Intentionally directing attacks against personnel, installations, material, units or vehicles involved in a humanitarian assistance or peacekeeping mission in accordance with the Charter of the United Nations, as long as they are entitled to the protection given to civilians or civilian objects under the international law of armed conflict;

(iv) Intentionally directing attacks against buildings dedicated to religion, education, art, science or charitable purposes, historic monuments, hospitals and places where the sick and wounded are collected, provided they are not military objectives;

(v) Pillaging a town or place, even when taken by assault;

(vi) Committing rape, sexual slavery, enforced prostitution, forced pregnancy, as defined in article 7, paragraph 2 (f), enforced sterilization, and any other form of sexual violence also constituting a serious violation of article 3 common to the four Geneva Conventions;

(vii) Conscripting or enlisting children under the age of fifteen years into armed forces or groups or using them to participate actively in hostilities;

(viii) Ordering the displacement of the civilian population for reasons related to the conflict, unless the security of the civilians involved or imperative military reasons so demand;

(ix) Killing or wounding treacherously a combatant adversary;

(x) Declaring that no quarter will be given;

(xi) Subjecting persons who are in the power of another party to the conflict to physical mutilation or to medical or scientific experiments of any kind which are neither justified by the medical, dental or hospital treatment of the person concerned nor carried out in his or her interest, and which cause death to or seriously endanger the health of such person or persons;

(xii) Destroying or seizing the property of an adversary unless such destruction or seizure be imperatively demanded by the necessities of the conflict;

(f) Paragraph 2 (e) applies to armed conflicts not of an international character and thus does not apply to situations of internal disturbances and tensions, such as riots, isolated and sporadic acts of violence or other acts of a similar nature. It applies to armed conflicts that take place in the territory of a State when there is protracted armed conflict between governmental authorities and organized armed groups or between such groups.

3. Nothing in paragraph 2 (c) and (e) shall affect the responsibility of a Government to maintain or re-establish law and order in the State or to defend the unity and territorial integrity of the State, by all legitimate means.

Article 9
Elements of Crimes

1. Elements of Crimes shall assist the Court in the interpretation and application of articles 6, 7 and 8. They shall be adopted by a two-thirds majority of the members of the Assembly of States Parties.

2. Amendments to the Elements of Crimes may be proposed by:

(a) Any State Party;

(b) The judges acting by an absolute majority;

(c) The Prosecutor.

Such amendments shall be adopted by a two-thirds majority of the members of the Assembly of States Parties.

3. The Elements of Crimes and amendments thereto shall be consistent with this Statute.

Article 10

Nothing in this Part shall be interpreted as limiting or prejudicing in any way existing or developing rules of international law for purposes other than this Statute.

Article 11
Jurisdiction Ratione Temporis

1. The Court has jurisdiction only with respect to crimes committed after the entry into force of this Statute.

2. If a State becomes a Party to this Statute after its entry into force, the Court may exercise its jurisdiction only with respect to crimes committed after the entry into force of this Statute for that State, unless that State has made a declaration under article 12, paragraph 3.

Article 12. Preconditions to the Exercise of Jurisdiction
* * *

Article 13. Exercise of Jurisdiction
* * *

Article 14. Referral of a Situation by a State Party
* * *

Article 15. Prosecutor
* * *

Article 17. Issues of Admissibility
* * *

Article 18. Preliminary Rulings Regarding Admissibility
* * *

Article 19. Challenges to the Jurisdiction of the Court or the Admissibility of a Case
* * *

Article 20. Ne Bis in Idem
* * *

Article 21. Applicable Law
* * *

PART 3.
GENERAL PRINCIPLES OF CRIMINAL LAW

Article 22. Nullum Crimen Sine Lege
* * *

Article 23. Nulla Poena Sine Lege
* * *

Article 24. Non-Retroactivity Ratione Personae
* * *

Article 25. Individual Criminal Responsibility
* * *

Article 26. Exclusion of Jurisdiction Over Persons Under Eighteen
* * *

Article 27. Irrelevance of Official Capacity
* * *

Article 28. Responsibility of Commanders and Other Superiors
* * *

Article 29. Non-Applicability of Statute of Limitations
* * *

Article 30. Mental Element
* * *

Article 31. Grounds for Excluding Criminal Responsibility
* * *

Article 32. Mistake of Fact or Mistake of Law
* * *

Article 33. Superior Orders and Prescription of Law

PART 4.
COMPOSITION AND ADMINISTRATION OF THE COURT
* * *

PART 5.
INVESTIGATION AND PROSECUTION
* * *

IN WITNESS WHEREOF, the undersigned, being duly authorized thereto by their respective Governments, have signed this Statute.

DONE at Rome, this 17th day of July 1998.

IV. HEALTH ASPECTS OF THE RIGHT TO AN ADEQUATE STANDARD OF LIVING (OTHER THAN THE RIGHT TO HEALTH)
A. The Right to an Adequate Standard of Living in General

Universal Declaration of Human Rights (1948)
Adopted and proclaimed by General Assembly
Resolution 217 A (III) of 10 December 1948.
[Available at http://www.ch/uchr/]

* * *

Article 25

1. Everyone has the right to a standard of living adequate for the health and well-being of himself and of his family, including food, clothing, housing and medical care and necessary social services, and the right to security in the event of unemployment, sickness, disability, widowhood, old age or other lack of livelihood in circumstances beyond his control.

2. Motherhood and childhood are entitled to special care and assistance. All children, whether born in or out of wedlock, shall enjoy the same social protection.

* * *

International Covenant on Economic, Social and Cultural Rights (1966)
General Assembly Resolution 2200A (XXI), on 16 December 1966.
Entered into force 3 January 1976.
[Available at http://www.unhchr.ch/html/menu3/b/a_cescr.htm]

* * *

Article 11

1. The States Parties to the present Covenant recognize the right of everyone to an adequate standard of living for himself and his family, including adequate food, clothing and housing, and to the continuous improvement of living conditions. The States Parties will take appropriate steps to ensure the realization of this right, recognizing to this effect the essential importance of international co-operation based on free consent.

2. The States Parties to the present Covenant, recognizing the fundamental right of everyone to be free from hunger, shall take, individually and through international co-operation, the measures, including specific programmes, which are needed:

(a) To improve methods of production, conservation and distribution of food by making full use of technical and scientific knowledge, by disseminating knowledge of the principles of nutrition and by developing or reforming agrarian systems in such a way as to achieve the most efficient development and utilization of natural resources;

(b) Taking into account the problems of both food-importing and food-exporting countries, to ensure an equitable distribution of world food supplies in relation to need.

* * *

United Nations Millennium Declaration (2000)

General Assembly Resolution 55/2 adopted 8 September 2000.
[Available at http://www.un.org/millennium/declaration/ares552e.htm]

[Footnotes omitted.]

The General Assembly Adopts the following Declaration:

United Nations Millennium Declaration

I. VALUES AND PRINCIPLES

1. We, heads of State and Government, have gathered at United Nations Headquarters in New York from 6 to 8 September 2000, at the dawn of a new millennium, to reaffirm our faith in the Organization and its Charter as indispensable foundations of a more peaceful, prosperous and just world.

2. We recognize that, in addition to our separate responsibilities to our individual societies, we have a collective responsibility to uphold the principles of human dignity, equality and equity at the global level. As leaders we have a duty therefore to all the world's people, especially the most vulnerable and, in particular, the children of the world, to whom the future belongs.

3. We reaffirm our commitment to the purposes and principles of the Charter of the United Nations, which have proved timeless and universal. Indeed, their relevance and capacity to inspire have increased, as nations and peoples have become increasingly interconnected and interdependent.

4. We are determined to establish a just and lasting peace all over the world in accordance with the purposes and principles of the Charter. We rededicate ourselves to support all efforts to uphold the sovereign equality of all States, respect for their territorial integrity and political independence, resolution of disputes by peaceful means and in conformity with the principles of justice and international law, the right to self-determination of peoples which remain under colonial domination and foreign occupation, non-interference in the internal affairs of States, respect for human rights and fundamental freedoms, respect for the equal rights of all without distinction as to race, sex, language or religion and international cooperation in solving international problems of an economic, social, cultural or humanitarian character.

5. We believe that the central challenge we face today is to ensure that globalization becomes a positive force for all the world's people. For while globalization offers great opportunities, at present its benefits are very unevenly shared, while its costs are unevenly distributed. We recognize that developing countries and countries with economies in transition face special difficulties in responding to this central challenge. Thus, only through broad and sustained efforts to create a shared future, based upon our common humanity in all its diversity, can globalization be made fully inclusive and equitable. These efforts must include policies and measures, at the global level, which correspond to the needs of developing countries and economies in transition and are formulated and implemented with their effective participation.

6. We consider certain fundamental values to be essential to international relations in the twenty-first century. These include:

• **Freedom**. Men and women have the right to live their lives and raise their children in dignity, free from hunger and from the fear of violence, oppression or injustice. Democratic and participatory governance based on the will of the people best assures these rights.

• **Equality**. No individual and no nation must be denied the opportunity to benefit from development. The equal rights and opportunities of women and men must be assured.

• **Solidarity**. Global challenges must be managed in a way that distributes the costs and burdens fairly in accordance with basic principles of equity and social justice. Those who suffer or who benefit least deserve help from those who benefit most.

• **Tolerance**. Human beings must respect one other,

in all their diversity of belief, culture and language. Differences within and between societies should be neither feared nor repressed, but cherished as a precious asset of humanity. A culture of peace and dialogue among all civilizations should be actively promoted.

• **Respect for nature.** Prudence must be shown in the management of all living species and natural resources, in accordance with the precepts of sustainable development. Only in this way can the immeasurable riches provided to us by nature be preserved and passed on to our descendants. The current unsustainable patterns of production and consumption must be changed in the interest of our future welfare and that of our descendants.

• **Shared responsibility.** Responsibility for managing worldwide economic and social development, as well as threats to international peace and security, must be shared among the nations of the world and should be exercised multilaterally. As the most universal and most representative organization in the world, the United Nations must play the central role.

7. In order to translate these shared values into actions, we have identified key objectives to which we assign special significance.

II. PEACE, SECURITY AND DISARMAMENT

8. We will spare no effort to free our peoples from the scourge of war, whether within or between States, which has claimed more than 5 million lives in the past decade. We will also seek to eliminate the dangers posed by weapons of mass destruction.

9. We Resolve Therefore:

• To strengthen respect for the rule of law in international and in national affairs and, in particular, to ensure compliance by Member States with the decisions of the International Court of Justice, in compliance with the Charter of the United Nations, in cases to which they are parties.

• To make the United Nations more effective in maintaining peace and security by giving it the resources and tools it needs for conflict prevention, peaceful resolution of disputes, peacekeeping, post-conflict peace-building and reconstruction. In this context, we take note of the report of the

Panel on United Nations Peace Operations 1 and request the General Assembly to consider its recommendations expeditiously.

• To strengthen cooperation between the United Nations and regional organizations, in accordance with the provisions of Chapter VIII of the Charter.

• To ensure the implementation, by States Parties, of treaties in areas such as arms control and disarmament and of international humanitarian law and human rights law, and call upon all States to consider signing and ratifying the Rome Statute of the International Criminal Court.

• To take concerted action against international terrorism, and to accede as soon as possible to all the relevant international conventions.

• To redouble our efforts to implement our commitment to counter the world drug problem.

• To intensify our efforts to fight transnational crime in all its dimensions, including trafficking as well as smuggling in human beings and money laundering.

• To minimize the adverse effects of United Nations economic sanctions on innocent populations, to subject such sanctions regimes to regular reviews and to eliminate the adverse effects of sanctions on third parties.

• To strive for the elimination of weapons of mass destruction, particularly nuclear weapons, and to keep all options open for achieving this aim, including the possibility of convening an international conference to identify ways of eliminating nuclear dangers.

• To take concerted action to end illicit traffic in small arms and light weapons, especially by making arms transfers more transparent and supporting regional disarmament measures, taking account of all the recommendations of the forthcoming United Nations Conference on Illicit Trade in Small Arms and Light Weapons.

• To call on all States to consider acceding to the Convention on the Prohibition of the Use, Stockpiling, Production and Transfer of Anti-personnel Mines and on Their Destruction, as well as the amended mines protocol to the Convention on conventional weapons.

10. We urge Member States to observe the Olympic Truce, individually and collectively, now and in the future, and to support the International

Olympic Committee in its efforts to promote peace and human understanding through sport and the Olympic Ideal.

III. DEVELOPMENT AND POVERTY ERADICATION

11. We will spare no effort to free our fellow men, women and children from the abject and dehumanizing conditions of extreme poverty, to which more than a billion of them are currently subjected. We are committed to making the right to development a reality for everyone and to freeing the entire human race from want.

12. We resolve therefore to create an environment — at the national and global levels alike — which is conducive to development and to the elimination of poverty.

13. Success in meeting these objectives depends, inter alia, on good governance within each country. It also depends on good governance at the international level and on transparency in the financial, monetary and trading systems. We are committed to an open, equitable, rule-based, predictable and non-discriminatory multilateral trading and financial system.

14. We are concerned about the obstacles developing countries face in mobilizing the resources needed to finance their sustained development. We will therefore make every effort to ensure the success of the High-level International and Intergovernmental Event on Financing for Development, to be held in 2001.

15. We also undertake to address the special needs of the least developed countries. In this context, we welcome the Third United Nations Conference on the Least Developed Countries to be held in May 2001 and will endeavour to ensure its success. We call on the industrialized countries:

• To adopt, preferably by the time of that Conference, a policy of duty- and quota-free access for essentially all exports from the least developed countries;

• To implement the enhanced programme of debt relief for the heavily indebted poor countries without further delay and to agree to cancel all of-ficial bilateral debts of those countries in return for their making demonstrable commitments to poverty reduction; and

• To grant more generous development assistance, especially to countries that are genuinely making an effort to apply their resources to poverty reduction.

16. We are also determined to deal comprehensively and effectively with the debt problems of low- and middle-income developing countries, through various national and international measures designed to make their debt sustainable in the long term.

17. We also resolve to address the special needs of small island developing States, by implementing the Barbados Programme of Action and the outcome of the twenty-second special session of the General Assembly rapidly and in full. We urge the international community to ensure that, in the development of a vulnerability index, the special needs of small island developing States are taken into account.

18. We recognize the special needs and problems of the landlocked developing countries, and urge both bilateral and multilateral donors to increase financial and technical assistance to this group of countries to meet their special development needs and to help them overcome the impediments of geography by improving their transit transport systems.

19. We Resolve Further:

• To halve, by the year 2015, the proportion of the world's people whose income is less than one dollar a day and the proportion of people who suffer from hunger and, by the same date, to halve the proportion of people who are unable to reach or to afford safe drinking water.

• To ensure that, by the same date, children everywhere, boys and girls alike, will be able to complete a full course of primary schooling and that girls and boys will have equal access to all levels of education.

• By the same date, to have reduced maternal mortality by three quarters, and under-five child mortality by two thirds, of their current rates.

• To have, by then, halted, and begun to reverse, the spread of HIV/AIDS, the scourge of malaria and other major diseases that afflict humanity.

• To provide special assistance to children orphaned by HIV/AIDS.

• By 2020, to have achieved a significant improvement in the lives of at least 100 million slum dwellers as proposed in the "Cities Without Slums" initiative.

20. We Also Resolve:

• To promote gender equality and the empowerment of women as effective ways to combat poverty, hunger and disease and to stimulate development that is truly sustainable.

• To develop and implement strategies that give young people everywhere a real chance to find decent and productive work.

• To encourage the pharmaceutical industry to make essential drugs more widely available and affordable to all who need them in developing countries.

• To develop strong partnerships with the private sector and with civil society organizations in pursuit of development and poverty eradication.

• To ensure that the benefits of new technologies, especially information and communication technologies, in conformity with recommendations contained in the ECOSOC 2000 Ministerial Declaration, are available to all.

IV. PROTECTING OUR COMMON ENVIRONMENT

21. We must spare no effort to free all of humanity, and above all our children and grandchildren, from the threat of living on a planet irredeemably spoilt by human activities, and whose resources would no longer be sufficient for their needs.

22. We reaffirm our support for the principles of sustainable development, including those set out in Agenda 21, agreed upon at the United Nations Conference on Environment and Development.

23. We resolve therefore to adopt in all our environmental actions a new ethic of conservation and stewardship and, as first steps, we resolve:

• To make every effort to ensure the entry into force of the Kyoto Protocol, preferably by the tenth anniversary of the United Nations Conference on Environment and Development in 2002, and to embark on the required reduction in emissions of greenhouse gases.

• To intensify our collective efforts for the management, conservation and sustainable development of all types of forests.

• To press for the full implementation of the Convention on Biological Diversity and the Convention to Combat Desertification in those Countries Experiencing Serious Drought and/or Desertification, particularly in Africa.

• To stop the unsustainable exploitation of water resources by developing water management strategies at the regional, national and local levels, which promote both equitable access and adequate supplies.

• To intensify cooperation to reduce the number and effects of natural and man-made disasters.

• To ensure free access to information on the human genome sequence.

V. HUMAN RIGHTS, DEMOCRACY AND GOOD GOVERNANCE

24. We will spare no effort to promote democracy and strengthen the rule of law, as well as respect for all internationally recognized human rights and fundamental freedoms, including the right to development.

25. We resolve therefore:

• To respect fully and uphold the Universal Declaration of Human Rights.

• To strive for the full protection and promotion in all our countries of civil, political, economic, social and cultural rights for all.

• To strengthen the capacity of all our countries to implement the principles and practices of democracy and respect for human rights, including minority rights.

• To combat all forms of violence against women and to implement the Convention on the Elimination of All Forms of Discrimination against Women.

• To take measures to ensure respect for and protection of the human rights of migrants, migrant workers and their families, to eliminate the increasing acts of racism and xenophobia in many societies and to promote greater harmony and tolerance in all societies.

• To work collectively for more inclusive political processes, allowing genuine participation by all citizens in all our countries.

• To ensure the freedom of the media to perform their essential role and the right of the public to have access to information.

VI. PROTECTING THE VULNERABLE

26. We will spare no effort to ensure that children and all civilian populations that suffer disproportionately the consequences of natural disasters, genocide, armed conflicts and other humanitarian emergencies are given every assistance and protection so that they can resume normal life as soon as possible.

We resolve therefore:

• To expand and strengthen the protection of civilians in complex emergencies, in conformity with international humanitarian law.

• To strengthen international cooperation, including burden sharing in, and the coordination of humanitarian assistance to, countries hosting refugees and to help all refugees and displaced persons to return voluntarily to their homes, in safety and dignity and to be smoothly reintegrated into their societies.

• To encourage the ratification and full implementation of the Convention on the Rights of the Child and its optional protocols on the involvement of children in armed conflict and on the sale of children, child prostitution and child pornography.

VII. MEETING THE SPECIAL NEEDS OF AFRICA

27. We will support the consolidation of democracy in Africa and assist Africans in their struggle for lasting peace, poverty eradication and sustainable development, thereby bringing Africa into the mainstream of the world economy.

28. We resolve therefore:

• To give full support to the political and institutional structures of emerging democracies in Africa.

• To encourage and sustain regional and subregional mechanisms for preventing conflict and promoting political stability, and to ensure a reliable flow of resources for peacekeeping operations on the continent.

• To take special measures to address the challenges of poverty eradication and sustainable development in Africa, including debt cancellation, improved market access, enhanced Official Development Assistance and increased flows of Foreign Direct Investment, as well as transfers of technology.

• To help Africa build up its capacity to tackle the spread of the HIV/AIDS pandemic and other infectious diseases.

VIII. STRENGTHENING THE UNITED NATIONS

29. We will spare no effort to make the United Nations a more effective instrument for pursuing all of these priorities: the fight for development for all the peoples of the world, the fight against poverty, ignorance and disease; the fight against injustice; the fight against violence, terror and crime; and the fight against the degradation and destruction of our common home.

30. We resolve therefore:

• To reaffirm the central position of the General Assembly as the chief deliberative, policy-making and representative organ of the United Nations, and to enable it to play that role effectively.

• To intensify our efforts to achieve a comprehensive reform of the Security Council in all its aspects.

• To strengthen further the Economic and Social Council, building on its recent achievements, to help it fulfill the role ascribed to it in the Charter.

• To strengthen the International Court of Justice, in order to ensure justice and the rule of law in international affairs.

• To encourage regular consultations and coordination among the principal organs of the United Nations in pursuit of their functions.

• To ensure that the Organization is provided on a timely and predictable basis with the resources it needs to carry out its mandates.

• To urge the Secretariat to make the best use of those resources, in accordance with clear rules and procedures agreed by the General Assembly, in the interests of all Member States, by adopting the best management practices and technologies available and by concentrating on those tasks that reflect the agreed priorities of Member States.

• To promote adherence to the Convention on the Safety of United Nations and Associated Personnel.

• To ensure greater policy coherence and better co-operation between the United Nations, its agencies, the Bretton Woods Institutions and the World Trade Organization, as well as other multilateral bodies, with a view to achieving a fully coordinated approach to the problems of peace and development.

• To strengthen further cooperation between the United Nations and national parliaments through their world organization, the Inter-Parliamentary Union, in various fields, including peace and security, economic and social development, international law and human rights and democracy and gender issues.

• To give greater opportunities to the private sector, non-governmental organizations and civil society, in general, to contribute to the realization of the Organization's goals and programmes.

31. We request the General Assembly to review on a regular basis the progress made in implementing the provisions of this Declaration, and ask the Secretary-General to issue periodic reports for consideration by the General Assembly and as a basis for further action.

32. We solemnly reaffirm, on this historic occasion, that the United Nations is the indispensable common house of the entire human family, through which we will seek to realize our universal aspirations for peace, cooperation and development. We therefore pledge our unstinting support for these common objectives and our determination to achieve them.

8th plenary meeting
8 September 2000

B. The Right to Adequate Food

Universal Declaration on the Eradication of Hunger and Malnutrition (1974)

Adopted on 16 November 1974 by the World Food Conference convened under General Assembly Resolution 3180 (XXVIII) of 17 December 1973; and endorsed by General Assembly Resolution 3348 (XXIX) of 17 December 1974.
[Available at http://www.unhchr.ch/html/menu3/b/69.htm]

The World Food Conference,

Convened by the General Assembly of the United Nations and entrusted with developing ways and means whereby the international community, as a whole, could take specific action to resolve the world food problem within the broader context of development and international economic co-operation,

Adopts the following Declaration:

UNIVERSAL DECLARATION ON THE ERADICATION OF HUNGER AND MALNUTRITION

Recognizing that:

(a) The grave food crisis that is afflicting the peoples of the developing countries where most of the world's hungry and ill-nourished live and where more than two thirds of the world's population produce about one third of the world's food — an imbalance which threatens to increase in the next 10 years — is not only fraught with grave economic and social implications, but also acutely jeopardizes the most fundamental principles and values associated with the right to life and human dignity as enshrined in the Universal Declaration of Human Rights;

(b) The elimination of hunger and malnutrition, included as one of the objectives in the United Nations Declaration on Social Progress and Development, and the elimination of the causes that determine this situation are the common objectives of all nations;

(c) The situation of the peoples afflicted by hunger and malnutrition arises from their historical circumstances, especially social inequalities, including in many cases alien and colonial domination, foreign occupation, racial discrimination, apartheid and neo-colonialism in all its forms, which continue to be among the greatest obstacles to the full emancipation and progress of the developing countries and all the peoples involved;

(d) This situation has been aggravated in recent years by a series of crises to which the world economy has been subjected, such as the deterioration in the international monetary system, the inflationary increase in import costs, the heavy burdens imposed by external debt on the balance of payments of many developing countries, a rising food demand partly due to demographic pressure, speculation, and a shortage of, and increased costs for, essential agricultural inputs;

(e) These phenomena should be considered within the framework of the on-going negotiations on the Charter of Economic Rights and Duties of States, and the General Assembly of the United Nations should be urged unanimously to agree upon, and to adopt, a Charter that will be an effective instrument for the establishment of new international economic relations based on principles of equity and justice;

(f) All countries, big or small, rich or poor, are equal. All countries have the full right to participate in the decisions on the food problem;

(g) The well-being of the peoples of the world largely depends on the adequate production and distribution of food as well as the establishment of a world food security system which would ensure adequate availability of, and reasonable prices for, food at all times, irrespective of periodic fluctuations and vagaries of weather and free of political and economic pressures, and should thus facilitate, amongst other things, the development process of developing countries;

(h) Peace and justice encompass an economic dimension helping the solution of the world economic problems, the liquidation of under-development, offering a lasting and definitive solution of the food problem for all peoples and guaranteeing to all countries the right to implement freely and effectively their development programmes. To this effect, it is necessary to eliminate threats and resort to force and to promote peaceful co-operation between States to the fullest extent possible, to apply the principles of non-interference in the internal affairs of other States, full equality of rights and respect of national independence and sovereignty, as well as to encourage the peaceful co-operation between all States, irrespective of their political, social and economic systems. The further improvement of international relations will create better conditions for international co-operation in all fields which should make possible large financial and material resources to be used, inter alia, for developing agricultural production and substantially improving world food security;

(i) For a lasting solution of the food problem all efforts should be made to eliminate the widening gaps which today separate developed and developing countries and to bring about a new international economic order. It should be possible for all countries to participate actively and effectively in the new international economic relations by the establishment of suitable international systems, where appropriate, capable of producing adequate action in order to establish just and equitable relations in international economic co-operation;

(j) Developing countries reaffirm their belief that the primary responsibility for ensuring their own rapid development rests with themselves. They declare, therefore, their readiness to continue to intensify their individual and collective efforts with a view to expanding their mutual co-operation in the field of agricultural development and food production, including the eradication of hunger and malnutrition;

(k) Since, for various reasons, many developing countries are not yet always able to meet their own food needs, urgent and effective international action should be taken to assist them, free of political pressures,

Consistent with the aims and objectives of the Declaration on the Establishment of a New International Economic Order and the Programme of Action adopted by the General Assembly at its sixth special session,

The Conference consequently solemnly proclaims:

1. Every man, woman and child has the inalienable right to be free from hunger and malnutrition in order to develop fully and maintain their physical and mental faculties. Society today already possesses sufficient resources, organizational ability and technology and hence the competence to achieve this objective. Accordingly, the eradication of hunger is a common objective of all the countries of the international community, especially of the developed countries and others in a position to help.

2. It is a fundamental responsibility of Governments to work together for higher food production and a more equitable and efficient distribution of food between countries and within countries. Governments should initiate immediately a greater concerted attack on chronic malnutrition and deficiency diseases among the vulnerable and lower income groups. In order to ensure adequate nutrition for all, Governments should formulate appropriate food and nutrition policies integrated in overall socio-economic and agricultural development plans based on adequate knowledge of available as well as potential food resources. The importance of human milk in this connection should be stressed on nutritional grounds.

3. Food problems must be tackled during the preparation and implementation of national plans and programmes for economic and social development, with emphasis on their humanitarian aspects.

4. It is a responsibility of each State concerned, in accordance with its sovereign judgement and internal legislation, to remove the obstacles to food production and to provide proper incentives to agricultural producers. Of prime importance for

the attainment of these objectives are effective measures of socio-economic transformation by agrarian, tax, credit and investment policy reform and the reorganization of rural structures, such as the reform of the conditions of ownership, the encouragement of producer and consumer co-operatives, the mobilization of the full potential of human resources, both male and female, in the developing countries for an integrated rural development and the involvement of small farmers, fishermen and landless workers in attaining the required food production and employment targets. Moreover, it is necessary to recognize the key role of women in agricultural production and rural economy in many countries, and to ensure that appropriate education, extension programmes and financial facilities are made available to women on equal terms with men.

5. Marine and inland water resources are today becoming more important than ever as a source of food and economic prosperity. Accordingly, action should be taken to promote a rational exploitation of these resources, preferably for direct consumption, in order to contribute to meeting the food requirements of all peoples.

6. The efforts to increase food production should be complemented by every endeavour to prevent wastage of food in all its forms.

7. To give impetus to food production in developing countries and in particular in the least developed and most seriously affected among them, urgent and effective international action should be taken, by the developed countries and other countries in a position to do so, to provide them with sustained additional technical and financial assistance on favourable terms and in a volume sufficient to their needs on the basis of bilateral and multilateral arrangements. This assistance must be free of conditions inconsistent with the sovereignty of the receiving States.

8. All countries, and primarily the highly industrialized countries, should promote the advancement of food production technology and should make all efforts to promote the transfer, adaptation and dissemination of appropriate food production technology for the benefit of the developing countries and, to that end, they should inter alia make all efforts to disseminate the results of their research work to Governments and scientific institutions of developing countries in order to enable them to promote a sustained agricultural development.

9. To assure the proper conservation of natural resources being utilized, or which might be utilized, for food production, all countries must collaborate in order to facilitate the preservation of the environment, including the marine environment.

10. All developed countries and others able to do so should collaborate technically and financially with the developing countries in their efforts to expand land and water resources for agricultural production and to assure a rapid increase in the availability, at fair costs, of agricultural inputs such as fertilizers and other chemicals, high-quality seeds, credit and technology. Co-operation among developing countries, in this connection, is also important.

11. All States should strive to the utmost to readjust, where appropriate, their agricultural policies to give priority to food production, recognizing, in this connection the interrelationship between the world food problem and international trade. In the determination of attitudes towards farm support programmes for domestic food production, developed countries should take into account, as far as possible, the interest of the food-exporting developing countries, in order to avoid detrimental effect on their exports. Moreover, all countries should co-operate to devise effective steps to deal with the problem of stabilizing world markets and promoting equitable and remunerative prices, where appropriate through international arrangements, to improve access to markets through reduction or elimination of tariff and non-tariff barriers on the products of interest to the developing countries, to substantially increase the export earnings of these countries, to contribute to the diversification of their exports, and apply to them, in the multilateral trade negotiations, the principles as agreed upon in the Tokyo Declaration, including the concept of non-reciprocity and more favourable treatment.

12. As it is the common responsibility of the entire international community to ensure the availability at all times of adequate world supplies of basic food-stuffs by way of appropriate reserves, including emergency reserves, all countries should

co-operate in the establishment of an effective system of world food security by:

Participating in and supporting the operation of the Global Information and Early Warning System on Food and Agriculture;

Adhering to the objectives, policies and guidelines of the proposed International Undertaking on World Food Security as endorsed by the World Food Conference;

Earmarking, where possible, stocks or funds for meeting international emergency food requirements as envisaged in the proposed International Undertaking on World Food Security and developing international guidelines to provide for the co-ordination and the utilization of such stocks;

Co-operating in the provision of food aid for meeting emergency and nutritional needs as well as for stimulating rural employment through development projects.

All donor countries should accept and implement the concept of forward planning of food aid and make all efforts to provide commodities and/or financial assistance that will ensure adequate quantities of grains and other food commodities.

Time is short. Urgent and sustained action is vital. The Conference, therefore, calls upon all peoples expressing their will as individuals, and through their Governments, and non-governmental organizations, to work together to bring about the end of the age-old scourge of hunger.

The Conference affirms:

The determination of the participating States to make full use of the United Nations system in the implementation of this Declaration and the other decisions adopted by the Conference.

General Comment 12: The Right to Adequate Food (1999)
Adopted by the Committee on Economic, Social and Cultural Rights on 12 May 1999.
UN Doc. E/C.12/1999/5. (General Comments)
[Available at http://www.unhchr.ch/tbs/doc.nsf/0/3d02758c707031d58025677f003b73b9?]

[Footnotes omitted.]

INTRODUCTION AND BASIC PREMISES

1. The human right to adequate food is recognized in several instruments under international law. The International Covenant on Economic, Social and Cultural Rights deals more comprehensively than any other instrument with this right. Pursuant to article 11.1 of the Covenant, States parties recognize "the right of everyone to an adequate standard of living for himself and his family, including adequate food, clothing and housing, and to the continuous improvement of living conditions", while pursuant to article 11.2 they recognize that more immediate and urgent steps may be needed to ensure "the fundamental right to freedom from hunger and malnutrition". The human right to adequate food is of crucial importance for the enjoyment of all rights. It applies to everyone; thus the reference in Article 11.1 to "himself and his family" does not imply any limitation upon the applicability of this right to individuals or to female-headed households.

2. The Committee has accumulated significant information pertaining to the right to adequate food through examination of State parties' reports over the years since 1979. The Committee has noted that while reporting guidelines are available relating to the right to adequate food, only a few States parties have provided information sufficient and precise enough to enable the Committee to determine the prevailing situation in the countries concerned with respect to this right and to identify the obstacles to its realization. This General Comment aims to identify some of the principal issues which the Committee considers to be important in relation to the right to adequate food. Its preparation was triggered by the request of Member States during the 1996 World Food

Summit, for a better definition of the rights relating to food in article 11 of the Covenant, and by a special request to the Committee to give particular attention to the Summit Plan of Action in monitoring the implementation of the specific measures provided for in article 11 of the Covenant.

3. In response to these requests, the Committee reviewed the relevant reports and documentation of the Commission on Human Rights and of the Sub-Commission on Prevention of Discrimination and Protection of Minorities on the right to adequate food as a human right; devoted a day of general discussion to this issue at its seventeenth session in 1997, taking into consideration the draft international code of conduct on the human right to adequate food prepared by international non-governmental organizations; participated in two expert consultations on the right to adequate food as a human right organized by the Office of the United Nations High Commissioner for Human Rights (OHCHR), in Geneva in December 1997, and in Rome in November 1998 co-hosted by the Food and Agriculture Organization of the United Nations (FAO), and noted their final reports. In April 1999 the Committee participated in a symposium on "The substance and politics of a human rights approach to food and nutrition policies and programmes", organized by the Administrative Committee on Co-ordination/Sub-Committee on Nutrition of the United Nations at its twenty-sixth session in Geneva and hosted by OHCHR.

4. The Committee affirms that the right to adequate food is indivisibly linked to the inherent dignity of the human person and is indispensable for the fulfillment of other human rights enshrined in the International Bill of Human Rights. It is also inseparable from social justice, requiring the adoption of appropriate economic, environmental and social policies, at both the national and international levels, oriented to the eradication of poverty and the fulfillment of all human rights for all.

5. Despite the fact that the international community has frequently reaffirmed the importance of full respect for the right to adequate food, a disturbing gap still exists between the standards set in article 11 of the Covenant and the situation prevailing in many parts of the world. More than 840 million people throughout the world, most of them in developing countries, are chronically hungry;

millions of people are suffering from famine as the result of natural disasters, the increasing incidence of civil strife and wars in some regions and the use of food as a political weapon. The Committee observes that while the problems of hunger and malnutrition are often particularly acute in developing countries, malnutrition, undernutrition and other problems which relate to the right to adequate food and the right to freedom from hunger, also exist in some of the most economically developed countries. Fundamentally, the roots of the problem of hunger and malnutrition are not lack of food but lack of *access to* available food, inter alia because of poverty, by large segments of the world's population.

NORMATIVE CONTENT OF ARTICLE 11, PARAGRAPHS 1 AND 2

6. The right to adequate food is realized when every man, woman and child, alone or in community with others, has physical and economic access at all times to adequate food or means for its procurement. The *right to adequate food* shall therefore not be interpreted in a narrow or restrictive sense which equates it with a minimum package of calories, proteins and other specific nutrients. The *right to adequate food* will have to be realized progressively. However, States have a core obligation to take the necessary action to mitigate and alleviate hunger as provided for in paragraph 2 of article 11, even in times of natural or other disasters.

Adequacy and Sustainability of Food Availability and Access

7. The concept of *adequacy* is particularly significant in relation to the right to food since it serves to underline a number of factors which must be taken into account in determining whether particular foods or diets that are accessible can be considered the most appropriate under given circumstances for the purposes of article 11 of the Covenant. The notion of *sustainability* is intrinsically linked to the notion of adequate food or food *security*, implying food being accessible for both present and future generations. The precise meaning of "adequacy" is to a large extent determined by prevailing social, economic, cultural, climatic, ecological and other conditions, while "sustainability" incorporates the notion of long-term availability and accessibility.

8. The Committee considers that the core content of the right to adequate food implies:

The availability of food in a quantity and quality sufficient to satisfy the dietary needs of individuals, free from adverse substances, and acceptable within a given culture;

The accessibility of such food in ways that are sustainable and that do not interfere with the enjoyment of other human rights.

9. *Dietary needs* implies that the diet as a whole contains a mix of nutrients for physical and mental growth, development and maintenance, and physical activity that are in compliance with human physiological needs at all stages throughout the life cycle and according to gender and occupation. Measures may therefore need to be taken to maintain, adapt or strengthen dietary diversity and appropriate consumption and feeding patterns, including breast-feeding, while ensuring that changes in availability and access to food supply as a minimum do not negatively affect dietary composition and intake.

10. *Free from adverse substances* sets requirements for food safety and for a range of protective measures by both public and private means to prevent contamination of foodstuffs through adulteration and/or through bad environmental hygiene or inappropriate handling at different stages throughout the food chain; care must also be taken to identify and avoid or destroy naturally occurring toxins.

11. *Cultural or consumer acceptability* implies the need also to take into account, as far as possible, perceived non nutrient-based values attached to food and food consumption and informed consumer concerns regarding the nature of accessible food supplies.

12. *Availability* refers to the possibilities either for feeding oneself directly from productive land or other natural resources, or for well functioning distribution, processing and market systems that can move food from the site of production to where it is needed in accordance with demand.

13. *Accessibility* encompasses both economic and physical accessibility:

Economic accessibility implies that personal or household financial costs associated with the acquisition of food for an adequate diet should be at a level such that the attainment and satisfaction of other basic needs are not threatened or compromised. Economic accessibility applies to any acquisition pattern or entitlement through which people procure their food and is a measure of the extent to which it is satisfactory for the enjoyment of the right to adequate food. Socially vulnerable groups such as landless persons and other particularly impoverished segments of the population may need attention through special programmes.

Physical accessibility implies that adequate food must be accessible to everyone, including physically vulnerable individuals, such as infants and young children, elderly people, the physically disabled, the terminally ill and persons with persistent medical problems, including the mentally ill. Victims of natural disasters, people living in disaster-prone areas and other specially disadvantaged groups may need special attention and sometimes priority consideration with respect to accessibility of food. A particular vulnerability is that of many indigenous population groups whose access to their ancestral lands may be threatened.

OBLIGATIONS AND VIOLATIONS

14. The nature of the legal obligations of States parties are set out in article 2 of the Covenant and has been dealt with in the Committee's General Comment No. 3 (1990). The principal obligation is to take steps to achieve *progressively* the full realization of the right to adequate food. This imposes an obligation to move as expeditiously as possible towards that goal. Every State is obliged to ensure for everyone under its jurisdiction access to the minimum essential food which is sufficient, nutritionally adequate and safe, to ensure their freedom from hunger.

15. The right to adequate food, like any other human right, imposes three types or levels of obligations on States parties: the obligations to *respect*, to *protect* and to *fulfill*. In turn, the obligation to fulfill incorporates both an obligation to *facilitate* and an obligation to *provide*. The obligation to *respect* existing access to adequate food requires States parties not to take any measures that result in preventing such access. The obligation to *protect* requires measures by the State to ensure

that enterprises or individuals do not deprive individuals of their access to adequate food. The obligation to *fulfill* (*facilitate*) means the State must pro-actively engage in activities intended to strengthen people's access to and utilization of resources and means to ensure their livelihood, including food security. Finally, whenever an individual or group is unable, for reasons beyond their control, to enjoy the right to adequate food by the means at their disposal, States have the obligation to *fulfill* (*provide*) that right directly. This obligation also applies for persons who are victims of natural or other disasters.

16. Some measures at these different levels of obligations of States parties are of a more immediate nature, while other measures are more of a long-term character, to achieve progressively the full realization of the right to food.

17. Violations of the Covenant occur when a State fails to ensure the satisfaction of, at the very least, the minimum essential level required to be free from hunger. In determining which actions or omissions amount to a violation of the right to food, it is important to distinguish the inability from the unwillingness of a State party to comply. Should a State party argue that resource constraints make it impossible to provide access to food for those who are unable by themselves to secure such access, the State has to demonstrate that every effort has been made to use all the resources at its disposal in an effort to satisfy, as a matter of priority, those minimum obligations. This follows from article 2.1 of the Covenant, which obliges a State party to take the necessary steps to the maximum of its available resources, as previously pointed out by the Committee in its General Comment No. 3, paragraph 10. A State claiming that it is unable to carry out its obligation for reasons beyond its control therefore has the burden of proving that this is the case and that it has unsuccessfully sought to obtain international support to ensure the availability and accessibility of the necessary food.

18. Furthermore, any discrimination in access to food, as well as to means and entitlements for its procurement, on the grounds of race, colour, sex, language, age, religion, political or other opinion, national or social origin, property, birth or other status with the purpose or effect of nullifying or impairing the equal enjoyment or exercise of economic, social and cultural rights constitutes a violation of the Covenant.

19. Violations of the right to food can occur through the direct action of States or other entities insufficiently regulated by States. These include: the formal repeal or suspension of legislation necessary for the continued enjoyment of the right to food; denial of access to food to particular individuals or groups, whether the discrimination is based on legislation or is pro-active; the prevention of access to humanitarian food aid in internal conflicts or other emergency situations; adoption of legislation or policies which are manifestly incompatible with pre-existing legal obligations relating to the right to food; and failure to regulate activities of individuals or groups so as to prevent them from violating the right to food of others, or the failure of a State to take into account its international legal obligations regarding the right to food when entering into agreements with other States or with international organizations.

20. While only States are parties to the Covenant and are thus ultimately accountable for compliance with it, all members of society — individuals, families, local communities, non-governmental organizations, civil society organizations, as well as the private business sector — have responsibilities in the realization of the right to adequate food. The State should provide an environment that facilitates implementation of these responsibilities. The private business sector — national and transnational — should pursue its activities within the framework of a code of conduct conducive to respect of the right to adequate food, agreed upon jointly with the Government and civil society.

IMPLEMENTATION AT THE NATIONAL LEVEL

21. The most appropriate ways and means of implementing the right to adequate food will inevitably vary significantly from one State party to another. Every State will have a margin of discretion in choosing its own approaches, but the Covenant clearly requires that each State party take whatever steps are necessary to ensure that everyone is free from hunger and as soon as possible can enjoy the right to adequate food. This will require the adoption of a national strategy to

ensure food and nutrition security for all, based on human rights principles that define the objectives, and the formulation of policies and corresponding benchmarks. It should also identify the resources available to meet the objectives and the most cost-effective way of using them.

22. The strategy should be based on a systematic identification of policy measures and activities relevant to the situation and context, as derived from the normative content of the right to adequate food and spelled out in relation to the levels and nature of State parties' obligations referred to in paragraph 15 of the present general comment. This will facilitate coordination between ministries and regional and local authorities and ensure that related policies and administrative decisions are in compliance with the obligations under article 11 of the Covenant.

23. The formulation and implementation of national strategies for the right to food requires full compliance with the principles of accountability, transparency, people's participation, decentralization, legislative capacity and the independence of the judiciary. Good governance is essential to the realization of all human rights, including the elimination of poverty and ensuring a satisfactory livelihood for all.

24. Appropriate institutional mechanisms should be devised to secure a representative process towards the formulation of a strategy, drawing on all available domestic expertise relevant to food and nutrition. The strategy should set out the responsibilities and time-frame for the implementation of the necessary measures.

25. The strategy should address critical issues and measures in regard to *all* aspects of the food system, including the production, processing, distribution, marketing and consumption of safe food, as well as parallel measures in the fields of health, education, employment and social security. Care should be taken to ensure the most sustainable management and use of natural and other resources for food at the national, regional, local and household levels.

26. The strategy should give particular attention to the need to prevent discrimination in access to food or resources for food. This should include:

guarantees of full and equal access to economic resources, particularly for women, including the right to inheritance and the ownership of land and other property, credit, natural resources and appropriate technology; measures to respect and protect self-employment and work which provides a remuneration ensuring a decent living for wage earners and their families (as stipulated in article 7 (a) (ii) of the Covenant); maintaining registries on rights in land (including forests).

27. As part of their obligations to protect people's resource base for food, States parties should take appropriate steps to ensure that activities of the private business sector and civil society are in conformity with the right to food.

28. Even where a State faces severe resource constraints, whether caused by a process of economic adjustment, economic recession, climatic conditions or other factors, measures should be undertaken to ensure that the right to adequate food is especially fulfilled for vulnerable population groups and individuals.

Benchmarks and Framework Legislation

29. In implementing the country-specific strategies referred to above, States should set verifiable benchmarks for subsequent national and international monitoring. In this connection, States should consider the adoption of a *framework law* as a major instrument in the implementation of the national strategy concerning the right to food. The framework law should include provisions on its purpose; the targets or goals to be achieved and the time-frame to be set for the achievement of those targets; the means by which the purpose could be achieved described in broad terms, in particular the intended collaboration with civil society and the private sector and with international organizations; institutional responsibility for the process; and the national mechanisms for its monitoring, as well as possible recourse procedures. In developing the benchmarks and framework legislation, States parties should actively involve civil society organizations.

30. Appropriate United Nations programmes and agencies should assist, upon request, in drafting the framework legislation and in reviewing the sectoral legislation. FAO, for example, has con-

siderable expertise and accumulated knowledge concerning legislation in the field of food and agriculture. The United Nations Children's Fund (UNICEF) has equivalent expertise concerning legislation with regard to the right to adequate food for infants and young children through maternal and child protection including legislation to enable breast-feeding, and with regard to the regulation of marketing of breast milk substitutes.

Monitoring

31. States parties shall develop and maintain mechanisms to monitor progress towards the realization of the right to adequate food for all, to identify the factors and difficulties affecting the degree of implementation of their obligations, and to facilitate the adoption of corrective legislation and administrative measures, including measures to implement their obligations under articles 2.1 and 23 of the Covenant.

Remedies and Accountability

32. Any person or group who is a victim of a violation of the right to adequate food should have access to effective judicial or other appropriate remedies at both national and international levels. All victims of such violations are entitled to adequate reparation, which may take the form of restitution, compensation, satisfaction or guarantees of non-repetition. National Ombudsmen and human rights commissions should address violations of the right to food.

33. The incorporation in the domestic legal order of international instruments recognizing the right to food, or recognition of their applicability, can significantly enhance the scope and effectiveness of remedial measures and should be encouraged in all cases. Courts would then be empowered to adjudicate violations of the core content of the right to food by direct reference to obligations under the Covenant.

34. Judges and other members of the legal profession are invited to pay greater attention to violations of the right to food in the exercise of their functions.

35. States parties should respect and protect the work of human rights advocates and other members of civil society who assist vulnerable groups in the realization of their right to adequate food.

INTERNATIONAL OBLIGATIONS

States Parties

36. In the spirit of article 56 of the Charter of the United Nations, the specific provisions contained in articles 11, 2.1, and 23 of the Covenant and the Rome Declaration of the World Food Summit, States parties should recognize the essential role of international cooperation and comply with their commitment to take joint and separate action to achieve the full realization of the right to adequate food. In implementing this commitment, States parties should take steps to respect the enjoyment of the right to food in other countries, to protect that right, to facilitate access to food and to provide the necessary aid when required. States parties should, in international agreements whenever relevant, ensure that the right to adequate food is given due attention and consider the development of further international legal instruments to that end.

37. States parties should refrain at all times from food embargoes or similar measures which endanger conditions for food production and access to food in other countries. Food should never be used as an instrument of political and economic pressure. In this regard, the Committee recalls its position, stated in its General Comment No. 8, on the relationship between economic sanctions and respect for economic, social and cultural rights.

States and International Organizations

38. States have a joint and individual responsibility, in accordance with the Charter of the United Nations, to cooperate in providing disaster relief and humanitarian assistance in times of emergency, including assistance to refugees and internally displaced persons. Each State should contribute to this task in accordance with its ability. The role of the World Food Programme (WFP) and the Office of the United Nations High Commissioner for Refugees (UNHCR), and increasingly that of UNICEF and FAO is of particular importance in this respect and should be strengthened. Priority in food aid should be given to the most vulnerable populations.

39. Food aid should, as far as possible, be provided in ways which do not adversely affect local producers and local markets, and should be organized in ways that facilitate the return to food self-reliance of the beneficiaries. Such aid should be

based on the needs of the intended beneficiaries. Products included in international food trade or aid programmes must be safe and culturally acceptable to the recipient population.

The United Nations and Other International Organizations

40. The role of the United Nations agencies, including through the United Nations Development Assistance Framework (UNDAF) at the country level, in promoting the realization of the right to food is of special importance. Coordinated efforts for the realization of the right to food should be maintained to enhance coherence and interaction among all the actors concerned, including the various components of civil society. The food organizations, FAO, WFP and the International Fund for Agricultural Development (IFAD) in conjunction with the United Nations Development Programme (UNDP), UNICEF, the World Bank and the regional development banks, should cooperate more effectively, building on their respective expertise, on the implementation of the right to food at the national level, with due respect to their individual mandates.

41. The international financial institutions, notably the International Monetary Fund (IMF) and the World Bank, should pay greater attention to the protection of the right to food in their lending policies and credit agreements and in international measures to deal with the debt crisis. Care should be taken, in line with the Committee's General Comment No. 2, paragraph 9, in any structural adjustment programme to ensure that the right to food is protected.

Voluntary Guidelines to Support the Progressive Realization of the Right to Adequate Food in the Context of National Food Security (2004)

Text approved during the Fourth Session the Intergovernmental Working Group for the Elaboration of a Set of Voluntary Guidelines to Support the Progressive Realization of the Right to Adequate Food in the Context of National Food Security (IGWG), a subsidiary body of the Committee on World Food Security (CFS) on 23 September 2004. Provisional text contained in FAO document IGWG RTFG/FINAL REPORT, Annex I, 23 September 2004.

[Footnotes omitted.]

SECTION I: PREFACE AND INTRODUCTION

PREFACE

* * *

INTRODUCTION

Basic Instruments

10. These Voluntary Guidelines have taken into account relevant international instruments, in particular those instruments in which the progressive realization of the right of everyone to an adequate standard of living, including adequate food, is enshrined.

* * *

13. These Voluntary Guidelines have taken into account the commitments contained in the Millennium Declaration, including the development goals, as well as the outcomes and commitments of the major UN conferences and summits in the economic, social and related fields.

* * *

The Right to Adequate Food and the Achievement of Food Security

15. Food security exists when all people, at all times, have physical and economic access to sufficient, safe and nutritious food to meet their dietary needs and food preferences for an active and healthy life. The four pillars of food security are availability, stability of supply, access and utilization.

16. The progressive realization of the right to adequate food requires States to fulfil their relevant human rights obligations under international law. These Voluntary Guidelines aim to guarantee the availability of food in quantity and quality suffi-

cient to satisfy the dietary needs of individuals; physical and economic accessibility for everyone, including vulnerable groups, to adequate food, free from unsafe substances and acceptable within a given culture; or the means of its procurement.

17. States have obligations under relevant international instruments relevant to the progressive realization of the right to adequate food. Notably, States Parties to the International Covenant on Economic, Social and Cultural Rights (ICESCR) have the obligation to respect, promote and protect and to take appropriate steps to achieve progressively the full realization of the right to adequate food. States Parties should respect existing access to adequate food by not taking any measures that result in preventing such access, and should protect the right of everyone to adequate food by taking steps so that enterprises and individuals do not deprive individuals of their access to adequate food. States Parties should promote policies intended to contribute to the progressive realization of people's right to adequate food by proactively engaging in activities intended to strengthen people's access to and utilization of resources and means to ensure their livelihood, including food security. States Parties should, to the extent that resources permit, establish and maintain safety nets or other assistance to protect those who are unable to provide for themselves.

* * *

SECTION II: ENABLING ENVIRONMENT, ASSISTANCE AND ACCOUNTABILITY

Guideline 1: Democracy, good governance, human rights and the rule of law

* * *

Guideline 2: Economic development policies

2.1 In order to achieve the progressive realization of the right to adequate food in the context of national food security, States should promote broad-based economic development that is supportive of their food security policies. States should establish policy goals and benchmarks based on the food security needs of the population.

2.2 States should assess, in consultation with key stakeholders, the economic and social situation, including the degree of food insecurity and its causes, the nutrition situation and food safety.

2.3 States should promote adequate and stable supplies of safe food through a combination of domestic production, trade, storage and distribution.

2.4 States should consider adopting a holistic and comprehensive approach to hunger and poverty reduction. Such an approach entails, inter alia, direct and immediate measures to ensure access to adequate food as part of a social safety net; investment in productive activities and projects to improve the livelihoods of the poor and hungry in a sustainable manner; the development of appropriate institutions, functioning markets, a conducive legal and regulatory framework; and access to employment, productive resources and appropriate services.

2.5 States should pursue inclusive, non-discriminatory and sound economic, agriculture, fisheries, forestry, land use, and, as appropriate, land reform policies — all of which will permit farmers, fishers, foresters and other food producers, particularly women, to earn a fair return from their labour, capital and management, and encourage conservation and sustainable management of natural resources including in marginal areas.

2.6 Where poverty and hunger are predominantly rural, States should focus on sustainable agricultural and rural development through measures to improve access to land, water, appropriate and affordable technologies, productive and financial resources, enhance the productivity of poor rural communities, promote the participation of the poor in economic policy decisions, share the benefits of productivity gains, conserve and protect natural resources, and invest in rural infrastructure, education and research. In particular, States should adopt policies that create conditions which encourage stable employment, especially in rural areas, including off-farm jobs.

2.7 In response to the growing problem of urban hunger and poverty, States should promote investments aimed at enhancing the livelihoods of the urban poor.

Guideline 3: Strategies

3.1 States, as appropriate and in consultation with relevant stakeholders and pursuant to their national laws, should consider adopting a national human-rights based strategy for the progressive realization of the right to adequate food in the context of national food security as part of an overarching national development strategy, including poverty reduction strategies, where they exist.

3.2 The elaboration of these strategies should begin with a careful assessment of existing national legislation, policy and administrative measures, current programmes, systematic identification of existing constraints and availability of existing resources. States should formulate the measures necessary to remedy any weakness, and propose an agenda for change and the means for its implementation and evaluation.

3.3 These strategies could include objectives, targets, benchmarks and time frames; and actions to formulate policies; identify and mobilize resources; define institutional mechanisms; allocate responsibilities; coordinate the activities of different actors; and provide for monitoring mechanisms. As appropriate, such strategies could address all aspects of the food system, including the production, processing, distribution, marketing and consumption of safe food. It could also address access to resources and to markets as well as parallel measures in other fields. These strategies should in particular address the needs of vulnerable and disadvantaged groups, as well as special situations such as natural disasters and emergencies.

3.4 Where necessary, States should consider adopting and, as appropriate, reviewing a national poverty reduction strategy that specifically addresses access to adequate food.

3.5 States, individually or in cooperation with relevant international organizations, should consider integrating into their poverty reduction strategy a human rights perspective based on the principle of non-discrimination. In raising the standard of living of those below the poverty line, due regard should be given to the need to ensure equality in practice to those who are traditionally disadvantaged and between women and men.

3.6 In their poverty reduction strategies, States also should give priority to providing basic services for the poorest, and investing in human resources by ensuring access to primary education for all, basic health care, capacity building in good practices, clean drinking water, adequate sanitation and justice and by supporting programmes in basic literacy, numeracy and good hygiene practices.

* * *

Guideline 4: Market systems

4.1 States should, in accordance with their national law and priorities, as well as their international commitments, improve the functioning of their markets, in particular their agricultural and food markets, in order to promote both economic growth and sustainable development, inter alia, by mobilizing domestic savings, both public and private, by developing appropriate credit policies, by generating sustainable adequate levels of national productive investment through credits in concessional terms and by increasing human capacity.

* * *

Guideline 5: Institutions

5.1 States, where appropriate, should assess the mandate and performance of relevant public institutions and, where necessary, establish, reform or improve their organization and structure to contribute to the progressive realization of the right to adequate food in the context of national food security.

* * *

Guideline 6: Stakeholders

6.1 Recognizing the primary responsibility of States for the progressive realisation of the right to adequate food, States are encouraged to apply a multi-stakeholder approach to national food security to identify the roles of and involve all relevant stakeholders, encompassing civil society and private sector, drawing together their know-how with a view to facilitate the efficient use of resources.

* * *

Guideline 7: Legal framework

7.1 States are invited to consider, in accordance with their domestic legal and policy frameworks, whether to include provisions in their domestic law, possibly including constitutional or legislative review that facilitates the progressive realization of the right to adequate food in the context of national food security.

7.2 States are invited to consider, in accordance with their domestic legal and policy frameworks, whether to include provisions in their domestic law, which may include their constitutions, bills of rights or legislation, to directly implement the progressive realization of the right to adequate food. Administrative, quasi-judicial and judicial mechanisms to provide adequate, effective and prompt remedies accessible, in particular, to members of vulnerable groups may be envisaged.

7.3 States that have established a right to adequate food under their legal system should inform the general public of all available rights and remedies to which they are entitled.

7.4 States should consider strengthening their domestic law and policies to accord access by women heads of households to poverty reduction and nutrition security programs and projects.

Guideline 8: Access to resources and assets
8.1 States should facilitate sustainable, non-discriminatory and secure access and utilization of resources consistent with their national law and with international law and protect the assets that are important for people's livelihoods. States should respect and protect the rights of individuals with respect to resources such as land, water, forests, fisheries, and livestock without any discrimination. Where necessary and appropriate, States should carry out land reforms and other policy reforms consistent with their human rights obligations and in accordance with the rule of law in order to secure efficient and equitable access to land and to strengthen pro-poor growth. Special attention may be given to groups such as pastoralists and indigenous people and their relation to natural resources.

8.2 States should take steps so that members of vulnerable groups can have access to opportunities and economic resources in order to participate fully and equally in the economy.

8.3 States should pay particular attention to the specific access problems of women and of vulnerable, marginalized and traditionally disadvantaged

groups, including all persons affected by HIV/AIDS. States should take measures to protect all people affected by HIV/AIDS from losing their access to resources and assets.

* * *

8.6 States should promote women's full and equal participation in the economy and, for this purpose, introduce, where it does not exist, and implement gender-sensitive legislation providing women with the right to inherit and possess land and other property. States should also provide women with secure and equal access to, control over, and benefits from productive resources, including credit, land, water, and appropriate technologies.

8.7 States should design and implement programs that include different mechanisms of access and appropriate use of agricultural land, directed to the poorest populations.

Guideline 8a: Labour
* * *
Guideline 8b: Land
* * *
Guideline 8c: Water
* * *
Guideline 8d: Genetic resources for food and agriculture
* * *
Guideline 8e: Sustainability
* * *
Guideline 8f: Services
* * *

Guideline 9: Food safety and consumer protection
9.1 States should take measures to ensure that all food, whether locally produced or imported, freely available or sold on markets, is safe and consistent with national food safety standards.

9.2 States should establish comprehensive and rational food-control systems that reduce risk of food borne disease using risk analysis and supervisory mechanisms to ensure food safety in the entire food chain including animal feed.

9.3 States are encouraged to take action to streamline institutional procedures for food control and food safety at national level and eliminate gaps and overlaps in inspection systems and in the legislative and regulatory framework for food. States are encouraged to adopt scientifically based food safety standards, including standards for additives, contaminants, residues of veterinary drugs and pesticides, and microbiological hazards, and establish standards for packaging, labelling and advertising of food. These standards should take into consideration internationally accepted food standards (Codex Alimentarius) in accordance with the WTO Sanitary and Phytosanitary Agreement (SPS). States should take action, to prevent contamination from industrial and other pollutants in the production, processing, storage, transport, distribution, handling and sale of food.

9.4 States may wish to establish a national coordinating committee for food to bring together both governmental and non-governmental actors involved in the food system and to act as liaison with the FAO/WHO Codex Alimentarius Commission. States should consider collaborating with private stakeholders in the food system, both by assisting them in exercising controls on their own production and handling practices, and by auditing those controls.

9.5 Where necessary, States should assist farmers and other primary producers to follow good agricultural practices, food processors to follow good manufacturing practices, and food handlers to follow good hygiene practices. States are encouraged to consider establishing food safety systems and supervisory mechanisms to ensure the provision of safe food to consumers.

9.6 States should ensure that education on safe practices is available for food business operators in order that their activities neither lead to harmful residues in food nor cause harm to the environment. States should also take measures to educate consumers about the safe storage, handling and utilization of food within the household. States should collect and disseminate information to the public regarding food-borne diseases and food safety matters, and should cooperate with regional and international organizations addressing food safety issues.

9.7 States should adopt measures to protect consumers from deception and misrepresentation in the packaging, labelling, advertising and sale of food and facilitate consumers' choice by ensuring appropriate information on marketed food, and provide recourse for any harm caused by unsafe or adulterated food, including food offered by street sellers. Such measures should not be used as unjustified barriers to trade and be in conformity with the WTO agreements (in particular SPS and TBT).

9.8 Developed countries are encouraged to provide technical assistance to developing countries through advice, credits, donations and grants for capacity building and training in food safety. When possible and appropriate, developing countries with more advanced capabilities in food safety-related areas are encouraged to lend assistance to less advanced developing countries.

9.9 States are encouraged to cooperate with all stakeholders, including regional and international consumer organizations, addressing food safety issues, and consider their participation in national and international fora where policies with impact on food production, processing, distribution, storage and marketing are discussed.

Guideline 10: Nutrition
10.1 If necessary, States should take measures to maintain, adapt or strengthen dietary diversity and healthy eating habits and food preparation, as well as feeding patterns, including breastfeeding, while ensuring that changes in availability and access to food supply do not negatively affect dietary composition and intake.

10.2 States are encouraged to take steps, in particular through education, information and labelling regulations, to prevent over-consumption and unbalanced diets which may lead to malnutrition, obesity and degenerative diseases.

10.3 States are encouraged to involve all relevant stakeholders, in particular communities and local government, in the design, implementation, management, monitoring and evaluation of programmes to increase the production and consumption of healthy and nutritious foods, especially those that are rich in micronutrients. States may wish to promote gardens at both home and school as a key element in combating micronutrient deficiencies and promoting healthy eating. States may also consider adopting regulations for fortifying foods to prevent and cure micronutrient deficiencies particularly iodine, iron and Vitamin A.

10.4 States should address the specific food and nutritional needs of people living with HIV/AIDS, or suffering from other epidemics.

10.5 States should take appropriate measures to promote and encourage breastfeeding, in line with their cultures, the International Code of Marketing of Breast-milk Substitutes and subsequent resolutions of the World Health Assembly, in accordance with the WHO/UNICEF recommendations.

10.6 States may wish to disseminate information on the feeding of infants and young children that is consistent and in line with current scientific knowledge and internationally accepted practices and to take steps to counteract misinformation on infant feeding. States should consider with utmost care issues regarding breastfeeding and human immunodeficiency virus (HIV) infection on the basis of the most up-to-date, authoritative scientific advice and referring to the latest WHO/UNICEF guidelines.

10.7 States are invited to take parallel action in the areas of health, education and sanitary infrastructure and promote intersectoral collaboration, so that necessary services and goods become available to people to enable them to make full use of the dietary value in the food they eat and thus achieve nutritional well-being.

10.8 States should adopt measures to eradicate any kind of discriminatory practices, especially in respect of gender, in order to achieve adequate levels of nutrition within the household.

10.9 States should recognize that food is a vital part of an individual's culture and are encouraged to take into account individuals' practices, customs and traditions on matters related to food.

10.10 States are reminded of the cultural values of dietary and eating habits in different cultures and should establish methods for promoting food safety, positive nutritional intake including fair distribution of food within communities and households with special emphasis on the needs and rights of both girls and boys and pregnant women and lactating mothers, in all cultures.

Guideline 11: Education and awareness raising

* * *

Guideline 13: Support for vulnerable groups
13.1 Consistent with the World Food Summit commitment, States should establish Food Insecurity and Vulnerability Information and Mapping Systems (FIVIMS), in order to identify groups and households particularly vulnerable to food insecurity along with the reasons for their food insecurity. States should develop and identify corrective measures to be implemented both immediately and progressively to provide access to adequate food.

* * *

Guideline 14: Safety nets
14.1 States should consider, to the extent that resources permit, establishing and maintaining social safety and food safety nets to protect those who are unable to provide for themselves. As far as possible, and with due regard to effectiveness and coverage, states should consider building on existing capacities within communities at risk to provide the necessary resources for social safety and food safety nets to fulfil the progressive realization of the right to adequate food states may wish to consider the benefits of procuring locally.

* * *

Guideline 15: Internationa food aid
15.1 Donor states should ensure that their food aid policies support national efforts by recipient States to achieve food security and base their food aid provisions on sound needs assessment targeting especially food insecure and vulnerable groups. In this context, donor states should provide assistance in a manner that takes into account food safety, the importance of not disrupting local food production and the nutritional and dietary needs and culture of recipient populations. Food aid should be provided with a clear exit strategy and avoid the creation of dependency. Donors should promote increased use of local and regional commercial markets to meet food needs in famine-prone countries and reduce dependence on food aid.

15.2 International food-aid transactions, including bilateral food aid which is monetized, should be carried out in a manner consistent with the FAO Principles of Surplus Disposal and Consultative Obligations, the Food Aid Convention and the WTO Agreement on Agriculture, and should meet the internationally agreed food safety standards, bearing in mind local circumstances, dietary traditions and cultures.

15.3 States and relevant non-state actors should ensure, in accordance with international law, safe and unimpeded access to the populations in need, as well as for international needs assessments and humanitarian agencies involved in the distribution of international food assistance.

15.4 The provision of international food aid in emergency situations should take particular account of longer term rehabilitation and development objectives in the recipient countries and should respect universally recognized humanitarian principles.

15.5 The assessment of needs and the planning, monitoring and evaluation of the provision of food aid should, as far as possible, be made in a participatory manner, and whenever possible, in close collaboration with recipient governments at the national and local level.

Guideline 16: Natural and human-made disasters

16.1 Food should never be used as a means of political and economic pressure.

16.2 States reaffirm the obligations they have assumed under international humanitarian law and, in particular, as parties to the 1949 Geneva Conventions and/or the 1977 Additional Protocols thereto with respect to the humanitarian needs of the civilian population, including their access to food in situations of armed conflict and occupation, inter alia,

— Additional Protocol I provides, inter alia, that "[t]he starvation of civilians as a method of warfare is prohibited" and that "[i]t is prohibited to attack, destroy, remove or render useless objects indispensable to the survival of the civilian population, such as foodstuffs, agricultural areas for the production of foodstuffs, crops, livestock,

drinking water installations and supplies and irrigation works, for the specific purpose of denying them, for their sustenance value to the civilian population or to the adverse party, whatever the motive, whether in order to starve out civilians, to cause them to move away, or for any other motive.", and that "these objects shall not be made the object of reprisals".

16.3 In situations of occupation, international humanitarian law provides, inter alia: that to the fullest extent of the means available to it, the Occupying Power has the duty of ensuring the food and medical supplies of the population; that it should, in particular, bring in the necessary foodstuffs, medical stores and other articles if the resources of the Occupied Territory are inadequate; and that if the whole or part of the population of an Occupied Territory is inadequately supplied, the Occupying Power shall agree to relief schemes on behalf of the said population, and shall facilitate them by all the means at its disposal.

16.4 States reaffirm the obligations they have assumed regarding the protection, safety and security of humanitarian personnel.

16.5 States should make every effort to ensure that refugees and internally displaced persons have access at all times to adequate food. In this respect, States and other relevant stakeholders should be encouraged to make use of the Guiding Principles on Internal Displacement when dealing with situations of internal displacement.

16.6 In the case of natural or human-made disasters, States should provide food assistance to those in need, may request international assistance if their own resources do not suffice, and should facilitate safe and unimpeded access for international assistance in accordance with international law and universally recognized humanitarian principles, bearing in mind local circumstances, dietary traditions and cultures.

16.7 States should put in place adequate and functioning mechanisms of early warning to prevent or mitigate the effects of natural or human-made disasters. Early warning systems should be based on international standards and cooperation, on reliable, disaggregated data and should be constantly monitored. States should take appropriate emergency preparedness measures, such as keeping food stocks for the acquisition of food and take steps to put in place adequate systems for distribution.

16.8 States are invited to consider establishing mechanisms to assess nutritional impact and to gain understanding of the coping strategies of affected households in the event of natural or human made disasters. This should inform the targeting, design, implementation and evaluation of relief, rehabilitation and resilience building programmes.

Guideline 17: Monitoring, indicators and benchmarks

17.1 States may wish to establish mechanisms to monitor and evaluate the implementation of these Guidelines towards the progressive realization of the right to adequate food in the context of national food security, in accordance with their capacity and by building on existing information systems and addressing information gaps.

17.2 States may wish to consider conducting "Right to Food Impact Assessments" in order to identify the impact of domestic policies, programmes and projects on the progressive realisation of the right to adequate food of the population at large and vulnerable groups in particular, and as a basis for the adoption of the necessary corrective measures.

17.3 States may also wish to develop a set of process, impact and outcome indicators, relying on indicators already in use and monitoring systems such as FIVIMS, so as to assess the implementation of the progressive realization of the right to adequate food. They may wish to establish appropriate benchmarks to be achieved in the short, medium and long term, which relate directly to meeting poverty and hunger reduction targets as a minimum, as well as other national and international goals including those adopted at the World Food Summit and the Millennium Summit.

17.4 In this evaluation process, process indicators could be so identified or designed that they explicitly relate and reflect the use of specific policy instruments and interventions with outcomes consistent with the progressive realization of the right to adequate food in the context of national food security. Such indicators could enable States to implement legal, policy and administrative measures, detect discriminatory practices and outcomes, and ascertain the extent of political and social participation in the process of realizing that right.

17.5 States should, in particular, monitor the food-security situation of vulnerable groups, in particular women, children and the elderly, and their nutritional status, including the prevalence of micronutrient deficiencies.

17.6 In this evaluation process, States should ensure a participatory approach to information gathering, management, analysis, interpretation and dissemination.

Guideline 18: National human rights institutions

18.1 States that have as a matter of national law or policy adopted a rights-based approach and which have national human rights institutions or ombudspersons, may wish to include the progressive realization of the right to adequate food in the context of national food security in their mandates. States which do not have national human rights institutions or ombudspersons are encouraged to establish them. Human rights institutions should be independent and autonomous from the government, in accordance with the Paris Principles. States should encourage civil society organizations and individuals to contribute to monitoring activities undertaken by national human rights institutions with respect to the progressive realization of the right to adequate food.

18.2 States are invited to encourage efforts by national institutions to establish partnerships and increase cooperation with civil society.

Guideline 19: International dimension

19.1 States should fulfil those measures, actions and commitments on the international dimension, as described in Section III below, in support of the implementation of the Voluntary Guidelines, which assist states in their national efforts in the progressive realization of the right to adequate food in the context of national food security as set forth by the World Food Summit and the World Food Summit: five years later within the context of the Millennium Declaration.

SECTION III: INTERNATIONAL MEASURES, ACTIONS AND COMMITMENTS

International Cooperation and Unilateral Measures
* * *

Role of the International Community
* * *

Technical Cooperation

5. Developed and developing countries should act in partnership to support their efforts to achieve the progressive realization of the right to adequate food in the context of national food security through technical cooperation, including institutional capacity building, and transfer of technology on mutually agreed terms, as committed in the major international conferences, in all areas covered in these guidelines, with special focus on impediments to food security such as HIV/AIDS.

International Trade
* * *

External Debt
* * *

Official Development Assistance
* * *

International Food Aid
* * *

Partnerships with NGOs/ CSOs/Private Sector

14. States, international organizations, civil society, private sector, and all relevant non-governmental organizations and other stakeholders should promote the strengthening of partnerships and coordinated action, including programs and capacity development efforts, with a view to strengthening the progressive realization of the right to adequate food in the context of national food security.

Promotion and Protection of the Right to Adequate Food

15. The organs and specialised agencies related to human rights should continue to enhance the coordination of their activities based on the consistent and objective application of international human right instruments including the promotion of the progressive realization of the right to adequate food. The promotion and protection of all human rights and fundamental freedoms must be considered a priority objective of the United Nations in accordance with its purposes and principles, in particular the purpose of international cooperation. In the framework of these purposes and principles, the promotion and protection of all human rights including the progressive realization of the right to adequate food, is a legitimate concern of all member states, the international community and civil society.

International Reporting

16. States may report on a voluntary basis on relevant activities and progress achieved in implementing the Voluntary Guidelines on the progressive realization of the right to adequate food in the context of national food security, to CFS within its reporting procedures.

C. The Right to Adequate Housing

General Comment 4: The Right to Adequate Housing (1991)

Adopted by the Committee on Economic, Social and Cultural Rights,
UN document E/1992/23 (13 December 1991).
[Available at http://www.unhchr.ch/tbs/doc.nsf/(symbol)/
CESCR+General+comment+4.En?OpenDocument]

1. Pursuant to article 11 (1) of the Covenant, States parties "recognize the right of everyone to an adequate standard of living for himself and his family, including adequate food, clothing and housing, and to the continuous improvement of living conditions". The human right to adequate housing, which is thus derived from the right to an adequate standard of living, is of central importance for the enjoyment of all economic, social and cultural rights.

2. The Committee has been able to accumulate a large amount of information pertaining to this right. Since 1979, the Committee and its predecessors have examined 75 reports dealing with the right to adequate housing. The Committee has also devoted a day of general discussion to the issue at each of its third (see E/1989/22, para. 312) and fourth sessions (E/1990/23, paras. 281-285). In addition, the Committee has taken careful note of information generated by the International Year of Shelter for the Homeless (1987) including the Global Strategy for Shelter to the Year 2000 adopted by the General Assembly in its resolution 42/191 of 11 December 1987.[1] The Committee has also reviewed relevant reports and other documentation of the Commission on Human Rights and the Sub-Commission on Prevention of Discrimination and Protection of Minorities.[2]

3. Although a wide variety of international instruments address the different dimensions of the right to adequate housing[3] article 11 (1) of the Covenant is the most comprehensive and perhaps the most important of the relevant provisions.

4. Despite the fact that the international community has frequently reaffirmed the importance of full respect for the right to adequate housing, there remains a disturbingly large gap between the standards set in article 11 (1) of the Covenant and the situation prevailing in many parts of the world.

While the problems are often particularly acute in some developing countries which confront major resource and other constraints, the Committee observes that significant problems of homelessness and inadequate housing also exist in some of the most economically developed societies. The United Nations estimates that there are over 100 million persons homeless worldwide and over 1 billion inadequately housed.[4] There is no indication that this number is decreasing. It seems clear that no State party is free of significant problems of one kind or another in relation to the right to housing.

5. In some instances, the reports of States parties examined by the Committee have acknowledged and described difficulties in ensuring the right to adequate housing. For the most part, however, the information provided has been insufficient to enable the Committee to obtain an adequate picture of the situation prevailing in the State concerned. This General Comment thus aims to identify some of the principal issues which the Committee considers to be important in relation to this right.

6. The right to adequate housing applies to everyone. While the reference to "himself and his family" reflects assumptions as to gender roles and economic activity patterns commonly accepted in 1966 when the Covenant was adopted, the phrase cannot be read today as implying any limitations upon the applicability of the right to individuals or to female-headed households or other such groups. Thus, the concept of "family" must be understood in a wide sense. Further, individuals, as well as families, are entitled to adequate housing regardless of age, economic status, group or other affiliation or status and other such factors. In particular, enjoyment of this right must, in accordance with article 2 (2) of the Covenant, not be subject to any form of discrimination.

7. In the Committee's view, the right to housing should not be interpreted in a narrow or restrictive sense which equates it with, for example, the shelter provided by merely having a roof over one's head or views shelter exclusively as a commodity. Rather it should be seen as the right to live somewhere in security, peace and dignity. This is appropriate for at least two reasons. In the first place, the right to housing is integrally linked to other human rights and to the fundamental principles upon which the Covenant is premised. This "the inherent dignity of the human person" from which the rights in the Covenant are said to derive requires that the term "housing" be interpreted so as to take account of a variety of other considerations, most importantly that the right to housing should be ensured to all persons irrespective of income or access to economic resources. Secondly, the reference in article 11 (1) must be read as referring not just to housing but to adequate housing. As both the Commission on Human Settlements and the Global Strategy for Shelter to the Year 2000 have stated: "Adequate shelter means ... adequate privacy, adequate space, adequate security, adequate lighting and ventilation, adequate basic infrastructure and adequate location with regard to work and basic facilities — all at a reasonable cost".

8. Thus the concept of adequacy is particularly significant in relation to the right to housing since it serves to underline a number of factors which must be taken into account in determining whether particular forms of shelter can be considered to constitute "adequate housing" for the purposes of the Covenant. While adequacy is determined in part by social, economic, cultural, climatic, ecological and other factors, the Committee believes that it is nevertheless possible to identify certain aspects of the right that must be taken into account for this purpose in any particular context. They include the following:

(a) Legal security of tenure:
Tenure takes a variety of forms, including rental (public and private) accommodation, cooperative housing, lease, owner-occupation, emergency housing and informal settlements, including occupation of land or property. Notwithstanding the type of tenure, all persons should possess a degree of security of tenure which guarantees legal protection against forced eviction, harassment and other threats. States parties should consequently take immediate measures aimed at conferring legal security of tenure upon those persons and households currently lacking such protection, in genuine consultation with affected persons and groups;

(b) Availability of services, materials, facilities and infrastructure:
An adequate house must contain certain facilities essential for health, security, comfort and nutrition. All beneficiaries of the right to adequate housing should have sustainable access to natural and common resources, safe drinking water, energy for cooking, heating and lighting, sanitation and washing facilities, means of food storage, refuse disposal, site drainage and emergency services;

(c) Affordability:
Personal or household financial costs associated with housing should be at such a level that the attainment and satisfaction of other basic needs are not threatened or compromised. Steps should be taken by States parties to ensure that the percentage of housing-related costs is, in general, commensurate with income levels. States parties should establish housing subsidies for those unable to obtain affordable housing, as well as forms and levels of housing finance which adequately reflect housing needs. In accordance with the principle of affordability, tenants should be protected by appropriate means against unreasonable rent levels or rent increases. In societies where natural materials constitute the chief sources of building materials for housing, steps should be taken by States parties to ensure the availability of such materials;

(d) Habitability:
Adequate housing must be habitable, in terms of providing the inhabitants with adequate space and protecting them from cold, damp, heat, rain, wind or other threats to health, structural hazards, and disease vectors. The physical safety of occupants must be guaranteed as well. The Committee encourages States parties to comprehensively apply the Health Principles of Housing[5] prepared by WHO which view housing as the environmental factor most frequently associated with conditions for disease in epidemiological analyses; i.e. inad-

equate and deficient housing and living conditions are invariably associated with higher mortality and morbidity rates;

(e) Accessibility:
Adequate housing must be accessible to those entitled to it. Disadvantaged groups must be accorded full and sustainable access to adequate housing resources. Thus, such disadvantaged groups as the elderly, children, the physically disabled, the terminally ill, HIV-positive individuals, persons with persistent medical problems, the mentally ill, victims of natural disasters, people living in disaster-prone areas and other groups should be ensured some degree of priority consideration in the housing sphere. Both housing law and policy should take fully into account the special housing needs of these groups. Within many States parties increasing access to land by landless or impoverished segments of the society should constitute a central policy goal. Discernible governmental obligations need to be developed aiming to substantiate the right of all to a secure place to live in peace and dignity, including access to land as an entitlement;

(f) Location:
Adequate housing must be in a location which allows access to employment options, health-care services, schools, child-care centres and other social facilities. This is true both in large cities and in rural areas where the temporal and financial costs of getting to and from the place of work can place excessive demands upon the budgets of poor households. Similarly, housing should not be built on polluted sites nor in immediate proximity to pollution sources that threaten the right to health of the inhabitants;

(g) Cultural adequacy:
The way housing is constructed, the building materials used and the policies supporting these must appropriately enable the expression of cultural identity and diversity of housing. Activities geared towards development or modernization in the housing sphere should ensure that the cultural dimensions of housing are not sacrificed, and that, inter alia, modern technological facilities, as appropriate are also ensured.

9. As noted above, the right to adequate housing cannot be viewed in isolation from other human rights contained in the two International Covenants and other applicable international instruments. Reference has already been made in this regard to the concept of human dignity and the principle of non-discrimination. In addition, the full enjoyment of other rights — such as the right to freedom of expression, the right to freedom of association (such as for tenants and other community-based groups), the right to freedom of residence and the right to participate in public decision-making — is indispensable if the right to adequate housing is to be realized and maintained by all groups in society. Similarly, the right not to be subjected to arbitrary or unlawful interference with one's privacy, family, home or correspondence constitutes a very important dimension in defining the right to adequate housing.

10. Regardless of the state of development of any country, there are certain steps which must be taken immediately. As recognized in the Global Strategy for Shelter and in other international analyses, many of the measures required to promote the right to housing would only require the abstention by the Government from certain practices and a commitment to facilitating "self-help" by affected groups. To the extent that any such steps are considered to be beyond the maximum resources available to a State party, it is appropriate that a request be made as soon as possible for international cooperation in accordance with articles 11 (1), 22 and 23 of the Covenant, and that the Committee be informed thereof.

11. States parties must give due priority to those social groups living in unfavourable conditions by giving them particular consideration. Policies and legislation should correspondingly not be designed to benefit already advantaged social groups at the expense of others. The Committee is aware that external factors can affect the right to a continuous improvement of living conditions, and that in many States parties overall living conditions declined during the 1980s. However, as noted by the Committee in its General Comment 2 (1990) (E/1990/23, annex III), despite externally caused problems, the obligations under the Covenant continue to apply and are perhaps even more pertinent during times of economic contraction. It would thus appear to the Committee that a general decline in living and housing conditions, directly attributable to policy and legislative decisions by States parties, and in the absence of ac-

companying compensatory measures, would be inconsistent with the obligations under the Covenant.

12. While the most appropriate means of achieving the full realization of the right to adequate housing will inevitably vary significantly from one State party to another, the Covenant clearly requires that each State party take whatever steps are necessary for that purpose. This will almost invariably require the adoption of a national housing strategy which, as stated in paragraph 32 of the Global Strategy for Shelter, "defines the objectives for the development of shelter conditions, identifies the resources available to meet these goals and the most cost-effective way of using them and sets out the responsibilities and time-frame for the implementation of the necessary measures". Both for reasons of relevance and effectiveness, as well as in order to ensure respect for other human rights, such a strategy should reflect extensive genuine consultation with, and participation by, all of those affected, including the homeless, the inadequately housed and their representatives. Furthermore, steps should be taken to ensure coordination between ministries and regional and local authorities in order to reconcile related policies (economics, agriculture, environment, energy, etc.) with the obligations under article 11 of the Covenant.

13. Effective monitoring of the situation with respect to housing is another obligation of immediate effect. For a State party to satisfy its obligations under article 11 (1) it must demonstrate, inter alia, that it has taken whatever steps are necessary, either alone or on the basis of international cooperation, to ascertain the full extent of homelessness and inadequate housing within its jurisdiction. In this regard, the revised general guidelines regarding the form and contents of reports adopted by the Committee (E/C.12/1991/1) emphasize the need to "provide detailed information about those groups within ... society that are vulnerable and disadvantaged with regard to housing". They include, in particular, homeless persons and families, those inadequately housed and without ready access to basic amenities, those living in "illegal" settlements, those subject to forced evictions and low-income groups.

14. Measures designed to satisfy a State party's obligations in respect of the right to adequate housing may reflect whatever mix of public and private sector measures considered appropriate. While in some States public financing of housing might most usefully be spent on direct construction of new housing, in most cases, experience has shown the inability of Governments to fully satisfy housing deficits with publicly built housing. The promotion by States parties of "enabling strategies", combined with a full commitment to obligations under the right to adequate housing, should thus be encouraged. In essence, the obligation is to demonstrate that, in aggregate, the measures being taken are sufficient to realize the right for every individual in the shortest possible time in accordance with the maximum of available resources.

15. Many of the measures that will be required will involve resource allocations and policy initiatives of a general kind. Nevertheless, the role of formal legislative and administrative measures should not be underestimated in this context. The Global Strategy for Shelter (paras. 66-67) has drawn attention to the types of measures that might be taken in this regard and to their importance.

16. In some States, the right to adequate housing is constitutionally entrenched. In such cases the Committee is particularly interested in learning of the legal and practical significance of such an approach. Details of specific cases and of other ways in which entrenchment has proved helpful should thus be provided.

17. The Committee views many component elements of the right to adequate housing as being at least consistent with the provision of domestic legal remedies. Depending on the legal system, such areas might include, but are not limited to: (a) legal appeals aimed at preventing planned evictions or demolitions through the issuance of court-ordered injunctions; (b) legal procedures seeking compensation following an illegal eviction; (c) complaints against illegal actions carried out or supported by landlords (whether public or private) in relation to rent levels, dwelling maintenance, and racial or other forms of discrimination; (d) allegations of any form of discrimination in the allocation and availability of access to housing; and (e) complaints against landlords concerning unhealthy or inadequate housing conditions. In some legal systems it would also be appropriate to explore the possibility of facilitating

class action suits in situations involving significantly increased levels of homelessness.

18. In this regard, the Committee considers that instances of forced eviction are prima facie incompatible with the requirements of the Covenant and can only be justified in the most exceptional circumstances, and in accordance with the relevant principles of international law.

19. Finally, article 11 (1) concludes with the obligation of States parties to recognize "the essential importance of international cooperation based on free consent". Traditionally, less than 5 per cent of all international assistance has been directed towards housing or human settlements, and often the manner by which such funding is provided does little to address the housing needs of disadvantaged groups. States parties, both recipients and providers, should ensure that a substantial proportion of financing is devoted to creating conditions leading to a higher number of persons being adequately housed. International financial institutions promoting measures of structural adjustment should ensure that such measures do not compromise the enjoyment of the right to adequate housing. States parties should, when contemplating international financial cooperation, seek to indicate areas relevant to the right to adequate housing where external financing would have the most effect. Such requests should take full account of the needs and views of the affected groups.

Notes

1. Official Records of the General Assembly, Forty-third Session, Supplement No. 8, addendum (A/43/8/Add.1).
2. Commission on Human Rights resolutions 1986/36 and 1987/22; reports by Mr. Danilo Türk, Special Rapporteur of the Sub-Commission (E/CN.4/Sub.2/1990/19, paras. 108-120; E/CN.4/Sub.2/1991/17, paras. 137-139); see also Sub-Commission resolution 1991/26.
3. See, for example, article 25 (1) of the Universal Declaration on Human Rights, article 5 (e) (iii) of the International Convention on the Elimination of All Forms of Racial Discrimination, article 14 (2) of the Convention on the Elimination of All Forms of Discrimination against Women, article 27 (3) of the Convention on the Rights of the Child, article 10 of the Declaration on Social Progress and Development, section III (8) of the Vancouver Declaration on Human Settlements, 1976 (Report of Habitat: United Nations Conference on Human Settlements (United Nations publication, Sales No. E.76.IV.7 and corrigendum), chap. I), article 8 (1) of the Declaration on the Right to Development and the ILO Recommendation Concerning Workers' Housing, 1961 (No. 115).
4. See footnote 1.
5. Geneva, World Health Organization, 1990.

D. The Right to Education

International Covenant on Economic, Social and Cultural Rights (1966)

Adopted and opened for signature, ratification and accession by General Assembly Resolution 2200A (XXI) of 16 December 1966. Entered into force 3 January 1976.
[Available at www.unhchr.ch/html/menu3/b/a_cescr.htm]

* * *

Article 13

1. The States Parties to the present Covenant recognize the right of everyone to education. They agree that education shall be directed to the full development of the human personality and the sense of its dignity, and shall strengthen the respect for human rights and fundamental freedoms. They further agree that education shall enable all persons to participate effectively in a free society, promote understanding, tolerance and friendship among all nations and all racial, ethnic or religious groups, and further the activities of the United Nations for the maintenance of peace.

2. The States Parties to the present Covenant recognize that, with a view to achieving the full realization of this right:

(a) Primary education shall be compulsory and available free to all;

(b) Secondary education in its different forms, including technical and vocational secondary education, shall be made generally available and accessible to all by every appropriate means, and in particular by the progressive introduction of free education;

(c) Higher education shall be made equally accessible to all, on the basis of capacity, by every appropriate means, and in particular by the progressive introduction of free education;

(d) Fundamental education shall be encouraged or intensified as far as possible for those persons who have not received or completed the whole period of their primary education;

(e) The development of a system of schools at all levels shall be actively pursued, an adequate fellowship system shall be established, and the material conditions of teaching staff shall be continuously improved.

3. The States Parties to the present Covenant undertake to have respect for the liberty of parents and, when applicable, legal guardians to choose for their children schools, other than those established by the public authorities, which conform to such minimum educational standards as may be laid down or approved by the State and to ensure the religious and moral education of their children in conformity with their own convictions.

4. No part of this article shall be construed so as to interfere with the liberty of individuals and bodies to establish and direct educational institutions, subject always to the observance of the principles set forth in paragraph 1 of this article and to the requirement that the education given in such institutions shall conform to such minimum standards as may be laid down by the State.

Article 14

Each State Party to the present Covenant which, at the time of becoming a Party, has not been able to secure in its metropolitan territory or other territories under its jurisdiction compulsory primary education, free of charge, undertakes, within two years, to work out and adopt a detailed plan of action for the progressive implementation, within a reasonable number of years, to be fixed in the plan, of the principle of compulsory education free of charge for all.

* * *

General Comment 13: The Right to Education (Article 13) (1999)

Committee on Economic, Social and Cultural Rights.
UN document E/C.12/1999/10 (8 December 1999)
[Available at www.unhchr.ch/tbs/doc.nsf/(symbol)/E.C.12.1999.10.En?OpenDocument]

[Footnotes omitted.]

THE RIGHT TO EDUCATION (ARTICLE 13)

1. Education is both a human right in itself and an indispensable means of realizing other human rights. As an empowerment right, education is the primary vehicle by which economically and socially marginalized adults and children can lift themselves out of poverty and obtain the means to participate fully in their communities. Education has a vital role in empowering women, safeguarding children from exploitative and hazardous labour and sexual exploitation, promoting human rights and democracy, protecting the environment, and controlling population growth. Increasingly, education is recognized as one of the best financial investments States can make. But the importance of education is not just practical: a well-educated, enlightened and active mind, able to wander freely and widely, is one of the joys and rewards of human existence.

2. The International Covenant on Economic, Social and Cultural Rights (ICESCR) devotes two articles to the right to education, articles 13 and 14. Article 13, the longest provision in the Covenant, is the most wide-ranging and comprehensive article on the right to education in international human rights law. The Committee has already adopted General Comment 11 on article 14 (plans of action for primary education); General Comment 11 and the present general comment are complementary and should be considered together. The Committee is aware that for millions of people throughout the world, the enjoyment of the right to education remains a distant goal. Moreover, in many cases, this goal is becoming increasingly remote. The Committee is also conscious of the formidable structural and other obstacles impeding the full implementation of article 13 in many States parties.

3. With a view to assisting States parties' implementation of the Covenant and the fulfillment of their reporting obligations, this general comment focuses on the normative content of article 13 (Part I, paras. 4-42), some of the obligations arising from it (Part II, paras. 43-57), and some illustrative violations (Part II, paras. 58-59). Part III briefly remarks upon the obligations of actors other than States parties. The general comment is based upon the Committee's experience in examining States parties, reports over many years.

I. NORMATIVE CONTENT OF ARTICLE 13

Article 13 (1)
Aims and Objectives of Education

4. States parties agree that all education, whether public or private, formal or non-formal, shall be directed towards the aims and objectives identified in article 13 (1). The Committee notes that these educational objectives reflect the fundamental purposes and principles of the United Nations as enshrined in Articles 1 and 2 of the Charter. For the most part, they are also found in article 26 (2) of the Universal Declaration of Human Rights, although article 13 (1) adds to the Declaration in three respects: education shall be directed to the human personality's "sense of dignity", it shall "enable all persons to participate effectively in a free society", and it shall promote understanding among all "ethnic" groups, as well as nations and racial and religious groups. Of those educational objectives which are common to article 26 (2) of the Universal Declaration of Human Rights and article 13 (1) of the Covenant, perhaps the most fundamental is that "education shall be directed to the full development of the human personality".

5. The Committee notes that since the General Assembly adopted the Covenant in 1966, other international instruments have further elaborated the objectives to which education should be directed. Accordingly, the Committee takes the view that States parties are required to ensure that education conforms to the aims and objectives identified in

article 13 (1), as interpreted in the light of the World Declaration on Education for All (Jomtien, Thailand, 1990) (art. 1), the Convention on the Rights of the Child (art. 29 (1)), the Vienna Declaration and Programme of Action (Part I, para. 33 and Part II, para. 80), and the Plan of Action for the United Nations Decade for Human Rights Education (para. 2). While all these texts closely correspond to article 13 (1) of the Covenant, they also include elements which are not expressly provided for in article 13 (1), such as specific references to gender equality and respect for the environment. These new elements are implicit in, and reflect a contemporary interpretation of article 13 (1). The Committee obtains support for this point of view from the widespread endorsement that the previously mentioned texts have received from all regions of the world.

Article 13 (2)
The Right to Receive an Education —
Some General Remarks

6. While the precise and appropriate application of the terms will depend upon the conditions prevailing in a particular State party, education in all its forms and at all levels shall exhibit the following interrelated and essential features:

(a) Availability — functioning educational institutions and programmes have to be available in sufficient quantity within the jurisdiction of the State party. What they require to function depends upon numerous factors, including the developmental context within which they operate; for example, all institutions and programmes are likely to require buildings or other protection from the elements, sanitation facilities for both sexes, safe drinking water, trained teachers receiving domestically competitive salaries, teaching materials, and so on; while some will also require facilities such as a library, computer facilities and information technology;

(b) Accessibility — educational institutions and programmes have to be accessible to everyone, without discrimination, within the jurisdiction of the State party. Accessibility has three overlapping dimensions:

Non-discrimination — education must be accessible to all, especially the most vulnerable groups,

in law and fact, without discrimination on any of the prohibited grounds (see paras. 31-37 on non-discrimination);

Physical accessibility — education has to be within safe physical reach, either by attendance at some reasonably convenient geographic location (e.g. a neighbourhood school) or via modern technology (e.g. access to a "distance learning" programme);

Economic accessibility — education has to be affordable to all. This dimension of accessibility is subject to the differential wording of article 13 (2) in relation to primary, secondary and higher education: whereas primary education shall be available "free to all", States parties are required to progressively introduce free secondary and higher education;

(c) Acceptability — the form and substance of education, including curricula and teaching methods, have to be acceptable (e.g. relevant, culturally appropriate and of good quality) to students and, in appropriate cases, parents; this is subject to the educational objectives required by article 13 (1) and such minimum educational standards as may be approved by the State (see art. 13 (3) and (4);

(d) Adaptability — education has to be flexible so it can adapt to the needs of changing societies and communities and respond to the needs of students within their diverse social and cultural settings.

7. When considering the appropriate application of these "interrelated and essential features" the best interests of the student shall be a primary consideration.

Article 13 (2) (a): The Right
to Primary Education
* * *

Article 13 (2) (b): The Right
to Secondary Education
* * *

Technical and Vocational Education
* * *

Article 13 (2) (c): The Right
to Higher Education
* * *

Article 13 (2) (d)
The Right to Fundamental Education

21. Fundamental education includes the elements of availability, accessibility, acceptability and adaptability which are common to education in all its forms and at all levels.

22. In general terms, fundamental education corresponds to basic education as set out in the World Declaration on Education For All. By virtue of article 13 (2) (d), individuals "who have not received or completed the whole period of their primary education" have a right to fundamental education, or basic education as defined in the World Declaration on Education For All.

23. Since everyone has the right to the satisfaction of their "basic learning needs" as understood by the World Declaration, the right to fundamental education is not confined to those "who have not received or completed the whole period of their primary education". The right to fundamental education extends to all those who have not yet satisfied their "basic learning needs".

24. It should be emphasized that enjoyment of the right to fundamental education is not limited by age or gender; it extends to children, youth and adults, including older persons. Fundamental education, therefore, is an integral component of adult education and life-long learning. Because fundamental education is a right of all age groups, curricula and delivery systems must be devised which are suitable for students of all ages.

Article 13 (2) (e): A School System; Adequate Fellowship System; Material Conditions of Teaching Staff

25. The requirement that the "development of a system of schools at all levels shall be actively pursued" means that a State party is obliged to have an overall developmental strategy for its school system. The strategy must encompass schooling at all levels, but the Covenant requires States parties to prioritize primary education (see para. 51). "[A]ctively pursued" suggests that the overall strategy should attract a degree of governmental priority and, in any event, must be implemented with vigour.

26. The requirement that "an adequate fellowship system shall be established" should be read with the Covenant's non-discrimination and equality provisions; the fellowship system should enhance equality of educational access for individuals from disadvantaged groups.

27. While the Covenant requires that "the material conditions of teaching staff shall be continuously improved", in practice the general working conditions of teachers have deteriorated, and reached unacceptably low levels, in many States parties in recent years. Not only is this inconsistent with article 13 (2) (e), but it is also a major obstacle to the full realization of students' right to education. The Committee also notes the relationship between articles 13 (2) (e), 2 (2), 3 and 6-8 of the Covenant, including the right of teachers to organize and bargain collectively; draws the attention of States parties to the joint UNESCO-ILO Recommendation Concerning the Status of Teachers (1966) and the UNESCO Recommendation Concerning the Status of Higher-Education Teaching Personnel (1997); and urges States parties to report on measures they are taking to ensure that all teaching staff enjoy the conditions and status commensurate with their role.

Article 13 (3) and (4)
The Right to Educational Freedom

28. Article 13 (3) has two elements, one of which is that States parties undertake to respect the liberty of parents and guardians to ensure the religious and moral education of their children in conformity with their own convictions.

The Committee is of the view that this element of article 13 (3) permits public school instruction in subjects such as the general history of religions and ethics if it is given in an unbiased and objective way, respectful of the freedoms of opinion, conscience and expression. It notes that public education that includes instruction in a particular religion or belief is inconsistent with article 13 (3) unless provision is made for non-discriminatory exemptions or alternatives that would accommodate the wishes of parents and guardians.

29. The second element of article 13 (3) is the liberty of parents and guardians to choose other than public schools for their children, provided the

schools conform to "such minimum educational standards as may be laid down or approved by the State". This has to be read with the complementary provision, article 13 (4), which affirms "the liberty of individuals and bodies to establish and direct educational institutions", provided the institutions conform to the educational objectives set out in article 13 (1) and certain minimum standards. These minimum standards may relate to issues such as admission, curricula and the recognition of certificates. In their turn, these standards must be consistent with the educational objectives set out in article 13 (1).

30. Under article 13 (4), everyone, including non-nationals, has the liberty to establish and direct educational institutions. The liberty also extends to "bodies", i.e. legal persons or entities. It includes the right to establish and direct all types of educational institutions, including nurseries, universities and institutions for adult education. Given the principles of non-discrimination, equal opportunity and effective participation in society for all, the State has an obligation to ensure that the liberty set out in article 13 (4) does not lead to extreme disparities of educational opportunity for some groups in society.

Article 13
Special Topics of Broad Application: Non-Discrimination and Equal Treatment

31. The prohibition against discrimination enshrined in article 2 (2) of the Covenant is subject to neither progressive realization nor the availability of resources; it applies fully and immediately to all aspects of education and encompasses all internationally prohibited grounds of discrimination. The Committee interprets articles 2 (2) and 3 in the light of the UNESCO Convention against Discrimination in Education, the relevant provisions of the Convention on the Elimination of All Forms of Discrimination against Women, the International Convention on the Elimination of All Forms of Racial Discrimination, the Convention on the Rights of the Child and the ILO Indigenous and Tribal Peoples Convention, 1989 (Convention No. 169), and wishes to draw particular attention to the following issues.

32. The adoption of temporary special measures intended to bring about de facto equality for men and women and for disadvantaged groups is not a violation of the right to non-discrimination with regard to education, so long as such measures do not lead to the maintenance of unequal or separate standards for different groups, and provided they are not continued after the objectives for which they were taken have been achieved.

33. In some circumstances, separate educational systems or institutions for groups defined by the categories in article 2 (2) shall be deemed not to constitute a breach of the Covenant. In this regard, the Committee affirms article 2 of the UNESCO Convention against Discrimination in Education (1960).

34. The Committee takes note of article 2 of the Convention on the Rights of the Child and article 3 (e) of the UNESCO Convention against Discrimination in Education and confirms that the principle of non-discrimination extends to all persons of school age residing in the territory of a State party, including non-nationals, and irrespective of their legal status.

35. Sharp disparities in spending policies that result in differing qualities of education for persons residing in different geographic locations may constitute discrimination under the Covenant.

36. The Committee affirms paragraph 35 of its General Comment 5, which addresses the issue of persons with disabilities in the context of the right to education, and paragraphs 36-42 of its General Comment 6, which address the issue of older persons in relation to articles 13-15 of the Covenant.

37. States parties must closely monitor education — including all relevant policies, institutions, programmes, spending patterns and other practices — so as to identify and take measures to redress any de facto discrimination. Educational data should be disaggregated by the prohibited grounds of discrimination.

Academic Freedom and Institutional Autonomy

38. In the light of its examination of numerous States parties' reports, the Committee has formed the view that the right to education can only be en-

joyed if accompanied by the academic freedom of staff and students. Accordingly, even though the issue is not explicitly mentioned in article 13, it is appropriate and necessary for the Committee to make some observations about academic freedom. The following remarks give particular attention to institutions of higher education because, in the Committee's experience, staff and students in higher education are especially vulnerable to political and other pressures which undermine academic freedom. The Committee wishes to emphasize, however, that staff and students throughout the education sector are entitled to academic freedom and many of the following observations have general application.

39. Members of the academic community, individually or collectively, are free to pursue, develop and transmit knowledge and ideas, through research, teaching, study, discussion, documentation, production, creation or writing. Academic freedom includes the liberty of individuals to express freely opinions about the institution or system in which they work, to fulfill their functions without discrimination or fear of repression by the State or any other actor, to participate in professional or representative academic bodies, and to enjoy all the internationally recognized human rights applicable to other individuals in the same jurisdiction. The enjoyment of academic freedom carries with it obligations, such as the duty to respect the academic freedom of others, to ensure the fair discussion of contrary views, and to treat all without discrimination on any of the prohibited grounds.

40. The enjoyment of academic freedom requires the autonomy of institutions of higher education. Autonomy is that degree of self-governance necessary for effective decision-making by institutions of higher education in relation to their academic work, standards, management and related activities. Self-governance, however, must be consistent with systems of public accountability, especially in respect of funding provided by the State. Given the substantial public investments made in higher education, an appropriate balance has to be struck between institutional autonomy and accountability. While there is no single model, institutional arrangements should be fair, just and equitable, and as transparent and participatory as possible.

Discipline in Schools

41. In the Committee's view, corporal punishment is inconsistent with the fundamental guiding principle of international human rights law enshrined in the Preambles to the Universal Declaration of Human Rights and both Covenants: the dignity of the individual. Other aspects of school discipline may also be inconsistent with human dignity, such as public humiliation. Nor should any form of discipline breach other rights under the Covenant, such as the right to food. A State party is required to take measures to ensure that discipline which is inconsistent with the Covenant does not occur in any public or private educational institution within its jurisdiction. The Committee welcomes initiatives taken by some States parties which actively encourage schools to introduce "positive", nonviolent approaches to school discipline.

Limitations on Article 13

42. The Committee wishes to emphasize that the Covenant's limitations clause, article 4, is primarily intended to be protective of the rights of individuals rather than permissive of the imposition of limitations by the State. Consequently, a State party which closes a university or other educational institution on grounds such as national security or the preservation of public order has the burden of justifying such a serious measure in relation to each of the elements identified in article 4.

II. STATES PARTIES' OBLIGATIONS AND VIOLATIONS
General Legal Obligations

43. While the Covenant provides for progressive realization and acknowledges the constraints due to the limits of available resources, it also imposes on States parties various obligations which are of immediate effect.

States parties have immediate obligations in relation to the right to education, such as the "guarantee" that the right "will be exercised without discrimination of any kind" (art. 2 (2)) and the obligation "to take steps" (art. 2 (1)) towards the full realization of article 13.

Such steps must be "deliberate, concrete and targeted" towards the full realization of the right to education.

44. The realization of the right to education over time, that is "progressively", should not be interpreted as depriving States parties' obligations of all meaningful content. Progressive realization means that States parties have a specific and continuing obligation "to move as expeditiously and effectively as possible" towards the full realization of article 13.

45. There is a strong presumption of impermissibility of any retrogressive measures taken in relation to the right to education, as well as other rights enunciated in the Covenant. If any deliberately retrogressive measures are taken, the State party has the burden of proving that they have been introduced after the most careful consideration of all alternatives and that they are fully justified by reference to the totality of the rights provided for in the Covenant and in the context of the full use of the State party's maximum available resources.

46. The right to education, like all human rights, imposes three types or levels of obligations on States parties: the obligations to respect, protect and fulfill. In turn, the obligation to fulfill incorporates both an obligation to facilitate and an obligation to provide.

47. The obligation to respect requires States parties to avoid measures that hinder or prevent the enjoyment of the right to education. The obligation to protect requires States parties to take measures that prevent third parties from interfering with the enjoyment of the right to education. The obligation to fulfill (facilitate) requires States to take positive measures that enable and assist individuals and communities to enjoy the right to education. Finally, States parties have an obligation to fulfill (provide) the right to education. As a general rule, States parties are obliged to fulfill (provide) a specific right in the Covenant when an individual or group is unable, for reasons beyond their control, to realize the right themselves by the means at their disposal. However, the extent of this obligation is always subject to the text of the Covenant.

48. In this respect, two features of article 13 require emphasis. First, it is clear that article 13 regards States as having principal responsibility for the direct provision of education in most circumstances; States parties recognize, for example, that

the "development of a system of schools at all levels shall be actively pursued" (art. 13 (2) (e)). Secondly, given the differential wording of article 13 (2) in relation to primary, secondary, higher and fundamental education, the parameters of a State party's obligation to fulfill (provide) are not the same for all levels of education. Accordingly, in light of the text of the Covenant, States parties have an enhanced obligation to fulfill (provide) regarding the right to education, but the extent of this obligation is not uniform for all levels of education. The Committee observes that this interpretation of the obligation to fulfill (provide) in relation to article 13 coincides with the law and practice of numerous States parties.

Specific Legal Obligations

49. States parties are required to ensure that curricula, for all levels of the educational system, are directed to the objectives identified in article 13 (1). They are also obliged to establish and maintain a transparent and effective system which monitors whether or not education is, in fact, directed to the educational objectives set out in article 13 (1).

50. In relation to article 13 (2), States have obligations to respect, protect and fulfill each of the "essential features" (availability, accessibility, acceptability, adaptability) of the right to education. By way of illustration, a State must respect the availability of education by not closing private schools; protect the accessibility of education by ensuring that third parties, including parents and employers, do not stop girls from going to school; fulfill (facilitate) the acceptability of education by taking positive measures to ensure that education is culturally appropriate for minorities and indigenous peoples, and of good quality for all; fulfill (provide) the adaptability of education by designing and providing resources for curricula which reflect the contemporary needs of students in a changing world; and fulfill (provide) the availability of education by actively developing a system of schools, including building classrooms, delivering programmes, providing teaching materials, training teachers and paying them domestically competitive salaries.

51. As already observed, the obligations of States parties in relation to primary, secondary, higher and fundamental education are not identical.

Given the wording of article 13 (2), States parties are obliged to prioritize the introduction of compulsory, free primary education. This interpretation of article 13 (2) is reinforced by the priority accorded to primary education in article 14. The obligation to provide primary education for all is an immediate duty of all States parties.

52. In relation to article 13 (2) (b)-(d), a State party has an immediate obligation "to take steps" (art. 2 (1)) towards the realization of secondary, higher and fundamental education for all those within its jurisdiction. At a minimum, the State party is required to adopt and implement a national educational strategy which includes the provision of secondary, higher and fundamental education in accordance with the Covenant. This strategy should include mechanisms, such as indicators and benchmarks on the right to education, by which progress can be closely monitored.

53. Under article 13 (2) (e), States parties are obliged to ensure that an educational fellowship system is in place to assist disadvantaged groups. The obligation to pursue actively the "development of a system of schools at all levels" reinforces the principal responsibility of States parties to ensure the direct provision of the right to education in most circumstances.

54. States parties are obliged to establish "minimum educational standards" to which all educational institutions established in accordance with article 13 (3) and (4) are required to conform. They must also maintain a transparent and effective system to monitor such standards. A State party has no obligation to fund institutions established in accordance with article 13 (3) and (4); however, if a State elects to make a financial contribution to private educational institutions, it must do so without discrimination on any of the prohibited grounds.

55. States parties have an obligation to ensure that communities and families are not dependent on child labour. The Committee especially affirms the importance of education in eliminating child labour and the obligations set out in article 7 (2) of the Worst Forms of Child Labour Convention, 1999 (Convention No. 182). Additionally, given article 2 (2), States parties are obliged to remove gender and other stereotyping which impedes the educational access of girls, women and other disadvantaged groups.

56. In its General Comment 3, the Committee drew attention to the obligation of all States parties to take steps, "individually and through international assistance and cooperation, especially economic and technical", towards the full realization of the rights recognized in the Covenant, such as the right to education. Articles 2 (1) and 23 of the Covenant, Article 56 of the Charter of the United Nations, article 10 of the World Declaration on Education for All, and Part I, paragraph 34 of the Vienna Declaration and Programme of Action all reinforce the obligation of States parties in relation to the provision of international assistance and cooperation for the full realization of the right to education. In relation to the negotiation and ratification of international agreements, States parties should take steps to ensure that these instruments do not adversely impact upon the right to education. Similarly, States parties have an obligation to ensure that their actions as members of international organizations, including international financial institutions, take due account of the right to education.

57. In its General Comment 3, the Committee confirmed that States parties have "a minimum core obligation to ensure the satisfaction of, at the very least, minimum essential levels" of each of the rights enunciated in the Covenant, including "the most basic forms of education". In the context of article 13, this core includes an obligation: to ensure the right of access to public educational institutions and programmes on a non-discriminatory basis; to ensure that education conforms to the objectives set out in article 13 (1); to provide primary education for all in accordance with article 13 (2) (a); to adopt and implement a national educational strategy which includes provision for secondary, higher and fundamental education; and to ensure free choice of education without interference from the State or third parties, subject to conformity with "minimum educational standards" (art. 13 (3) and (4)).

Violations

58. When the normative content of article 13 (Part I) is applied to the general and specific obligations of States parties (Part II), a dynamic process is set in motion which facilitates identification of viola-

tions of the right to education. Violations of article 13 may occur through the direct action of States parties (acts of commission) or through their failure to take steps required by the Covenant (acts of omission).

59. By way of illustration, violations of article 13 include: the introduction or failure to repeal legislation which discriminates against individuals or groups, on any of the prohibited grounds, in the field of education; the failure to take measures which address de facto educational discrimination; the use of curricula inconsistent with the educational objectives set out in article 13 (1); the failure to maintain a transparent and effective system to monitor conformity with article 13 (1); the failure to introduce, as a matter of priority, primary education which is compulsory and available free to all; the failure to take "deliberate, concrete and targeted" measures towards the progressive realization of secondary, higher and fundamental education in accordance with article 13 (2) (b)-(d); the prohibition of private educational institutions; the failure to ensure private educational institutions conform to the "minimum educational standards" required by article 13 (3) and (4); the denial of academic freedom of staff and students; the closure of educational institutions in times of political tension in non-conformity with article 4.

III. OBLIGATIONS OF ACTORS OTHER THAN STATES PARTIES

60. Given article 22 of the Covenant, the role of the United Nations agencies, including at the country level through the United Nations Development Assistance Framework (UNDAF), is of special importance in relation to the realization of article 13. Coordinated efforts for the realization of the right to education should be maintained to improve coherence and interaction among all the actors concerned, including the various components of civil society. UNESCO, the United Nations Development Programme, UNICEF, ILO, the World Bank, the regional development banks, the International Monetary Fund and other relevant bodies within the United Nations system should enhance their cooperation for the implementation of the right to education at the national level, with due respect to their specific mandates, and building on their respective expertise. In particular, the international financial institutions, notably the World Bank and IMF, should pay greater attention to the protection of the right to education in their lending policies, credit agreements, structural adjustment programmes and measures taken in response to the debt crisis. When examining the reports of States parties, the Committee will consider the effects of the assistance provided by all actors other than States parties on the ability of States to meet their obligations under article 13. The adoption of a human rights-based approach by United Nations specialized agencies, programmes and bodies will greatly facilitate implementation of the right to education.

The Dakar Framework for Action — Education for All:
Meeting Our Collective Commitments (2000)
Text adopted by the World Education Forum, Dakar, Senegal, on 28 April 2000.
[Available at http://www.unesco.org/education/efa/ed_for_all/dakfram_eng.shtml]

1. Meeting in Dakar, Senegal, in April 2000, we, the participants in the World Education Forum, commit ourselves to the achievement of education for all (EFA) goals and targets for every citizen and for every society.

2. The Dakar Framework is a collective commitment to action. Governments have an obligation to ensure that EFA goals and targets are reached and sustained. This is a responsibility that will be met most effectively through broad-based partnerships within countries, supported by cooperation with regional and international agencies and institutions.

3. We re-affirm the vision of the World Declaration on Education for All (Jomtien 1990), supported by the Universal Declaration of Human Rights and the Convention on the Rights of the Child, that all children, young people and adults have the human right to benefit from an education that will meet their basic learning needs in the best and fullest sense of the term, an education that includes learning to know, to do, to live together and to be. It is an education geared to tapping each individual's talents and potential, and developing learners' personalities, so that they can improve their lives and transform their societies.

4. We welcome the commitments made by the international community to basic education throughout the 1990s, notably at the World Summit for Children (1990), the Conference on Environment and Development (1992), the World Conference on Human Rights (1993), the World Conference on Special Needs Education: Access and Quality (1994), the International Conference on Population and Development (1994), the World Summit for Social Development (1995), the Fourth World Conference on Women (1995), the Mid-Term Meeting of the International Consultative Forum on Education for All (1996), the Fifth International Conference on Adult Education (1997), and the International

Conference on Child Labour (1997). The challenge now is to deliver on these commitments.

5. The EFA 2000 Assessment demonstrates that there has been significant progress in many countries. But it is unacceptable in the year 2000 that more than 113 million children have no access to primary education, 880 million adults are illiterate, gender discrimination continues to permeate education systems, and the quality of learning and the acquisition of human values and skills fall far short of the aspirations and needs of individuals and societies. Youth and adults are denied access to the skills and knowledge necessary for gainful employment and full participation in their societies. Without accelerated progress towards education for all, national and internationally agreed targets for poverty reduction will be missed, and inequalities between countries and within societies will widen.

6. Education is a fundamental human right. It is the key to sustainable development and peace and stability within and among countries, and thus an indispensable means for effective participation in the societies and economies of the twenty-first century, which are affected by rapid globalization. Achieving EFA goals should be postponed no longer. The basic learning needs of all can and must be met as a matter of urgency.

7. We hereby collectively commit ourselves to the attainment of the following goals:

(i) expanding and improving comprehensive early childhood care and education, especially for the most vulnerable and disadvantaged children;

(ii) ensuring that by 2015 all children, particularly girls, children in difficult circumstances and those belonging to ethnic minorities, have access to and complete free and compulsory primary education of good quality;

(iii) ensuring that the learning needs of all young people and adults are met through equitable access to appropriate learning and life skills programmes;

(iv) achieving a 50 per cent improvement in levels of adult literacy by 2015, especially for women, and equitable access to basic and continuing education for all adults;

(v) eliminating gender disparities in primary and secondary education by 2005, and achieving gender equality in education by 2015, with a focus on ensuring girls' full and equal access to and achievement in basic education of good quality;

(vi) improving all aspects of the quality of education and ensuring excellence of all so that recognized and measurable learning outcomes are achieved by all, especially in literacy, numeracy and essential life skills.

8. To achieve these goals, we the governments, organizations, agencies, groups and associations represented at the World Education Forum pledge ourselves to:

(i) mobilize strong national and international political commitment for education for all, develop national action plans and enhance significantly investment in basic education;

(ii) promote EFA policies within a sustainable and well-integrated sector framework clearly linked to poverty elimination and development strategies;

(iii) ensure the engagement and participation of civil society in the formulation, implementation and monitoring of strategies for educational development;

(iv) develop responsive, participatory and accountable systems of educational governance and management;

(v) meet the needs of education systems affected by conflict, national calamities and instability and conduct educational programmes in ways that promote mutual understanding, peace and tolerance, and help to prevent violence and conflict;

(vi) implement integrated strategies for gender equality in education which recognize the need for changes in attitudes, values and practices;

(vii) implement as a matter of urgency education programmes and actions to combat the HIV/AIDS pandemic;

(viii) create safe, healthy, inclusive and equitably resourced educational environments conducive to excellence in learning with clearly defined levels of achievement for all;

(ix) enhance the status, morale and professionalism of teachers;

(x) harness new information and communication technologies to help achieve EFA goals;

(xi) systematically monitor progress towards EFA goals and strategies at the national, regional and international levels; and

(xii) build on existing mechanisms to accelerate progress towards education for all.

9. Drawing on the evidence accumulated during the national and regional EFA assessments, and building on existing national sector strategies, all States will be requested to develop or strengthen existing national plans of action by 2002 at the latest. These plans should be integrated into a wider poverty reduction and development framework, and should be developed through more transparent and democratic processes, involving stakeholders, especially peoples' representatives, community leaders, parents, learners, non-governmental organizations (NGOs) and civil society. The plans will address problems associated with the chronic under-financing of basic education by establishing budget priorities that reflect a commitment to achieving EFA goals and targets at the earliest possible date, and no later than 2015. They will also set out clear strategies for overcoming the special problems facing those currently excluded from educational opportunities, with a clear commitment to girls' education and gender equity. The plans will give substance and form to the goals and strategies set out in this Framework, and to the commitments made during a succession of international conferences in the 1990s.

Regional activities to support national strategies will be based on strengthened regional and subregional organizations, networks and initiatives.

10. Political will and stronger national leadership are needed for the effective and successful implementation of national plans in each of the countries concerned. However, political will must be underpinned by resources. The international community acknowledges that many countries currently lack the resources to achieve education for all within an acceptable time-frame. New financial resources, preferably in the form of grants and concessional assistance, must therefore be mobilized by bilateral and multilateral funding agencies, including the World Bank and regional development banks, and the private sector. We affirm that no countries seriously committed to education for all will be thwarted in their achievement of this goal by a lack of resources.

11. The international community will deliver on this collective commitment by launching with immediate effect a global initiative aimed at developing the strategies and mobilizing the resources needed to provide effective support to national efforts. Options to be considered under this initiative will include:

(i) increasing external finance for education, in particular basic education;

(ii) ensuring greater predictability in the flow of external assistance;

(iii) facilitating more effective donor coordination;

(iv) strengthening sector-wide approaches;

(v) providing earlier, more extensive and broader debt relief and/or debt cancellation for poverty reduction, with a strong commitment to basic education; and

(vi) undertaking more effective and regular monitoring of progress towards EFA goals and targets, including periodic assessments.

12. There is already evidence from many countries of what can be achieved through strong national strategies supported by effective development cooperation. Progress under these strategies could — and must — be accelerated through increased international support. At the same time, countries with less developed strategies — including countries in transition, countries affected by conflict, and post-crisis countries — must be given the support they need to achieve more rapid progress towards education for all.

13. We will strengthen accountable international and regional mechanisms to give clear expression to these commitments and to ensure that the Dakar Framework for Action is on the agenda of every international and regional organization, every national legislature and every local decision-making forum.

14. The EFA 2000 Assessment highlights that the challenge of education for all is greatest in sub-Saharan Africa, in South Asia, and in the least developed countries. Accordingly, while no country in need should be denied international assistance, priority should be given to these regions and countries. Countries in conflict or undergoing reconstruction should also be given special attention in building up their education systems to meet the needs of all learners.

15. Implementation of the preceding goals and strategies will require national, regional and international mechanisms to be galvanized immediately. To be most effective these mechanisms will be participatory and, wherever possible, build on what already exists. They will include representatives of all stakeholders and partners and they will operate in transparent and accountable ways. They will respond comprehensively to the word and spirit of the Jomtien Declaration and this Dakar Framework for Action. The functions of these mechanisms will include, to varying degrees, advocacy, resource mobilization, monitoring, and EFA knowledge generation and sharing.

16. The heart of EFA activity lies at the country level. National EFA Forums will be strengthened or established to support the achievement of EFA. All relevant ministries and national civil society organizations will be systematically represented in these Forums. They should be transparent and democratic and should constitute a framework for implementation at subnational levels. Countries will prepare comprehensive National EFA Plans by 2002 at the latest. For those countries with sig-

nificant challenges, such as complex crises or natural disasters, special technical support will be provided by the international community. Each National EFA Plan will:

(i) be developed by government leadership in direct and systematic consultation with national civil society;

(ii) attract co-ordinated support of all development partners;

(iii) specify reforms addressing the six EFA goals;

(iv) establish a sustainable financial framework;

(v) be time-bound and action-oriented;

(vi) include mid-term performance indicators; and

(vii) achieve a synergy of all human development efforts, through its inclusion within the national development planning framework and process.

17. Where these processes and a credible plan are in place, partner members of the international community undertake to work in a consistent, co-ordinated and coherent manner. Each partner will contribute according to its comparative advantage in support of the National EFA Plans to ensure that resource gaps are filled.

18. Regional activities to support national efforts will be based on existing regional and subregional organizations, networks and initiatives, augmented where necessary. Regions and subregions will decide on a lead EFA network that will become the Regional or Subregional Forum with an explicit EFA mandate. Systematic involvement of, and co-ordination with, all relevant civil society and other regional and subregional organizations are essential. These Regional and Subregional EFA Forums will be linked organically with, and be accountable to, National EFA Forums. Their functions will be: co-ordination with all relevant networks; setting and monitoring regional/subregional targets; advocacy; policy dialogue; the promotion of partnerships and technical cooperation;

the sharing of best practices and lessons learned; monitoring and reporting for accountability; and promoting resource mobilization. Regional and international support will be available to strengthen Regional and Subregional Forums and relevant EFA capacities, especially within Africa and South Asia.

19. UNESCO will continue its mandated role in co-ordinating EFA partners and maintaining their collaborative momentum. In line with this, UNESCO's Director-General will convene annually a high-level, small and flexible group. It will serve as a lever for political commitment and technical and financial resource mobilization. Informed by a monitoring report from the UNESCO International Institute for Educational Planning (IIEP), the UNESCO International Bureau of Education (IBE), the UNESCO Institute for Education (UIE) and, in particular, the UNESCO Institute of Statistics, and inputs from Regional and Subregional EFA Forums, it will also be an opportunity to hold the global community to account for commitments made in Dakar. It will be composed of highest-level leaders from governments and civil society of developing and developed countries, and from development agencies.

20. UNESCO will serve as the Secretariat. It will refocus its education programme in order to place the outcomes and priorities of Dakar at the heart of its work. This will involve working groups on each of the six goals adopted at Dakar. This Secretariat will work closely with other organizations and may include staff seconded from them.

21. Achieving Education for All will require additional financial support by countries and increased development assistance and debt relief for education by bilateral and multilateral donors, estimated to cost in the order of $8 billion a year. It is therefore essential that new, concrete financial commitments be made by national governments and also by bilateral and multilateral donors including the World Bank and the regional development banks, by civil society and by foundations.

V. HEALTH AND HUMAN RIGHTS OF VULNERABLE POPULATIONS
A. Women and Reproductive Health

General Recommendation 14: Female Circumcision (1990)

Adopted by the Committee on the Elimination of Discrimination against Women on 2 February 1990. UN Document CEDAW, A/45/38. (General Comments) [Available at http://www.unhchr.ch/tbs/doc.nsf/0/bad3a652ca102401c 12563ee0062e685?Opendocument]

The Committee on the Elimination of Discrimination against Women,

Concerned about the continuation of the practice of female circumcision and other traditional practices harmful to the health of women,

Noting with satisfaction that Governments, where such practices exist, national women's organizations, non-governmental organizations, specialized agencies, such as the World Health Organization, the United Nations Children's Fund, as well as the Commission on Human Rights and its Sub-Commission on Prevention of Discrimination and Protection of Minorities, remain seized of the issue having particularly recognized that such traditional practices as female circumcision have serious health and other consequences for women and children,

Noting with interest the study of the Special Rapporteur on Traditional Practices Affecting the Health of Women and Children, as well as the study of the Special Working Group on Traditional Practices,

Recognizing that women are taking important action themselves to identify and to combat practices that are prejudicial to the health and well-being of women and children,

Convinced that the important action that is being taken by women and by all interested groups needs to be supported and encouraged by Governments,

Noting with grave concern that there are contin-

uing cultural, traditional and economic pressures which help to perpetuate harmful practices, such as female circumcision,

Recommends to States Parties:

(a) That States parties take appropriate and effective measures with a view to eradicating the practice of female circumcision. Such measures could include:

(i) The collection and dissemination by universities, medical or nursing associations, national women's organizations or other bodies of basic data about such traditional practices;

(ii) The support of women's organizations at the national and local levels working for the elimination of female circumcision and other practices harmful to women;

(iii) The encouragement of politicians, professionals, religious and community leaders at all levels including the media and the arts to cooperate in influencing attitudes towards the eradication of female circumcision;

(iv) The introduction of appropriate educational and training programmes and seminars based on research findings about the problems arising from female circumcision;

(b) That States parties include in their national health policies appropriate strategies aimed at eradicating female circumcision in public health care. Such strategies could include the special responsibility of health personnel including traditional birth attendants to explain the harmful effects of female circumcision;

(c) That States parties invite assistance, information and advice from the appropriate organizations of the United Nations system to support and assist efforts being deployed to eliminate harmful traditional practices;

(d) That States parties include in their reports to the Committee under articles 10 and 12 of the Convention on the Elimination of All Forms of Discrimination against Women information about measures taken to eliminate female circumcision.

General Recommendation 15: Avoidance of Discrimination against Women in National Strategies for the Prevention and Control of Acquired Immunodeficiency Syndrome (AIDS) (1990)

Adopted by the Committee on the Elimination of Discrimination against Women on 2 February 1990. UN Document CEDAW, A/45/38. (General Comments) [Available at http://www.unhchr.ch/tbs/doc.nsf/0/bad3a652ca102401c 12563ee0062e685!Opendocument]

The Committee on the Elimination of Discrimination against Women,

Having considered information brought to its attention on the potential effects of both the global pandemic of acquired immunodeficiency syndrome (AIDS) and strategies to control it on the exercise of the rights of women,

Having regard to the reports and materials prepared by the World Health Organization and other United Nations organizations, organs and bodies in relation to human immunodeficiency virus (HIV), and, in particular, the note by the Secretary-General to the Commission on the Status of Women on the effects of AIDS on the advancement of women and the Final Document of the International Consultation on AIDS and Human Rights, held at Geneva from 26 to 28 July 1989,

Noting World Health Assembly resolution WHA 41.24 on the avoidance of discrimination in relation to HIV-infected people and people with AIDS of 13 May 1988, resolution 1989/11 of the Commission on Human Rights on non-discrimination in the field of health, of 2 March 1989, and in particular the Paris Declaration on Women, Children and AIDS, of 30 November 1989,

Noting that the World Health Organization has announced that the theme of World Aids Day, 1 December 1990, will be "Women and Aids",

Recommends:

(a) That States parties intensify efforts in disseminating information to increase public awareness of the risk of HIV infection and AIDS, especially in women and children, and of its effects on them;

(b) That programmes to combat AIDS should give special attention to the rights and needs of women and children, and to the factors relating to the reproductive role of women and their subordinate position in some societies which make them especially vulnerable to HIV infection;

(c) That States parties ensure the active participation of women in primary health care and take measures to enhance their role as care providers, health workers and educators in the prevention of infection with HIV;

(d) That all States parties include in their reports under article 12 of the Convention information on the effects of AIDS on the situation of women and on the action taken to cater to the needs of those women who are infected and to prevent specific discrimination against women in response to AIDS.

Programme of Action of the International Conference on Population and Development (1994)

Report of the International Conference on Population and Development (Cairo, 5-13 September 1994). UN Document A/CONF.171.13 (18 October 1994). [Available at http://www.unfpa.org/icpd/icpd_poa.htm#ch4]

[Footnotes omitted.]

* * *

CHAPTER IV

GENDER EQUALITY, EQUITY AND EMPOWERMENT OF WOMEN

A. Empowerment and Status of Women

Basis for Action

4.1. The empowerment and autonomy of women and the improvement of their political, social, economic and health status is a highly important end in itself. In addition, it is essential for the achievement of sustainable development. The full participation and partnership of both women and men is required in productive and reproductive life, including shared responsibilities for the care and nurturing of children and maintenance of the household. In all parts of the world, women are facing threats to their lives, health and well- being as a result of being overburdened with work and of their lack of power and influence. In most regions of the world, women receive less formal education than men, and at the same time, women's own knowledge, abilities and coping mechanisms often go unrecognized. The power relations that impede women's attainment of healthy and fulfilling lives operate at many levels of society, from the most personal to the highly public. Achieving change requires policy and programme actions that will improve women's access to secure livelihoods and economic resources, alleviate their extreme responsibilities with regard to housework, remove legal impediments to their participation in public life, and raise social awareness through effective programmes of education and mass communication. In addition, improving the status of women also enhances their decision-making capacity at all levels in all spheres of life, especially in the area of sexuality and reproduc-tion. This, in turn, is essential for the long-term success of population programmes. Experience shows that population and development programmes are most effective when steps have simultaneously been taken to improve the status of women.

4.2. Education is one of the most important means of empowering women with the knowledge, skills and self-confidence necessary to participate fully in the development process. More than 40 years ago, the Universal Declaration of Human Rights asserted that "everyone has the right to educa-tion". In 1990, Governments meeting at the World Conference on Education for All in Jomtien, Thailand, committed themselves to the goal of universal access to basic education. But despite notable efforts by countries around the globe that have appreciably expanded access to basic educa-tion, there are approximately 960 million illiterate adults in the world, of whom two thirds are women. More than one third of the world's adults, most of them women, have no access to printed knowledge, to new skills or to technologies that would improve the quality of their lives and help them shape and adapt to social and economic change. There are 130 million children who are not enrolled in primary school and 70 per cent of them are girls.

Objectives

4.3. The objectives are:

(a) To achieve equality and equity based on harmonious partnership between men and women and enable women to realize their full potential;

(b) To ensure the enhancement of women's contributions to sustainable development through their full involvement in policy- and decision-making processes at all stages and participation in all aspects of production, employment, income-generating activities, education, health, science and technology, sports, culture and population-related activities and other areas, as active decision makers, participants and beneficiaries;

(c) To ensure that all women, as well as men, are provided with the education necessary for them to meet their basic human needs and to exercise their human rights.

* * *

4.5. All countries should make greater efforts to promulgate, implement and enforce national laws and international conventions to which they are party, such as the Convention on the Elimination of All Forms of Discrimination against Women, that protect women from all types of economic discrimination and from sexual harassment, and to implement fully the Declaration on the Elimination of Violence against Women and the Vienna Declaration and Programme of Action adopted at the World Conference on Human Rights in 1993. Countries are urged to sign, ratify and implement all existing agreements that promote women's rights.

4.6. Governments at all levels should ensure that women can buy, hold and sell property and land equally with men, obtain credit and negotiate contracts in their own name and on their own behalf and exercise their legal rights to inheritance.

4.7. Governments and employers are urged to eliminate gender discrimination in hiring, wages, benefits, training and job security with a view to eliminating gender-based disparities in income.

4.8. Governments, international organizations and non-governmental organizations should ensure that their personnel policies and practices comply with the principle of equitable representation of both sexes, especially at the managerial and policy-making levels, in all programmes, including population and development programmes. Specific procedures and indicators should be devised for gender-based analysis of development programmes and for assessing the impact of those programmes on women's social, economic and health status and access to resources.

4.9. Countries should take full measures to eliminate all forms of exploitation, abuse, harassment and violence against women, adolescents and children. This implies both preventive actions and rehabilitation of victims. Countries should prohibit degrading practices, such as trafficking in women, adolescents and children and exploitation through prostitution, and pay special attention to protecting the rights and safety of those who suffer from these crimes and those in potentially exploitable situations, such as migrant women, women in domestic service and schoolgirls. In this regard, international safeguards and mechanisms for cooperation should be put in place to ensure that these measures are implemented.

4.10. Countries are urged to identify and condemn the systematic practice of rape and other forms of inhuman and degrading treatment of women as a deliberate instrument of war and ethnic cleansing and take steps to assure that full assistance is provided to the victims of such abuse for their physical and mental rehabilitation.

4.11. The design of family health and other development interventions should take better account of the demands on women's time from the responsibilities of child-rearing, household work and income-generating activities. Male responsibilities should be emphasized with respect to child-rearing and housework. Greater investments should be made in appropriate measures to lessen the daily burden of domestic responsibilities, the greatest share of which falls on women. Greater attention should be paid to the ways in which environmental degradation and changes in land use adversely affect the allocation of women's time. Women's domestic working environments should not adversely affect their health.

4.12. Every effort should be made to encourage the expansion and strengthening of grass-roots, community-based and activist groups for women. Such groups should be the focus of national campaigns to foster women's awareness of the full range of their legal rights, including their rights within the family, and to help women organize to achieve those rights.

4.13. Countries are strongly urged to enact laws and to implement programmes and policies which will enable employees of both sexes to organize their family and work responsibilities through flexible work-hours, parental leave, day-care facilities, maternity leave, policies that enable working mothers to breast-feed their children, health insurance and other such measures. Similar rights should be ensured to those working in the informal sector.

4.14. Programmes to meet the needs of growing numbers of elderly people should fully take into account that women represent the larger proportion of the elderly and that elderly women generally have a lower socio-economic status than elderly men.

CHAPTER VII

A. REPRODUCTIVE RIGHTS AND REPRODUCTIVE HEALTH

7.1. This chapter is especially guided by the principles contained in chapter II and in particular the introductory paragraphs.

Basis for Action

7.2. Reproductive health is a state of complete physical, mental and social well-being and not merely the absence of disease or infirmity, in all matters relating to the reproductive system and to its functions and processes. Reproductive health therefore implies that people are able to have a satisfying and safe sex life and that they have the capability to reproduce and the freedom to decide if, when and how often to do so. Implicit in this last condition are the right of men and women to be informed and to have access to safe, effective, affordable and acceptable methods of family planning of their choice, as well as other methods of their choice for regulation of fertility which are not against the law, and the right of access to appropriate health-care services that will enable women to go safely through pregnancy and childbirth and provide couples with the best chance of having a healthy infant. In line with the above definition of reproductive health, reproductive health care is defined as the constellation of methods, techniques and services that contribute to reproductive health and well-being by preventing and solving reproductive health problems. It also includes sexual health, the purpose of which is the enhancement of life and personal relations, and not merely counselling and care related to reproduction and sexually transmitted diseases.

7.3. Bearing in mind the above definition, reproductive rights embrace certain human rights that are already recognized in national laws, international human rights documents and other consensus documents. These rights rest on the recognition of the basic right of all couples and individuals to decide freely and responsibly the number, spacing and timing of their children and to have the information and means to do so, and the right to attain the highest standard of sexual and reproductive health. It also includes their right to make decisions concerning reproduction free of discrimination, coercion and violence, as expressed in human rights documents. In the exercise of this right, they should take into account the needs of their living and future children and their responsibilities towards the community. The promotion of the responsible exercise of these rights for all people should be the fundamental basis for government- and community-supported policies and programmes in the area of reproductive health, including family planning. As part of their commitment, full attention should be given to the promotion of mutually respectful and equitable gender relations and particularly to meeting the educational and service needs of adolescents to enable them to deal in a positive and responsible way with their sexuality. Reproductive health eludes many of the world's people because of such factors as: inadequate levels of knowledge about human sexuality and inappropriate or poor-quality reproductive health information and services; the prevalence of high-risk sexual behaviour; discriminatory social practices; negative attitudes towards women and girls; and the limited power many women and girls have over their sexual and reproductive lives. Adolescents are particularly vulnerable because of their lack of information and access to relevant services in most countries. Older women and men have distinct reproductive and sexual health issues which are often inadequately addressed.

7.4. The implementation of the present Programme of Action is to be guided by the above comprehensive definition of reproductive health, which includes sexual health.

Objectives

7.5. The objectives are:

(a) To ensure that comprehensive and factual information and a full range of reproductive health-care services, including family planning, are accessible, affordable, acceptable and convenient to all users;

(b) To enable and support responsible voluntary decisions about child-bearing and methods of family planning of their choice, as well as other methods of their choice for regulation of fertility which are not against the law and to have the information, education and means to do so;

(c) To meet changing reproductive health needs over the life cycle and to do so in ways sensitive to the diversity of circumstances of local communities.

* * *

B. FAMILY PLANNING

Basis for Action

7.12. The aim of family-planning programmes must be to enable couples and individuals to decide freely and responsibly the number and spacing of their children and to have the information and means to do so and to ensure informed choices and make available a full range of safe and effective methods. The success of population education and family-planning programmes in a variety of settings demonstrates that informed individuals everywhere can and will act responsibly in the light of their own needs and those of their families and communities. The principle of informed free choice is essential to the long-term success of family-planning programmes. Any form of coercion has no part to play. In every society there are many social and economic incentives and disincentives that affect individual decisions about child-bearing and family size. Over the past century, many Governments have experimented with such schemes, including specific incentives and disincentives, in order to lower or raise fertility. Most such schemes have had only marginal impact on fertility and in some cases have been counterproductive. Governmental goals for family planning should be defined in terms of unmet needs for information and services. Demographic goals, while legitimately the subject of government development strategies, should not be imposed on family-planning providers in the form of targets or quotas for the recruitment of clients.

7.13. Over the past three decades, the increasing availability of safer methods of modern contraception, although still in some respects inadequate, has permitted greater opportunities for individual choice and responsible decision-making in matters of reproduction throughout much of the world. Currently, about 55 per cent of couples in developing regions use some method of family planning. This figure represents nearly a fivefold increase since the 1960s. Family-planning programmes have contributed considerably to the decline in average fertility rates for developing countries, from about six to seven children per woman in the 1960s to about three to four children at present. However, the full range of modern family-planning methods still remains unavailable to at least 350 million couples world wide, many of whom say they want to space or prevent another pregnancy. Survey data suggest that approximately 120 million additional women world wide would be currently using a modern family-planning method if more accurate information and affordable services were easily available, and if partners, extended families and the community were more supportive. These numbers do not include the substantial and growing numbers of sexually active unmarried individuals wanting in and need of information and services. During the decade of the 1990s, the number of couples of reproductive age will grow by about 18 million per annum. To meet their needs and close the existing large gaps in services, family planning and contraceptive supplies will need to expand very rapidly over the next several years. The quality of family-planning programmes is often directly related to the level and continuity of contraceptive use and to the growth in demand for services. Family-planning programmes work best when they are part of or linked to broader reproductive health programmes that address closely related health needs and when women are fully involved in the design, provision, management and evaluation of services.

Objectives

7.14. The objectives are:

(a) To help couples and individuals meet their reproductive goals in a framework that promotes optimum health, responsibility and family well-being, and respects the dignity of all persons and their right to choose the number, spacing and timing of the birth of their children;

(b) To prevent unwanted pregnancies and reduce the incidence of high-risk pregnancies and morbidity and mortality;

(c) To make quality family-planning services affordable, acceptable and accessible to all who need and want them, while maintaining confidentiality;

(d) To improve the quality of family-planning advice, information, education, communication, counselling and services;

(e) To increase the participation and sharing of responsibility of men in the actual practice of family planning;

(f) To promote breast-feeding to enhance birth spacing.

* * *

C. SEXUALLY TRANSMITTED DISEASES AND PREVENTION OF HUMAN IMMUNODEFICIENCY VIRUS (HIV)

Basis for Action

7.27. The world-wide incidence of sexually transmitted diseases is high and increasing. The situation has worsened considerably with the emergence of the HIV epidemic. Although the incidence of some sexually transmitted diseases has stabilized in parts of the world, there have been increasing cases in many regions.

7.28. The social and economic disadvantages that women face make them especially vulnerable to sexually transmitted infections, including HIV, as illustrated, for example, by their exposure to the high-risk sexual behaviour of their partners. For women, the symptoms of infections from sexually transmitted diseases are often hidden, making them more difficult to diagnose than in men, and the health consequences are often greater, including increased risk of infertility and ectopic pregnancy. The risk of transmission from infected men to women is also greater than from infected

women to men, and many women are powerless to take steps to protect themselves.

Objective

7.29. The objective is to prevent, reduce the incidence of, and provide treatment for, sexually transmitted diseases, including HIV/AIDS, and the complications of sexually transmitted diseases such as infertility, with special attention to girls and women.

* * *

D. HUMAN SEXUALITY AND GENDER RELATIONS

Basis for Action

7.34. Human sexuality and gender relations are closely interrelated and together affect the ability of men and women to achieve and maintain sexual health and manage their reproductive lives. Equal relationships between men and women in matters of sexual relations and reproduction, including full respect for the physical integrity of the human body, require mutual respect and willingness to accept responsibility for the consequences of sexual behaviour. Responsible sexual behaviour, sensitivity and equity in gender relations, particularly when instilled during the formative years, enhance and promote respectful and harmonious partnerships between men and women.

7.35. Violence against women, particularly domestic violence and rape, is widespread, and rising numbers of women are at risk from AIDS and other sexually transmitted diseases as a result of high-risk sexual behaviour on the part of their partners. In a number of countries, harmful practices meant to control women's sexuality have led to great suffering. Among them is the practice of female genital mutilation, which is a violation of basic rights and a major lifelong risk to women's health.

Objectives

7.36. The objectives are:

(a) To promote adequate development of responsible sexuality, permitting relations of equity and mutual respect between the genders and contributing to improving the quality of life of individuals;

(b) To ensure that women and men have access to the information, education and services needed to achieve good sexual health and exercise their reproductive rights and responsibilities.

* * *

E. ADOLESCENTS

Basis for Action

7.41. The reproductive health needs of adolescents as a group have been largely ignored to date by existing reproductive health services. The response of societies to the reproductive health needs of adolescents should be based on information that helps them attain a level of maturity required to make responsible decisions. In particular, information and services should be made available to adolescents to help them understand their sexuality and protect them from unwanted pregnancies, sexually transmitted diseases and subsequent risk of infertility. This should be combined with the education of young men to respect women's self-determination and to share responsibility with women in matters of sexuality and reproduction. This effort is uniquely important for the health of young women and their children, for women's self-determination and, in many countries, for efforts to slow the momentum of population growth. Motherhood at a very young age entails a risk of maternal death that is much greater than average, and the children of young mothers have higher levels of morbidity and mortality. Early child-bearing continues to be an impediment to improvements in the educational, economic and social status of women in all parts of the world. Overall for young women, early marriage and early motherhood can severely curtail educational and employment opportunities and are likely to have a long-term, adverse impact on their and their children's quality of life.

7.42. Poor educational and economic opportunities and sexual exploitation are important factors in the high levels of adolescent child-bearing. In both developed and developing countries, adolescents faced with few apparent life choices have little incentive to avoid pregnancy and childbearing.

7.43. In many societies, adolescents face pressures to engage in sexual activity. Young women, particularly low-income adolescents, are especially vulnerable. Sexually active adolescents of both sexes are increasingly at high risk of contracting and transmitting sexually transmitted diseases, including HIV/AIDS, and they are typically poorly informed about how to protect themselves. Programmes for adolescents have proven most effective when they secure the full involvement of adolescents in identifying their reproductive and sexual health needs and in designing programmes that respond to those needs.

Objectives

7.44. The objectives are:

(a) To address adolescent sexual and reproductive health issues, including unwanted pregnancy, unsafe abortion and sexually transmitted diseases, including HIV/AIDS, through the promotion of responsible and healthy reproductive and sexual behaviour, including voluntary abstinence, and the provision of appropriate services and counselling specifically suitable for that age group;

(b) To substantially reduce all adolescent pregnancies.

Platform of Action of the Fourth World Conference on Women (1995)

Report of the Fourth World Conference on Women (Beijing, China, 4-15 September 1995).
UN Document A/CONF.177/20 (17 October 1995)
[Available at http://www.un.org/esa/gopher-data/conf/fwcw/off/a—20.en]

[Footnotes omitted.]

* * *

C. WOMEN AND HEALTH*

[*The Holy See expressed a general reservation on this section. The reservation is to be interpreted in terms of the statement made by the representative of the Holy See at the 4th meeting of the Main Committee, on 14 September 1995.]

89. Women have the right to the enjoyment of the highest attainable standard of physical and mental health. The enjoyment of this right is vital to their life and well-being and their ability to participate in all areas of public and private life. Health is a state of complete physical, mental and social well-being and not merely the absence of disease or infirmity. Women's health involves their emotional, social and physical well-being and is determined by the social, political and economic context of their lives, as well as by biology. However, health and well-being elude the majority of women. A major barrier for women to the achievement of the highest attainable standard of health is inequality, both between men and women and among women in different geographical regions, social classes and indigenous and ethnic groups. In national and international forums, women have emphasized that to attain optimal health throughout the life cycle, equality, including the sharing of family responsibilities, development and peace are necessary conditions.

90. Women have different and unequal access to and use of basic health resources, including primary health services for the prevention and treatment of childhood diseases, malnutrition, anaemia, diarrhoeal diseases, communicable diseases, malaria and other tropical diseases and tuberculosis, among others. Women also have different and unequal opportunities for the protection, promotion and maintenance of their health. In many developing countries, the lack of emergency obstetric services is also of particular concern.

Health policies and programmes often perpetuate gender stereotypes and fail to consider socio-economic disparities and other differences among women and may not fully take account of the lack of autonomy of women regarding their health. Women's health is also affected by gender bias in the health system and by the provision of inadequate and inappropriate medical services to women.

91. In many countries, especially developing countries, in particular the least developed countries, a decrease in public health spending and, in some cases, structural adjustment, contribute to the deterioration of public health systems. In addition, privatization of health-care systems without appropriate guarantees of universal access to affordable health care further reduces health-care availability. This situation not only directly affects the health of girls and women, but also places disproportionate responsibilities on women, whose multiple roles, including their roles within the family and the community, are often not acknowledged; hence they do not receive the necessary social, psychological and economic support.

92. Women's right to the enjoyment of the highest standard of health must be secured throughout the whole life cycle in equality with men. Women are affected by many of the same health conditions as men, but women experience them differently. The prevalence among women of poverty and economic dependence, their experience of violence, negative attitudes towards women and girls, racial and other forms of discrimination, the limited power many women have over their sexual and reproductive lives and lack of influence in decision-making are social realities which have an adverse impact on their health. Lack of food and inequitable distribution of food for girls and women in the household, inadequate access to safe water, sanitation facilities and fuel supplies, particularly in rural and poor urban areas, and deficient housing conditions, all overburden women and their families and have a negative effect on their

health. Good health is essential to leading a productive and fulfilling life, and the right of all women to control all aspects of their health, in particular their own fertility, is basic to their empowerment.

93. Discrimination against girls, often resulting from son preference, in access to nutrition and health-care services endangers their current and future health and well-being. Conditions that force girls into early marriage, pregnancy and child-bearing and subject them to harmful practices, such as female genital mutilation, pose grave health risks. Adolescent girls need, but too often do not have, access to necessary health and nutrition services as they mature. Counselling and access to sexual and reproductive health information and services for adolescents are still inadequate or lacking completely, and a young woman's right to privacy, confidentiality, respect and informed consent is often not considered. Adolescent girls are both biologically and psychosocially more vulnerable than boys to sexual abuse, violence and prostitution, and to the consequences of unprotected and premature sexual relations. The trend towards early sexual experience, combined with a lack of information and services, increases the risk of unwanted and too early pregnancy, HIV infection and other sexually transmitted diseases, as well as unsafe abortions. Early child-bearing continues to be an impediment to improvements in the educational, economic and social status of women in all parts of the world. Overall, for young women early marriage and early motherhood can severely curtail educational and employment opportunities and are likely to have a long-term, adverse impact on the quality of their lives and the lives of their children. Young men are often not educated to respect women's self-determination and to share responsibility with women in matters of sexuality and reproduction.

94. Reproductive health is a state of complete physical, mental and social well-being and not merely the absence of disease or infirmity, in all matters relating to the reproductive system and to its functions and processes. Reproductive health therefore implies that people are able to have a satisfying and safe sex life and that they have the capability to reproduce and the freedom to decide if, when and how often to do so. Implicit in this last condition are the right of men and women to be informed and to have access to safe, effective, affordable and acceptable methods of family planning of their choice, as well as other methods of their choice for regulation of fertility which are not against the law, and the right of access to appropriate health-care services that will enable women to go safely through pregnancy and childbirth and provide couples with the best chance of having a healthy infant. In line with the above definition of reproductive health, reproductive health care is defined as the constellation of methods, techniques and services that contribute to reproductive health and well-being by preventing and solving reproductive health problems. It also includes sexual health, the purpose of which is the enhancement of life and personal relations, and not merely counselling and care related to reproduction and sexually transmitted diseases.

95. Bearing in mind the above definition, reproductive rights embrace certain human rights that are already recognized in national laws, international human rights documents and other consensus documents. These rights rest on the recognition of the basic right of all couples and individuals to decide freely and responsibly the number, spacing and timing of their children and to have the information and means to do so, and the right to attain the highest standard of sexual and reproductive health. It also includes their right to make decisions concerning reproduction free of discrimination, coercion and violence, as expressed in human rights documents. In the exercise of this right, they should take into account the needs of their living and future children and their responsibilities towards the community. The promotion of the responsible exercise of these rights for all people should be the fundamental basis for government- and community-supported policies and programmes in the area of reproductive health, including family planning. As part of their commitment, full attention should be given to the promotion of mutually respectful and equitable gender relations and particularly to meeting the educational and service needs of adolescents to enable them to deal in a positive and responsible way with their sexuality. Reproductive health eludes many of the world's people because of such factors as: inadequate levels of knowledge about human sexuality and inappropriate or poor-quality reproductive health information and services; the prevalence of high-risk sexual behaviour; discrim-

inatory social practices; negative attitudes towards women and girls; and the limited power many women and girls have over their sexual and reproductive lives. Adolescents are particularly vulnerable because of their lack of information and access to relevant services in most countries. Older women and men have distinct reproductive and sexual health issues which are often inadequately addressed.

96. The human rights of women include their right to have control over and decide freely and responsibly on matters related to their sexuality, including sexual and reproductive health, free of coercion, discrimination and violence.

Equal relationships between women and men in matters of sexual relations and reproduction, including full respect for the integrity of the person, require mutual respect, consent and shared responsibility for sexual behaviour and its consequences.

97. Further, women are subject to particular health risks due to inadequate responsiveness and lack of services to meet health needs related to sexuality and reproduction. Complications related to pregnancy and childbirth are among the leading causes of mortality and morbidity of women of reproductive age in many parts of the developing world. Similar problems exist to a certain degree in some countries with economies in transition. Unsafe abortions threaten the lives of a large number of women, representing a grave public health problem as it is primarily the poorest and youngest who take the highest risk. Most of these deaths, health problems and injuries are preventable through improved access to adequate health-care services, including safe and effective family planning methods and emergency obstetric care, recognizing the right of women and men to be informed and to have access to safe, effective, affordable and acceptable methods of family planning of their choice, as well as other methods of their choice for regulation of fertility which are not against the law, and the right of access to appropriate health-care services that will enable women to go safely through pregnancy and childbirth and provide couples with the best chance of having a healthy infant. These problems and means should be addressed on the basis of the report of the International Conference on Population

and Development, with particular reference to relevant paragraphs of the Programme of Action of the Conference. In most countries, the neglect of women's reproductive rights severely limits their opportunities in public and private life, including opportunities for education and economic and political empowerment. The ability of women to control their own fertility forms an important basis for the enjoyment of other rights. Shared responsibility between women and men in matters related to sexual and reproductive behaviour is also essential to improving women's health.

98. HIV/AIDS and other sexually transmitted diseases, the transmission of which is sometimes a consequence of sexual violence, are having a devastating effect on women's health, particularly the health of adolescent girls and young women. They often do not have the power to insist on safe and responsible sex practices and have little access to information and services for prevention and treatment. Women, who represent half of all adults newly infected with HIV/AIDS and other sexually transmitted diseases, have emphasized that social vulnerability and the unequal power relationships between women and men are obstacles to safe sex, in their efforts to control the spread of sexually transmitted diseases. The consequences of HIV/AIDS reach beyond women's health to their role as mothers and caregivers and their contribution to the economic support of their families. The social, developmental and health consequences of HIV/AIDS and other sexually transmitted diseases need to be seen from a gender perspective.

99. Sexual and gender-based violence, including physical and psychological abuse, trafficking in women and girls, and other forms of abuse and sexual exploitation place girls and women at high risk of physical and mental trauma, disease and unwanted pregnancy. Such situations often deter women from using health and other services.

100. Mental disorders related to marginalization, powerlessness and poverty, along with overwork and stress and the growing incidence of domestic violence as well as substance abuse, are among other health issues of growing concern to women. Women throughout the world, especially young women, are increasing their use of tobacco with serious effects on their health and that of their

children. Occupational health issues are also growing in importance, as a large number of women work in low-paid jobs in either the formal or the informal labour market under tedious and unhealthy conditions, and the number is rising. Cancers of the breast and cervix and other cancers of the reproductive system, as well as infertility affect growing numbers of women and may be preventable, or curable, if detected early.

101. With the increase in life expectancy and the growing number of older women, their health concerns require particular attention. The long-term health prospects of women are influenced by changes at menopause, which, in combination with life-long conditions and other factors, such as poor nutrition and lack of physical activity, may increase the risk of cardiovascular disease and osteoporosis. Other diseases of ageing and the inter-relationships of ageing and disability among women also need particular attention.

102. Women, like men, particularly in rural areas and poor urban areas, are increasingly exposed to environmental health hazards owing to environmental catastrophes and degradation. Women have a different susceptibility to various environmental hazards, contaminants and substances and they suffer different consequences from exposure to them.

103. The quality of women's health care is often deficient in various ways, depending on local circumstances. Women are frequently not treated with respect, nor are they guaranteed privacy and confidentiality, nor do they always receive full information about the options and services available. Furthermore, in some countries, over-medicating of women's life events is common, leading to unnecessary surgical intervention and inappropriate medication.

104. Statistical data on health are often not systematically collected, disaggregated and analysed by age, sex and socio-economic status and by established demographic criteria used to serve the interests and solve the problems of subgroups, with particular emphasis on the vulnerable and marginalized and other relevant variables. Recent and reliable data on the mortality and morbidity of women and conditions and diseases particularly affecting women are not available in many coun-

tries. Relatively little is known about how social and economic factors affect the health of girls and women of all ages, about the provision of health services to girls and women and the patterns of their use of such services, and about the value of disease prevention and health promotion programmes for women. Subjects of importance to women's health have not been adequately researched and women's health research often lacks funding. Medical research, on heart disease, for example, and epidemiological studies in many countries are often based solely on men; they are not gender specific. Clinical trials involving women to establish basic information about dosage, side-effects and effectiveness of drugs, including contraceptives, are noticeably absent and do not always conform to ethical standards for research and testing. Many drug therapy protocols and other medical treatments and interventions administered to women are based on research on men without any investigation and adjustment for gender differences.

105. In addressing inequalities in health status and unequal access to and inadequate health-care services between women and men, Governments and other actors should promote an active and visible policy of mainstreaming a gender perspective in all policies and programmes, so that, before decisions are taken, an analysis is made of the effects for women and men, respectively.

Strategic objective C.1. Increase women's access throughout the life cycle to appropriate, affordable and quality health care, information and related services
* * *

Strategic objective C.2. Strengthen preventive programmes that promote women's health
* * *

Strategic objective C.3. Undertake gender-sensitive initiatives that address sexually transmitted diseases, HIV/AIDS, and sexual and reproductive health issues
* * *

Strategic objective C.4. Promote research and disseminate information on women's health
* * *

Strategic objective C.5. Increase resources and monitor follow-up for women's health
* * *

E. WOMEN AND ARMED CONFLICT

An environment that maintains world peace and promotes and protects human rights, democracy and the peaceful settlement of disputes, in accordance with the principles of non-threat or use of force against territorial integrity or political independence and of respect for sovereignty as set forth in the Charter of the United Nations, is an important factor for the advancement of women. Peace is inextricably linked with equality between women and men and development. Armed and other types of conflicts and terrorism and hostage-taking still persist in many parts of the world. Aggression, foreign occupation, ethnic and other types of conflicts are an ongoing reality affecting women and men in nearly every region. Gross and systematic violations and situations that constitute serious obstacles to the full enjoyment of human rights continue to occur in different parts of the world. Such violations and obstacles include, as well as torture and cruel, inhuman and degrading treatment or punishment, summary and arbitrary executions, disappearances, arbitrary detentions, all forms of racism and racial discrimination, foreign occupation and alien domination, xenophobia, poverty, hunger and other denials of economic, social and cultural rights, religious intolerance, terrorism, discrimination against women and lack of the rule of law. International humanitarian law, prohibiting attacks on civilian populations, as such, is at times systematically ignored and human rights are often violated in connection with situations of armed conflict, affecting the civilian population, especially women, children, the elderly and the disabled. Violations of the human rights of women in situations of armed conflict are violations of the fundamental principles of international human rights and humanitarian law. Massive violations of human rights, especially in the form of genocide, ethnic cleansing as a strategy of war and its consequences, and rape, including systematic rape of women in war situations, creating a mass exodus of refugees and displaced persons, are abhorrent practices that are strongly condemned and must be stopped immediately, while perpetrators of such crimes must be punished. Some of these situations of armed conflict have their origin in the conquest or colonialization of a country by another State and the perpetuation of that colonization through state and military repression.

The Geneva Convention relative to the Protection of Civilian Persons in Time of War, of 1949, and the Additional Protocols of 1977 provide that women shall especially be protected against any attack on their honour, in particular against humiliating and degrading treatment, rape, enforced prostitution or any form of indecent assault. The Vienna Declaration and Programme of Action, adopted by the World Conference on Human Rights, states that "violations of the human rights of women in situations of armed conflict are violations of the fundamental principles of international human rights and humanitarian law". All violations of this kind, including in particular murder, rape, including systematic rape, sexual slavery and forced pregnancy require a particularly effective response. Gross and systematic violations and situations that constitute serious obstacles to the full enjoyment of human rights continue to occur in different parts of the world. Such violations and obstacles include, as well as torture and cruel, inhuman and degrading treatment or summary and arbitrary detention, all forms of racism, racial discrimination, xenophobia, denial of economic, social and cultural rights and religious intolerance.

Violations of human rights in situations of armed conflict and military occupation are violations of the fundamental principles of international human rights and humanitarian law as embodied in international human rights instruments and in the Geneva Conventions of 1949 and the Additional Protocols thereto. Gross human rights violations and policies of ethnic cleansing in war-torn and occupied areas continue to be carried out. These practices have created, inter alia, a mass flow of refugees and other displaced persons in need of international protection and internally displaced persons, the majority of whom are women, adolescent girls and children. Civilian victims, mostly women and children, often outnumber casualties among combatants. In addition, women often become caregivers for injured combatants and find themselves, as a result of conflict, unexpectedly cast as sole manager of household, sole parent, and caretaker of elderly relatives.

In a world of continuing instability and violence, the implementation of cooperative approaches to peace and security is urgently needed. The equal access and full participation of women in power structures and their full involvement in all efforts for the prevention and resolution of conflicts are essential for the maintenance and promotion of peace and security. Although women have begun to play an important role in conflict resolution, peace-keeping and defence and foreign affairs mechanisms, they are still underrepresented in decision-making positions. If women are to play an equal part in securing and maintaining peace, they must be empowered politically and economically and represented adequately at all levels of decision-making.

While entire communities suffer the consequences of armed conflict and terrorism, women and girls are particularly affected because of their status in society and their sex. Parties to conflict often rape women with impunity, sometimes using systematic rape as a tactic of war and terrorism. The impact of violence against women and violation of the human rights of women in such situations is experienced by women of all ages, who suffer displacement, loss of home and property, loss or involuntary disappearance of close relatives, poverty and family separation and disintegration, and who are victims of acts of murder, terrorism, torture, involuntary disappearance, sexual slavery, rape, sexual abuse and forced pregnancy in situations of armed conflict, especially as a result of policies of ethnic cleansing and other new and emerging forms of violence. This is compounded by the life-long social, economic and psychologically traumatic consequences of armed conflict and foreign occupation and alien domination.

Women and children constitute some 80 per cent of the world's millions of refugees and other displaced persons, including internally displaced persons. They are threatened by deprivation of property, goods and services and deprivation of their right to return to their homes of origin as well as by violence and insecurity. Particular attention should be paid to sexual violence against uprooted women and girls employed as a method of persecution in systematic campaigns of terror and intimidation and forcing members of a particular ethnic, cultural or religious group to flee their homes. Women may also be forced to flee as a result of a well-founded fear of persecution for reasons enumerated in the 1951 Convention relating to the Status of Refugees and the 1967 Protocol, including persecution through sexual violence or other gender-related persecution, and they continue to be vulnerable to violence and exploitation while in flight, in countries of asylum and resettlement and during and after repatriation. Women often experience difficulty in some countries of asylum in being recognized as refugees when the claim is based on such persecution.

Refugee, displaced and migrant women in most cases display strength, endurance and resourcefulness and can contribute positively to countries of resettlement or to their country of origin on their return. They need to be appropriately involved in decisions that affect them.

Many women's non-governmental organizations have called for reductions in military expenditures world wide, as well as in international trade and trafficking in and the proliferation of weapons. Those affected most negatively by conflict and excessive military spending are people living in poverty, who are deprived because of the lack of investment in basic services. Women living in poverty, particularly rural women, also suffer because of the use of arms that are particularly injurious or have indiscriminate effects. There are more than 100 million anti-personnel land-mines scattered in 64 countries globally. The negative impact on development of excessive military expenditures, the arms trade, and investment for arms production and acquisition must be addressed. At the same time, maintenance of national security and peace is an important factor for economic growth and development and the empowerment of women.

During times of armed conflict and the collapse of communities, the role of women is crucial. They often work to preserve social order in the midst of armed and other conflicts. Women make an important but often unrecognized contribution as peace educators both in their families and in their societies.

Education to foster a culture of peace that upholds justice and tolerance for all nations and peoples is essential to attaining lasting peace and should be begun at an early age. It should include elements of conflict resolution, mediation, reduction of prejudice and respect for diversity.

In addressing armed or other conflicts, an active and visible policy of mainstreaming a gender perspective into all policies and programmes should be promoted so that before decisions are taken an analysis is made of the effects on women and men, respectively.

Strategic objective E.1.
Increase the participation of women in conflict resolution at decision-making levels and protect women living in situations of armed and other conflicts or under foreign occupation.
* * *

Strategic objective E.2. Reduce excessive military expenditures and control the availability of armaments.
* * *

Strategic objective E.3. Promote non-violent forms of conflict resolution and reduce the incidence of human rights abuse in conflict.
* * *

Strategic objective E.4. Promote women's contribution to fostering a culture of peace.
* * *

Strategic objective E.5. Provide protection, assistance and training to refugee women, other displaced women in need of international protection and internally displaced women. Actions to be taken.
* * *

Strategic objective E.6. Provide assistance to the women of the colonies and non-self-governing territories.
* * *

Plan of Action for the Elimination of Harmful Traditional Practices Affecting the Health of Women and Children (1994)

Based on seminars held in Ouagadougou, Burkina Faso, from 29 April to 3 May 1991, and in Colombo, Sri Lanka, from 4 to 8 July 1994.E/CN.4/Sub.2/1994/10/Add.1 and corr.1, 22 July 1994. [Available at http://ods-dds ny.un.org/doc/UNDOC/GEN/G94/ 132/66/PDF/G9413266.pdf?OpenElement12563ee0062e685?Opendocument]

A. NATIONAL ACTION

(1) A clear expression of political will and an undertaking to put an end to traditional practices affecting the health of women and girl children, particularly female circumcision, is required on the part of the Governments of countries concerned.

(2) International instruments, including those relating to the protection of women and children, should be ratified and effectively implemented.

(3) Legislation prohibiting practices harmful to the health of women and children, particularly female circumcision, should be drafted.

(4) Governmental bodies should be created to implement the official policy adopted.

(5) Governmental agencies established to ensure the implementation of the Forward-looking Strategies for the Advancement of Women adopted at Nairobi in 1985 by the World Conference to Review and Appraise the Achievements of the United Nations Decade for Women: Equality, Development and

Peace, should be involved in activities undertaken to combat harmful traditional practices affecting the health of women and children.

(6) National committees should be established to combat traditional practices affecting the health of young girls and women, particularly female circumcision, and governmental financial assistance provided to those committees.

(7) A survey and review of school curricula and textbooks should be undertaken with a view to eliminating prejudices against women.

(8) Courses on the ill effects of female circumcision and other traditional practices should be included in training programmes for medical and paramedical personnel.

(9) Instruction on the harmful effects of such practices should be included in health and sex education programmes.

(10) Topics relating to traditional practices af-

fecting the health of women and children should be introduced into functional literacy campaigns.

(11) Audio-visual programmes (sketches, plays, etc.) should be prepared and articles published in the press on traditional practices adversely affecting the health of young girls and children, particularly female circumcision.

(12) Cooperation with religious institutions and their leaders and with traditional authorities is required in order to eliminate traditional practices such as female circumcision which are harmful to the health of women and children.

(13) All persons able to contribute directly or indirectly to the elimination of such practices should be mobilized.

Son Preference

(14) The family being the basic institution from where gender biases emanate, wide-ranging motivational campaigns should be launched to educate parents to value the worth of a girl child, so as to eliminate such biases.

(15) In view of the scientific fact that male chromosomes determine the sex of children, it is necessary to emphasize that the mother is not responsible for selection. Governments must, therefore, actively attempt to change the misconceptions regarding the responsibilities of the mother in determining the sex of the child.

(16) Non-discriminatory legislation on succession and inheritance should be introduced.

(17) In the light of the dominant role religion plays in shaping the image of women in each society, efforts should be made to remove misconceptions in religious teachings which reinforce the unequal status of women.

(18) Governments should mobilize all educational institutions and the media to change negative attitudes and values towards the female gender and project a positive image of women in general, and the girl-child in particular.

(19) Immediate measures should be taken by Governments to introduce and implement compulsory primary education and free secondary education and to increase the access of girls to technical education. Affirmative action in this field should be adopted in favour of the promotion of girls' education to achieve gender equity. Parents should be motivated to ensure the education of their daughters.

(20) Considering the importance of promoting self-esteem as a prerequisite for their higher status of women in the family and the community, Governments should take effective measures to ensure that women have access to and have control over economic resources, including land, credit, employment and other institutional facilities.

(21) Measures must be taken to provide free health care and services to women and children (in particular, girls) and to promote health consciousness among women with emphasis on their own basic health needs.

(22) Governments should regularly conduct nutritional surveys, identify nutritional gender disparities and undertake special nutritional programmes in areas where malnutrition in various forms is manifested.

(23) Governments should also undertake nutritional education programmes to address, inter alia, the special nutritional needs of women at various stages of their life cycle.

(24) As son preference is often associated with future security, Governments should take measures to introduce a social security system especially for widows, women-headed families and the aged.

(25) Governments are urged to take measures to eliminate gender stereotyping in the educational system, including removing gender bias from the curricula and other teaching materials.

(26) Governments should encourage by all means the activities of non-governmental organizations concerned with this problem.

(27) Women's organizations should mobilize all efforts to eradicate prejudicial and internalized values which project a diminished image of women. They should take action towards raising awareness among women about their potential

and self-esteem, the lack of which is one of the factors for perpetuating discrimination.

(28) Public opinion makers, national institutions, religious leaders, political parties, trade unions, legislators, educators, medical practitioners and all other organizations should be actively involved in combating all forms of discrimination against women and girls.

(29) Gender disaggregated data on morbidity, mortality, education, health, employment and political participation should be collected regularly, analysed and utilized for the formulation of policy and programmes for girls and women.

Early Marriage

(30) Governments are urged to adopt legislative measures fixing a minimum age for marriage for boys and girls. As recommended by the World Health Organization, the minimum age for girls should be 18 years. Such legislative measures should be reinforced with necessary mechanisms for its implementation.

(31) Registration of births and deaths, marriages and divorces should be made compulsory.

(32) Health issues relating to sex and family life education should be included in the school curricula to promote responsible and harmonious parenthood and to create awareness among young people about the harmful effects of early marriage, as well as the need for education about sexually transmitted diseases, especially AIDS.

(33) The media should be mobilized to raise public awareness on the consequences of child marriage and other such practices and the need to combat them. Government and women's activist groups could monitor the role of the mass media in this regard. All Governments should adopt and work towards "safe motherhood" initiatives.

(34) Effective training programmes should be ensured for traditional birth attendants and paramedical personnel to equip them with the necessary skills and knowledge, including concerning the effects of harmful traditional practices, to provide care

and services during the ante-natal, child delivery and post-natal periods, especially for rural mothers.

(35) Governments should promote male contraception, as well as female contraception.

(36) To discourage the early marriage of girls, the Government should make provision to increase vocational training, retraining and apprenticeship programmes for young women to empower them economically. A certain percentage of the places in existing training institutions should be reserved for women and girls.

(37) Governments should recognize and promote the reproductive rights of women, including their right to decide on the number and spacing of their children.

(38) Considering that non-governmental organizations have an effective role in urging Governments to enhance women's health status and in keeping the international organizations informed about the trends relating to traditional practices affecting the health of women and children, they should continue to report on the progress made and obstacles encountered in this area.

Child Delivery Practices

(39) Contraception should be encouraged as a means of promoting the health of women and children rather than as a means of achieving demographic goals.

(40) Governments should eliminate through educational and legislative measures and the creation of monitoring mechanisms, all forms of harmful traditional childbirth practices.

(41) Governments should expand and improve health services and introduce training programmes for traditional birth attendants to upgrade their positive traditional skills, as well as to give them new skills on a priority basis.

(42) Research and documentation is essential to assess the harmful effects of certain traditional birth related practices and to identify and continue some positive traditions like breast-feeding.

Violence Against Women and Girl Children

(43) Violence against women and girl children is a global phenomenon which cuts across geographical, cultural and political boundaries and varies only in its manifestations and severity. Gender violence has existed from time immemorial and continues up to the present day. It takes covert and overt forms including physical and mental abuse. Violence against women, including female genital mutilation, wife-burning, dowry-related violence, rape, incest, wife battering, female foeticide and female infanticide, trafficking and prostitution, is a human rights violation and not only a moral issue. It has serious negative implications on the economic and social development of women and society, and is an expression of the societal gender subordination of women.

(44) Governments should openly condemn all forms of violence against women and children, in particular girls, and commit themselves to confronting and eliminating such violence.

(45) To stop all forms of violence against women, all available media should be mobilized to cultivate a social attitude and climate against such totally unacceptable human behaviour.

(46) Governments should set up monitoring mechanisms to control depiction of any form of violence against women in the media.

(47) Violence being a form of social aberration, Governments should advocate the cultivation of a social attitude so that victims of violence do not suffer any continuing disability, feelings of guilt, or low self-esteem.

(48) Governments should enact and regularly review legislation for effectively combating all forms of violence, including rape, against women and children. In this connection, more severe penalties for acts of rape and trafficking should be introduced and specialized courts should be established to process such cases speedily and to create a climate of deterrence.

(49) Female infanticide and female foeticide should be openly condemned by all Governments as a flagrant violation of the basic right to life of the girl-child.

(50) The hearing of cases of rape should be in camera and the details not publicized, and legal assistance should be provided to the victims.

(51) Traditional practices of dowry and bride price should be condemned by Governments and made illegal. Acts of bride-burning should likewise be condemned and a heavy penalty inflicted on the guilty.

(52) Families, medical personnel and the public should be encouraged to report and have registered all forms of violence.

(53) More and more women should be inducted in law enforcement machinery as police officers, judiciary, medical personnel and counsellors.

(54) Gender sensitization training should be organized for all law enforcement personnel and such training should be incorporated in all induction and refresher courses in police training institutions.

(55) Mechanisms for networking and exchanges of information on violence should be established and strengthened.

(56) Governments should provide shelters, counselling and rehabilitation centres for victims of all forms of violence. They should also provide free legal assistance to victims.

(57) Governments must develop and implement a legal literacy campaign to improve the legal awareness of women, including dissemination of information through all available means, particularly NGO programmes, adult literacy courses and school curricula.

(58) Governments must promote research on violence against women and create and update databases on this subject.

(59) Community-based vigilance should be promoted regarding gender violence, including domestic violence.

(60) At the national level, Governments should promote and set up independent, autonomous and vigilant institutions to monitor and inquire into violations of women's rights, such as national com-

missions for women consisting of individuals and experts from outside the Governments.

(61) Governments which have not done so are urged to ratify the Convention on the Elimination of All Forms of Discrimination against Women and the Convention on the Rights of the Child, to ensure full gender equality in all spheres of life. The States Parties to these Conventions must comply with their provisions in order to achieve their ultimate objectives, including the eradication of all harmful traditional practices.

(62) NGOs should be active in bringing all available information on systematic and massive violence against women and children, in particular girls, to the attention of all relevant bodies of the United Nations, such as the Centre for Human Rights, the Commission on the Status of Women, and specialized agencies for the necessary intervention. Such information should also be shared with the Governments concerned, womens' commissions and human rights organizations.

(63) Women's organizations should mobilize all efforts, including action research, to eradicate prejudicial and internalized values which project a diminished image of women. They should take action towards raising awareness among women about their potential and self-esteem, the lack of which is one of the factors for perpetuating discrimination.

B. INTERNATIONAL ACTION

* * *

Other Measures

(74) Health workers should be required to dissociate themselves completely from harmful traditional practices.

(75) All women aware of the problem should be called on to react against traditional practices affecting the health of women and children and to mobilize other women.

(76) Women engaged in combating traditional practices affecting the health of women and children should exchange their experiences.

* * *

General Recommendation No. 24: Women and Health (1999)

*Adopted by the Committee on the Elimination of Discrimination
Against Women at its 20th session in 1999.
[Available at http://www.unhchr.ch/tbs/doc.nsf/(symbol)/
cedaw+General+recom.+24.En?OpenDocument]*

[Footnotes omitted.]

* * *

KEY ELEMENTS

Article 12 (1)

9. States parties are in the best position to report on the most critical health issues affecting women in that country. Therefore, in order to enable the Committee to evaluate whether measures to eliminate discrimination against women in the field of health care are appropriate, States parties must report on their health legislation, plans and policies for women with reliable data disaggregated by sex on the incidence and severity of diseases and conditions hazardous to women's health and nutrition and on the availability and cost-effectiveness of preventive and curative measures. Reports to the Committee must demonstrate that health legislation, plans and policies are based on scientific and ethical research and assessment of the health status and needs of women in that country and take into account any ethnic, regional or community variations or practices based on religion, tradition or culture.

10. States parties are encouraged to include in their reports information on diseases, health conditions and conditions hazardous to health that affect women or certain groups of women differently from men, as well as information on possible intervention in this regard.

11. Measures to eliminate discrimination against women are considered to be inappropriate if a health care system lacks services to prevent, detect and treat illnesses specific to women. It is discriminatory for a State party to refuse to legally provide for the performance of certain reproductive health services for women. For instance, if health service providers refuse to perform such services based on conscientious objection, measures should be introduced to ensure that women are referred to alternative health providers.

12. States parties should report on their understanding of how policies and measures on health care address the health rights of women from the perspective of women's needs and interests and how it addresses distinctive features and factors which differ for women in comparison to men, such as:

(a) Biological factors which differ for women in comparison with men, such as their menstrual cycle and their reproductive function and menopause. Another example is the higher risk of exposure to sexually transmitted diseases which women face;

(b) Socio-economic factors that vary for women in general and some groups of women in particular. For example, unequal power relationships between women and men in the home and workplace may negatively affect women's nutrition and health. They may also be exposed to different forms of violence which can affect their health. Girl children and adolescent girls are often vulnerable to sexual abuse by older men and family members, placing them at risk of physical and psychological harm and unwanted and early pregnancy. Some cultural or traditional practices such as female genital mutilation also carry a high risk of death and disability;

(c) Psychosocial factors which vary between women and men include depression in general and post-partum depression in particular as well as other psychological conditions, such as those that lead to eating disorders such as anorexia and bulimia;

(d) While lack of respect for the confidentiality of patients will affect both men and women, it may deter women from seeking advice and treatment and thereby adversely affect their health and well-being. Women will be less willing, for that reason, to seek medical care for diseases of the genital tract, for contraception or for incomplete abortion and in cases where they have suffered sexual or physical violence.

13. The duty of States parties to ensure, on a basis of equality between men and women, access to health care services, information and education implies an obligation to respect, protect and fulfil women's rights to health care. States parties have the responsibility to ensure that legislation and executive action and policy comply with these three obligations. They must also put in place a system which ensures effective judicial action. Failure to do so will constitute a violation of article 12.

14. The obligation to respect rights requires States parties to refrain from obstructing action taken by women in pursuit of their health goals. States parties should report on how public and private health care providers meet their duties to respect women's rights to have access to health care. For example, States parties should not restrict women's access to health services or to the clinics that provide those services on the ground that women do not have the authorization of husbands, partners, parents or health authorities, because they are unmarried or because they are women. Other barriers to women's access to appropriate health care include laws that criminalize medical procedures only needed by women and that punish women who undergo those procedures.

15. The obligation to protect rights relating to women's health requires States parties, their agents and officials to take action to prevent and impose sanctions for violations of rights by private persons and organizations. Since gender-based violence is a critical health issue for women, States parties should ensure:

(a) The enactment and effective enforcement of laws and the formulation of policies, including health care protocols and hospital procedures to address violence against women and abuse of girl children and the provision of appropriate health services;

(b) Gender-sensitive training to enable health care workers to detect and manage the health consequences of gender-based violence;

(c) Fair and protective procedures for hearing complaints and imposing appropriate sanctions on health care professionals guilty of sexual abuse of women patients;

(d) The enactment and effective enforcement of laws that prohibit female genital mutilation and marriage of girl children.

16. States parties should ensure that adequate protection and health services, including trauma treatment and counselling, are provided for women in especially difficult circumstances, such as those trapped in situations of armed conflict and women refugees.

17. The duty to fulfil rights places an obligation on States parties to take appropriate legislative, judicial, administrative, budgetary, economic and other measures to the maximum extent of their available resources to ensure that women realize their rights to health care. Studies such as those which emphasize the high maternal mortality and morbidity rates worldwide and the large numbers of couples who would like to limit their family size but lack access to or do not use any form of contraception provide an important indication for States parties of possible breaches of their duties to ensure women's access to health care. The Committee asks States parties to report on what they have done to address the magnitude of women's ill-health, in particular when it arises from preventable conditions, such as tuberculosis and HIV/AIDS. The Committee is concerned at the growing evidence that States are relinquishing these obligations as they transfer State health functions to private agencies. States parties cannot absolve themselves of responsibility in these areas by delegating or transferring these powers to private sector agencies. States parties should therefore report on what they have done to organize governmental processes and all structures through which public power is exercised to promote and protect women's health. They should include information on positive measures taken to curb violations of women's rights by third parties, to protect their health and the measures they have taken to ensure the provision of such services.

18. The issues of HIV/AIDS and other sexually transmitted disease are central to the rights of women and adolescent girls to sexual health.

Adolescent girls and women in many countries lack adequate access to information and services necessary to ensure sexual health. As a consequence of unequal power relations based on gender, women and adolescent girls are often unable to refuse sex or insist on safe and responsible sex practices. Harmful traditional practices, such as female genital mutilation, polygamy, as well as marital rape, may also expose girls and women to the risk of contracting HIV/AIDS and other sexually transmitted diseases. Women in prostitution are also particularly vulnerable to these diseases. States parties should ensure, without prejudice and discrimination, the right to sexual health information, education and services for all women and girls, including those who have been trafficked, even if they are not legally resident in the country. In particular, States parties should ensure the rights of female and male adolescents to sexual and reproductive health education by properly trained personnel in specially designed programmes that respect their rights to privacy and confidentiality.

19. In their reports States parties should identify the test by which they assess whether women have access to health care on a basis of equality of men and women in order to demonstrate compliance with article 12. In applying these tests, States parties should bear in mind the provisions of article 1 of the Convention. Reports should therefore include comments on the impact that health policies, procedures, laws and protocols have on women when compared with men.

20. Women have the right to be fully informed, by properly trained personnel, of their options in agreeing to treatment or research, including likely benefits and potential adverse effects of proposed procedures and available alternatives.

21. States parties should report on measures taken to eliminate barriers that women face in gaining access to health care services and what measures they have taken to ensure women timely and affordable access to such services. Barriers include requirements or conditions that prejudice women's access such as high fees for health care services, the requirement for preliminary authorization by spouse, parent or hospital authorities, distance from health facilities and absence of convenient and affordable public transport.

22. States parties should also report on measures taken to ensure access to quality health care services, for example, by making them acceptable to women. Acceptable services are those which are delivered in a way that ensures that a woman gives her fully informed consent, respects her dignity, guarantees her confidentiality and is sensitive to her needs and perspectives. States parties should not permit forms of coercion, such as non-consensual sterilization, mandatory testing for sexually transmitted diseases or mandatory pregnancy testing as a condition of employment that violate women's rights to informed consent and dignity.

23. In their reports, States parties should state what measures they have taken to ensure timely access to the range of services which are related to family planning, in particular, and to sexual and reproductive health in general. Particular attention should be paid to the health education of adolescents, including information and counselling on all methods of family planning.

24. The Committee is concerned about the conditions of health care services for older women, not only because women often live linger than men and are more likely than men to suffer from disabling and degenerative chronic diseases, such as osteoporosis and dementia, but because they often have the responsibility for their ageing spouses. Therefore, States parties should take appropriate measures to ensure the access of older women to health services that address the handicaps and disabilities associated with ageing.

25. Women with disabilities, of all ages, often have difficulty with physical access to health services. Women with mental disabilities are particularly vulnerable, while there is limited understanding, in general, of the broad range of risks to mental health to which women are disproportionately susceptible as a result of gender discrimination, violence, poverty, armed conflict, dislocation and other forms of social deprivation. States parties should take appropriate measures to ensure that health services are sensitive to the needs of women with disabilities and are respectful of their human rights and dignity.

Article 12 (2)

* * *

Declaration on the Elimination of Violence Against Women (1993)

General Assembly Resolution 48/104 of 20 December 1993.
[Available at http://www.unhchr.ch/huridocda/huridoca.nsf/7dec5261b3c5d5
dac12565cc0037502c?OpenNavigator]

[Footnotes omitted.]

The General Assembly,

Recognizing the urgent need for the universal application to women of the rights and principles with regard to equality, security, liberty, integrity and dignity of all human beings,

Noting that those rights and principles are enshrined in international instruments, including the Universal Declaration of Human Rights, the International Covenant on Civil and Political Rights, the International Covenant on Economic, Social and Cultural Rights, the Convention on the Elimination of All Forms of Discrimination against Women and the Convention against Torture and Other Cruel, Inhuman or Degrading Treatment or Punishment,

Recognizing that effective implementation of the Convention on the Elimination of All Forms of Discrimination against Women would contribute to the elimination of violence against women and that the Declaration on the Elimination of Violence against Women, set forth in the present resolution, will strengthen and complement that process,

Concerned that violence against women is an obstacle to the achievement of equality, development and peace, as recognized in the Nairobi Forward-looking Strategies for the Advancement of Women, in which a set of measures to combat violence against women was recommended, and to the full implementation of the Convention on the Elimination of All Forms of Discrimination against Women,

Affirming that violence against women constitutes a violation of the rights and fundamental freedoms of women and impairs or nullifies their enjoyment of those rights and freedoms, and concerned about the long-standing failure to protect and promote those rights and freedoms in the case of violence against women,

Recognizing that violence against women is a manifestation of historically unequal power relations between men and women, which have led to domination over and discrimination against women by men and to the prevention of the full advancement of women, and that violence against women is one of the crucial social mechanisms by which women are forced into a subordinate position compared with men,

Concerned that some groups of women, such as women belonging to minority groups, indigenous women, refugee women, migrant women, women living in rural or remote communities, destitute women, women in institutions or in detention, female children, women with disabilities, elderly women and women in situations of armed conflict, are especially vulnerable to violence,

Recalling the conclusion in paragraph 23 of the annex to Economic and Social Council resolution 1990/15 of 24 May 1990 that the recognition that violence against women in the family and society was pervasive and cut across lines of income, class and culture had to be matched by urgent and effective steps to eliminate its incidence,

Recalling also Economic and Social Council resolution 1991/18 of 30 May 1991, in which the Council recommended the development of a framework for an international instrument that would address explicitly the issue of violence against women,

Welcoming the role that women's movements are playing in drawing increasing attention to the nature, severity and magnitude of the problem of violence against women,

Alarmed that opportunities for women to achieve legal, social, political and economic equality in society are limited, inter alia, by continuing and endemic violence,

Convinced that in the light of the above there is a need for a clear and comprehensive definition of violence against women, a clear statement of the rights to be applied to ensure the elimination of violence against women in all its forms, a commitment by States in respect of their responsibilities, and a commitment by the international community at large to the elimination of violence against women,

Solemnly proclaims the following Declaration on the Elimination of Violence against Women and urges that every effort be made so that it becomes generally known and respected:

Article 1

For the purposes of this Declaration, the term "violence against women" means any act of gender-based violence that results in, or is likely to result in, physical, sexual or psychological harm or suffering to women, including threats of such acts, coercion or arbitrary deprivation of liberty, whether occurring in public or in private life.

Article 2

Violence against women shall be understood to encompass, but not be limited to, the following:

(a) Physical, sexual and psychological violence occurring in the family, including battering, sexual abuse of female children in the household, dowry-related violence, marital rape, female genital mutilation and other traditional practices harmful to women, non-spousal violence and violence related to exploitation;

(b) Physical, sexual and psychological violence occurring within the general community, including rape, sexual abuse, sexual harassment and intimidation at work, in educational institutions and elsewhere, trafficking in women and forced prostitution;

(c) Physical, sexual and psychological violence perpetrated or condoned by the State, wherever it occurs.

Article 3

Women are entitled to the equal enjoyment and protection of all human rights and fundamental freedoms in the political, economic, social, cultural, civil or any other field. These rights include, inter alia:

(a) The right to life;

(b) The right to equality;

(c) The right to liberty and security of person;

(d) The right to equal protection under the law;

(e) The right to be free from all forms of discrimination;

(f) The right to the highest standard attainable of physical and mental health;

(g) The right to just and favourable conditions of work;

(h) The right not to be subjected to torture, or other cruel, inhuman or degrading treatment or punishment.

Article 4

States should condemn violence against women and should not invoke any custom, tradition or religious consideration to avoid their obligations with respect to its elimination. States should pursue by all appropriate means and without delay a policy of eliminating violence against women and, to this end, should:

(a) Consider, where they have not yet done so, ratifying or acceding to the Convention on the Elimination of All Forms of Discrimination against Women or withdrawing reservations to that Convention;

(b) Refrain from engaging in violence against women;

(c) Exercise due diligence to prevent, investigate and, in accordance with national legislation, punish acts of violence against women, whether those acts are perpetrated by the State or by private persons;

(d) Develop penal, civil, labour and administrative sanctions in domestic legislation to punish and redress the wrongs caused to women who are subjected to violence; women who are subjected to violence should be provided with access to the mechanisms of justice and, as provided for by national legislation, to just and effective remedies for the harm that they have suffered; States should also inform women of their rights in seeking redress through such mechanisms;

(e) Consider the possibility of developing national plans of action to promote the protection of women against any form of violence, or to include provisions for that purpose in plans already existing, taking into account, as appropriate, such cooperation as can be provided by non-governmental organizations, particularly those concerned with the issue of violence against women;

(f) Develop, in a comprehensive way, preventive approaches and all those measures of a legal, political, administrative and cultural nature that promote the protection of women against any form of violence, and ensure that the re-victimization of women does not occur because of laws insensitive to gender considerations, enforcement practices or other interventions;

(g) Work to ensure, to the maximum extent feasible in the light of their available resources and, where needed, within the framework of international cooperation, that women subjected to violence and, where appropriate, their children have specialized assistance, such as rehabilitation, assistance in child care and maintenance, treatment, counselling, and health and social services, facilities and programmes, as well as support structures, and should take all other appropriate measures to promote their safety and physical and psychological rehabilitation;

(h) Include in government budgets adequate resources for their activities related to the elimination of violence against women;

(i) Take measures to ensure that law enforcement officers and public officials responsible for implementing policies to prevent, investigate and punish violence against women receive training to sensitize them to the needs of women;

(j) Adopt all appropriate measures, especially in the field of education, to modify the social and cultural patterns of conduct of men and women and to eliminate prejudices, customary practices and all other practices based on the idea of the inferiority or superiority of either of the sexes and on stereotyped roles for men and women;

(k) Promote research, collect data and compile statistics, especially concerning domestic violence, relating to the prevalence of different forms of violence against women and encourage research on the causes, nature, seriousness and consequences of violence against women and on the effectiveness of measures implemented to prevent and redress violence against women; those statistics and findings of the research will be made public;

(l) Adopt measures directed towards the elimination of violence against women who are especially vulnerable to violence;

(m) Include, in submitting reports as required under relevant human rights instruments of the United Nations, information pertaining to violence against women and measures taken to implement the present Declaration;

(n) Encourage the development of appropriate guidelines to assist in the implementation of the principles set forth in the present Declaration;

(o) Recognize the important role of the women's movement and non-governmental organizations world wide in raising awareness and alleviating the problem of violence against women;

(p) Facilitate and enhance the work of the women's movement and non-governmental organizations and cooperate with them at local, national and regional levels;

(q) Encourage intergovernmental regional organizations of which they are members to include the elimination of violence against women in their programmes, as appropriate.

Article 5

The organs and specialized agencies of the United Nations system should, within their respective fields of competence, contribute to the recognition and realization of the rights and the principles set forth in the present Declaration and, to this end, should, inter alia:

(a) Foster international and regional cooperation with a view to defining regional strategies for combating violence, exchanging experiences and financing programmes relating to the elimination of violence against women;

(b) Promote meetings and seminars with the aim of creating and raising awareness among all persons of the issue of the elimination of violence against women;

(c) Foster coordination and exchange within the United Nations system between human rights treaty bodies to address the issue of violence against women effectively;

(d) Include in analyses prepared by organizations and bodies of the United Nations system of social trends and problems, such as the periodic reports on the world social situation, examination of trends in violence against women;

(e) Encourage coordination between organizations and bodies of the United Nations system to incorporate the issue of violence against women into ongoing programmes, especially with reference to groups of women particularly vulnerable to violence;

(f) Promote the formulation of guidelines or manuals relating to violence against women, taking into account the measures referred to in the present Declaration;

(g) Consider the issue of the elimination of violence against women, as appropriate, in fulfilling their mandates with respect to the implementation of human rights instruments;

(h) Cooperate with non-governmental organizations in addressing the issue of violence against women.

Article 6

Nothing in the present Declaration shall affect any provision that is more conducive to the elimination of violence against women that may be contained in the legislation of a State or in any international convention, treaty or other instrument in force in a State.

B. Children

Convention on the Rights of the Child (1989)

Adopted and opened for signature, ratification and accession by General Assembly Resolution 44/25 of 20 November 1989. Entered into force 2 September 1990. [Available at www.unhchr.ch/tbs/doc.nsf/ (symbol)/E.C.12.1999.10.En!OpenDocument]

PREAMBLE

The States Parties to the present Convention,

Considering that, in accordance with the principles proclaimed in the Charter of the United Nations, recognition of the inherent dignity and of the equal and inalienable rights of all members of the human family is the foundation of freedom, justice and peace in the world,

Bearing in mind that the peoples of the United Nations have, in the Charter, reaffirmed their faith in fundamental human rights and in the dignity and worth of the human person, and have determined to promote social progress and better standards of life in larger freedom,

Recognizing that the United Nations has, in the Universal Declaration of Human Rights and in the International Covenants on Human Rights, proclaimed and agreed that everyone is entitled to all the rights and freedoms set forth therein, without distinction of any kind, such as race, colour, sex, language, religion, political or other opinion, national or social origin, property, birth or other status,

Recalling that, in the Universal Declaration of Human Rights, the United Nations has proclaimed that childhood is entitled to special care and assistance,

Convinced that the family, as the fundamental group of society and the natural environment for the growth and well-being of all its members and particularly children, should be afforded the necessary protection and assistance so that it can fully assume its responsibilities within the community,

Recognizing that the child, for the full and harmonious development of his or her personality, should grow up in a family environment, in an atmosphere of happiness, love and understanding,

Considering that the child should be fully prepared to live an individual life in society, and brought up in the spirit of the ideals proclaimed in the Charter of the United Nations, and in particular in the spirit of peace, dignity, tolerance, freedom, equality and solidarity,

Bearing in mind that the need to extend particular care to the child has been stated in the Geneva Declaration of the Rights of the Child of 1924 and in the Declaration of the Rights of the Child adopted by the General Assembly on 20 November 1959 and recognized in the Universal Declaration of Human Rights, in the International Covenant on Civil and Political Rights (in particular in articles 23 and 24), in the International Covenant on Economic, Social and Cultural Rights (in particular in article 10) and in the statutes and relevant instruments of specialized agencies and international organizations concerned with the welfare of children,

Bearing in mind that, as indicated in the Declaration of the Rights of the Child, "the child, by reason of his physical and mental immaturity, needs special safeguards and care, including appropriate legal protection, before as well as after birth",

Recalling the provisions of the Declaration on Social and Legal Principles relating to the Protection and Welfare of Children, with Special Reference to Foster Placement and Adoption Nationally and Internationally; the United Nations Standard Minimum Rules for the Administration of Juvenile Justice (The Beijing Rules) ; and the Declaration on the Protection of Women and Children in Emergency and Armed Conflict,

Recognizing that, in all countries in the world, there are children living in exceptionally difficult conditions, and that such children need special consideration,

Taking due account of the importance of the traditions and cultural values of each people for the protection and harmonious development of the child,

Recognizing the importance of international co-operation for improving the living conditions of children in every country, in particular in the developing countries,

Have agreed as follows:

PART I

Article 1

For the purposes of the present Convention, a child means every human being below the age of eighteen years unless under the law applicable to the child, majority is attained earlier.

Article 2

1. States Parties shall respect and ensure the rights set forth in the present Convention to each child within their jurisdiction without discrimination of any kind, irrespective of the child's or his or her parent's or legal guardian's race, colour, sex, language, religion, political or other opinion, national, ethnic or social origin, property, disability, birth or other status.

2. States Parties shall take all appropriate measures to ensure that the child is protected against all forms of discrimination or punishment on the basis of the status, activities, expressed opinions, or beliefs of the child's parents, legal guardians, or family members.

Article 3

1. In all actions concerning children, whether undertaken by public or private social welfare institutions, courts of law, administrative authorities or legislative bodies, the best interests of the child shall be a primary consideration.

2. States Parties undertake to ensure the child such protection and care as is necessary for his or her well-being, taking into account the rights and duties of his or her parents, legal guardians, or other individuals legally responsible for him or her, and, to this end, shall take all appropriate legislative and administrative measures.

3. States Parties shall ensure that the institutions, services and facilities responsible for the care or protection of children shall conform with the standards established by competent authorities, particularly in the areas of safety, health, in the number and suitability of their staff, as well as competent supervision.

Article 4

States Parties shall undertake all appropriate legislative, administrative, and other measures for the implementation of the rights recognized in the present Convention. With regard to economic, social and cultural rights, States Parties shall undertake such measures to the maximum extent of their available resources and, where needed, within the framework of international co-operation.

Article 5

States Parties shall respect the responsibilities, rights and duties of parents or, where applicable, the members of the extended family or community as provided for by local custom, legal guardians or other persons legally responsible for the child, to provide, in a manner consistent with the evolving capacities of the child, appropriate direction and guidance in the exercise by the child of the rights recognized in the present Convention.

Article 6

1. States Parties recognize that every child has the inherent right to life.

2. States Parties shall ensure to the maximum extent possible the survival and development of the child.

Article 7

1. The child shall be registered immediately after birth and shall have the right from birth to a name, the right to acquire a nationality and, as far as possible, the right to know and be cared for by his or her parents.

2. States Parties shall ensure the implementation of these rights in accordance with their national law and their obligations under the relevant international instruments in this field, in particular where the child would otherwise be stateless.

Article 8

1. States Parties undertake to respect the right of the child to preserve his or her identity, including nationality, name and family relations as recognized by law without unlawful interference.

2. Where a child is illegally deprived of some or all of the elements of his or her identity, States Parties shall provide appropriate assistance and protection, with a view to re-establishing speedily his or her identity.

Article 9

1. States Parties shall ensure that a child shall not be separated from his or her parents against their will, except when competent authorities subject to judicial review determine, in accordance with applicable law and procedures, that such separation is necessary for the best interests of the child. Such determination may be necessary in a particular case such as one involving abuse or neglect of the child by the parents, or one where the parents are living separately and a decision must be made as to the child's place of residence.

2. In any proceedings pursuant to paragraph 1 of the present article, all interested parties shall be given an opportunity to participate in the proceedings and make their views known.

3. States Parties shall respect the right of the child who is separated from one or both parents to maintain personal relations and direct contact with both parents on a regular basis, except if it is contrary to the child's best interests.

4. Where such separation results from any action initiated by a State Party, such as the detention, imprisonment, exile, deportation or death (including death arising from any cause while the person is in the custody of the State) of one or both parents or of the child, that State Party shall, upon request, provide the parents, the child or, if appropriate, another member of the family with the essential information concerning the whereabouts of the absent member(s) of the family unless the provision of the information would be detrimental to the well-being of the child. States Parties shall further ensure that the submission of such a request shall of itself entail no adverse consequences for the person(s) concerned.

Article 10

1. In accordance with the obligation of States Parties under article 9, paragraph 1, applications by a child or his or her parents to enter or leave a State Party for the purpose of family reunification shall be dealt with by States Parties in a positive, humane and expeditious manner. States Parties shall further ensure that the submission of such a request shall entail no adverse consequences for the applicants and for the members of their family.

2. A child whose parents reside in different States shall have the right to maintain on a regular basis, save in exceptional circumstances personal relations and direct contacts with both parents. Towards that end and in accordance with the obligation of States Parties under article 9, paragraph 1, States Parties shall respect the right of the child and his or her parents to leave any country, including their own, and to enter their own country. The right to leave any country shall be subject only to such restrictions as are prescribed by law and which are necessary to protect the national security, public order (ordre public), public health or morals or the rights and freedoms of others and are consistent with the other rights recognized in the present Convention.

Article 11

1. States Parties shall take measures to combat the illicit transfer and non-return of children abroad.

2. To this end, States Parties shall promote the conclusion of bilateral or multilateral agreements or accession to existing agreements.

Article 12

1. States Parties shall assure to the child who is capable of forming his or her own views the right to express those views freely in all matters affecting the child, the views of the child being given due weight in accordance with the age and maturity of the child.

2. For this purpose, the child shall in particular be provided the opportunity to be heard in any judicial and administrative proceedings affecting the child, either directly, or through a representative or an appropriate body, in a manner consistent with the procedural rules of national law.

Article 13

1. The child shall have the right to freedom of expression; this right shall include freedom to seek, receive and impart information and ideas of all kinds, regardless of frontiers, either orally, in writing or in print, in the form of art, or through any other media of the child's choice.

2. The exercise of this right may be subject to certain restrictions, but these shall only be such as are provided by law and are necessary:

(a) For respect of the rights or reputations of others; or

(b) For the protection of national security or of public order (ordre public), or of public health or morals.

Article 14

1. States Parties shall respect the right of the child to freedom of thought, conscience and religion.

2. States Parties shall respect the rights and duties of the parents and, when applicable, legal guardians, to provide direction to the child in the exercise of his or her right in a manner consistent with the evolving capacities of the child.

3. Freedom to manifest one's religion or beliefs may be subject only to such limitations as are prescribed by law and are necessary to protect public safety, order, health or morals, or the fundamental rights and freedoms of others.

Article 15

1. States Parties recognize the rights of the child to freedom of association and to freedom of peaceful assembly.

2. No restrictions may be placed on the exercise of these rights other than those imposed in conformity with the law and which are necessary in a democratic society in the interests of national security or public safety, public order (ordre public), the protection of public health or morals or the protection of the rights and freedoms of others.

Article 16

1. No child shall be subjected to arbitrary or unlawful interference with his or her privacy, family, home or correspondence, nor to unlawful attacks on his or her honour and reputation.

2. The child has the right to the protection of the law against such interference or attacks.

Article 17

States Parties recognize the important function performed by the mass media and shall ensure that the child has access to information and material from a diversity of national and international sources, especially those aimed at the promotion of his or her social, spiritual and moral well-being and physical and mental health. To this end, States Parties shall:

(a) Encourage the mass media to disseminate information and material of social and cultural benefit to the child and in accordance with the spirit of article 29;

(b) Encourage international co-operation in the production, exchange and dissemination of such information and material from a diversity of cultural, national and international sources;

(c) Encourage the production and dissemination of children's books;

(d) Encourage the mass media to have particular regard to the linguistic needs of the child who belongs to a minority group or who is indigenous;

(e) Encourage the development of appropriate guidelines for the protection of the child from information and material injurious to his or her well-being, bearing in mind the provisions of articles 13 and 18.

Article 18

1. States Parties shall use their best efforts to ensure recognition of the principle that both parents have common responsibilities for the upbringing and development of the child. Parents or, as the case may be, legal guardians, have the primary responsibility for the upbringing and development of the child. The best interests of the child will be their basic concern.

2. For the purpose of guaranteeing and promoting the rights set forth in the present Convention,

States Parties shall render appropriate assistance to parents and legal guardians in the performance of their child-rearing responsibilities and shall ensure the development of institutions, facilities and services for the care of children.

3. States Parties shall take all appropriate measures to ensure that children of working parents have the right to benefit from child-care services and facilities for which they are eligible.

Article 19

1. States Parties shall take all appropriate legislative, administrative, social and educational measures to protect the child from all forms of physical or mental violence, injury or abuse, neglect or negligent treatment, maltreatment or exploitation, including sexual abuse, while in the care of parent(s), legal guardian(s) or any other person who has the care of the child.

2. Such protective measures should, as appropriate, include effective procedures for the establishment of social programmes to provide necessary support for the child and for those who have the care of the child, as well as for other forms of prevention and for identification, reporting, referral, investigation, treatment and follow-up of instances of child maltreatment described heretofore, and, as appropriate, for judicial involvement.

Article 20

1. A child temporarily or permanently deprived of his or her family environment, or in whose own best interests cannot be allowed to remain in that environment, shall be entitled to special protection and assistance provided by the State.

2. States Parties shall in accordance with their national laws ensure alternative care for such a child.

3. Such care could include, inter alia, foster placement, kafalah of Islamic law, adoption or if necessary placement in suitable institutions for the care of children. When considering solutions, due regard shall be paid to the desirability of continuity in a child's upbringing and to the child's ethnic, religious, cultural and linguistic background.

Article 21

States Parties that recognize and/or permit the system of adoption shall ensure that the best interests of the child shall be the paramount consideration and they shall:

(a) Ensure that the adoption of a child is authorized only by competent authorities who determine, in accordance with applicable law and procedures and on the basis of all pertinent and reliable information, that the adoption is permissible in view of the child's status concerning parents, relatives and legal guardians and that, if required, the persons concerned have given their informed consent to the adoption on the basis of such counselling as may be necessary;

(b) Recognize that inter-country adoption may be considered as an alternative means of child's care, if the child cannot be placed in a foster or an adoptive family or cannot in any suitable manner be cared for in the child's country of origin;

(c) Ensure that the child concerned by inter-country adoption enjoys safeguards and standards equivalent to those existing in the case of national adoption;

(d) Take all appropriate measures to ensure that, in inter-country adoption, the placement does not result in improper financial gain for those involved in it;

(e) Promote, where appropriate, the objectives of the present article by concluding bilateral or multilateral arrangements or agreements, and endeavour, within this framework, to ensure that the placement of the child in another country is carried out by competent authorities or organs.

Article 22

1. States Parties shall take appropriate measures to ensure that a child who is seeking refugee status or who is considered a refugee in accordance with applicable international or domestic law and procedures shall, whether unaccompanied or accompanied by his or her parents or by any other person, receive appropriate protection and humanitarian assistance in the enjoyment of applicable rights set forth in the present Convention and in other international human rights or humanitarian instruments to which the said States are Parties.

2. For this purpose, States Parties shall provide, as they consider appropriate, co-operation in any efforts by the United Nations and other competent intergovernmental organizations or non-governmental organizations co-operating with the United Nations to protect and assist such a child and to trace the parents or other members of the family of any refugee child in order to obtain information necessary for reunification with his or her family. In cases where no parents or other members of the family can be found, the child shall be accorded the same protection as any other child permanently or temporarily deprived of his or her family environment for any reason, as set forth in the present Convention.

Article 23

1. States Parties recognize that a mentally or physically disabled child should enjoy a full and decent life, in conditions which ensure dignity, promote self-reliance and facilitate the child's active participation in the community.

2. States Parties recognize the right of the disabled child to special care and shall encourage and ensure the extension, subject to available resources, to the eligible child and those responsible for his or her care, of assistance for which application is made and which is appropriate to the child's condition and to the circumstances of the parents or others caring for the child.

3. Recognizing the special needs of a disabled child, assistance extended in accordance with paragraph 2 of the present article shall be provided free of charge, whenever possible, taking into account the financial resources of the parents or others caring for the child, and shall be designed to ensure that the disabled child has effective access to and receives education, training, health care services, rehabilitation services, preparation for employment and recreation opportunities in a manner conducive to the child's achieving the fullest possible social integration and individual development, including his or her cultural and spiritual development.

4. States Parties shall promote, in the spirit of international cooperation, the exchange of appropriate information in the field of preventive health care and of medical, psychological and functional treatment of disabled children, including dissemination of and access to information concerning methods of rehabilitation, education and vocational services, with the aim of enabling States Parties to improve their capabilities and skills and to widen their experience in these areas. In this regard, particular account shall be taken of the needs of developing countries.

Article 24

1. States Parties recognize the right of the child to the enjoyment of the highest attainable standard of health and to facilities for the treatment of illness and rehabilitation of health. States Parties shall strive to ensure that no child is deprived of his or her right of access to such health care services.

2. States Parties shall pursue full implementation of this right and, in particular, shall take appropriate measures:

(a) To diminish infant and child mortality;

(b) To ensure the provision of necessary medical assistance and health care to all children with emphasis on the development of primary health care;

(c) To combat disease and malnutrition, including within the framework of primary health care, through, inter alia, the application of readily available technology and through the provision of adequate nutritious foods and clean drinking-water, taking into consideration the dangers and risks of environmental pollution;

(d) To ensure appropriate pre-natal and post-natal health care for mothers;

(e) To ensure that all segments of society, in particular parents and children, are informed, have access to education and are supported in the use of basic knowledge of child health and nutrition, the advantages of breastfeeding, hygiene and environmental sanitation and the prevention of accidents;

(f) To develop preventive health care, guidance for parents and family planning education and services.

3. States Parties shall take all effective and appropriate measures with a view to abolishing traditional practices prejudicial to the health of children.

4. States Parties undertake to promote and encourage international co-operation with a view to achieving progressively the full realization of the right recognized in the present article. In this regard, particular account shall be taken of the needs of developing countries.

Article 25

States Parties recognize the right of a child who has been placed by the competent authorities for the purposes of care, protection or treatment of his or her physical or mental health, to a periodic review of the treatment provided to the child and all other circumstances relevant to his or her placement.

Article 26

1. States Parties shall recognize for every child the right to benefit from social security, including social insurance, and shall take the necessary measures to achieve the full realization of this right in accordance with their national law.

2. The benefits should, where appropriate, be granted, taking into account the resources and the circumstances of the child and persons having responsibility for the maintenance of the child, as well as any other consideration relevant to an application for benefits made by or on behalf of the child.

Article 27

1. States Parties recognize the right of every child to a standard of living adequate for the child's physical, mental, spiritual, moral and social development.

2. The parent(s) or others responsible for the child have the primary responsibility to secure, within their abilities and financial capacities, the conditions of living necessary for the child's development.

3. States Parties, in accordance with national conditions and within their means, shall take appropriate measures to assist parents and others responsible for the child to implement this right and shall in case of need provide material assistance and support programmes, particularly with regard to nutrition, clothing and housing.

4. States Parties shall take all appropriate measures to secure the recovery of maintenance for the child from the parents or other persons having financial responsibility for the child, both within the State Party and from abroad. In particular, where the person having financial responsibility for the child lives in a State different from that of the child, States Parties shall promote the accession to international agreements or the conclusion of such agreements, as well as the making of other appropriate arrangements.

Article 28

1. States Parties recognize the right of the child to education, and with a view to achieving this right progressively and on the basis of equal opportunity, they shall, in particular:

(a) Make primary education compulsory and available free to all;

(b) Encourage the development of different forms of secondary education, including general and vocational education, make them available and accessible to every child, and take appropriate measures such as the introduction of free education and offering financial assistance in case of need;

(c) Make higher education accessible to all on the basis of capacity by every appropriate means;

(d) Make educational and vocational information and guidance available and accessible to all children;

(e) Take measures to encourage regular attendance at schools and the reduction of drop-out rates.

2. States Parties shall take all appropriate measures to ensure that school discipline is administered in a manner consistent with the child's human dignity and in conformity with the present Convention.

3. States Parties shall promote and encourage international cooperation in matters relating to education, in particular with a view to contributing to the elimination of ignorance and illiteracy throughout the world and facilitating access to scientific and technical knowledge and modern teaching methods. In this regard, particular account shall be taken of the needs of developing countries.

Article 29

1. States Parties agree that the education of the child shall be directed to:

(a) The development of the child's personality, talents and mental and physical abilities to their fullest potential;

(b) The development of respect for human rights and fundamental freedoms, and for the principles enshrined in the Charter of the United Nations;

(c) The development of respect for the child's parents, his or her own cultural identity, language and values, for the national values of the country in which the child is living, the country from which he or she may originate, and for civilizations different from his or her own;

(d) The preparation of the child for responsible life in a free society, in the spirit of understanding, peace, tolerance, equality of sexes, and friendship among all peoples, ethnic, national and religious groups and persons of indigenous origin;

(e) The development of respect for the natural environment.

2. No part of the present article or article 28 shall be construed so as to interfere with the liberty of individuals and bodies to establish and direct educational institutions, subject always to the observance of the principle set forth in paragraph 1 of the present article and to the requirements that the education given in such institutions shall conform to such minimum standards as may be laid down by the State.

Article 30

In those States in which ethnic, religious or linguistic minorities or persons of indigenous origin exist, a child belonging to such a minority or who is indigenous shall not be denied the right, in community with other members of his or her group, to enjoy his or her own culture, to profess and practice his or her own religion, or to use his or her own language.

Article 31

1. States Parties recognize the right of the child to rest and leisure, to engage in play and recreational activities appropriate to the age of the child and to participate freely in cultural life and the arts.

2. States Parties shall respect and promote the right of the child to participate fully in cultural and artistic life and shall encourage the provision of appropriate and equal opportunities for cultural, artistic, recreational and leisure activity.

Article 32

1. States Parties recognize the right of the child to be protected from economic exploitation and from performing any work that is likely to be hazardous or to interfere with the child's education, or to be harmful to the child's health or physical, mental, spiritual, moral or social development.

2. States Parties shall take legislative, administrative, social and educational measures to ensure the implementation of the present article. To this end, and having regard to the relevant provisions of other international instruments, States Parties shall in particular:

(a) Provide for a minimum age or minimum ages for admission to employment;

(b) Provide for appropriate regulation of the hours and conditions of employment;

(c) Provide for appropriate penalties or other sanctions to ensure the effective enforcement of the present article.

Article 33

States Parties shall take all appropriate measures, including legislative, administrative, social and educational measures, to protect children from the illicit use of narcotic drugs and psychotropic substances as defined in the relevant international treaties, and to prevent the use of children in the illicit production and trafficking of such substances.

Article 34

States Parties undertake to protect the child from all forms of sexual exploitation and sexual abuse. For these purposes, States Parties shall in particular take all appropriate national, bilateral and multilateral measures to prevent:

(a) The inducement or coercion of a child to engage in any unlawful sexual activity;

(b) The exploitative use of children in prostitution or other unlawful sexual practices;

(c) The exploitative use of children in pornographic performances and materials.

Article 35

States Parties shall take all appropriate national, bilateral and multilateral measures to prevent the abduction of, the sale of or traffic in children for any purpose or in any form.

Article 36

States Parties shall protect the child against all other forms of exploitation prejudicial to any aspects of the child's welfare.

Article 37

States Parties shall ensure that:

(a) No child shall be subjected to torture or other cruel, inhuman or degrading treatment or punishment. Neither capital punishment nor life imprisonment without possibility of release shall be imposed for offences committed by persons below eighteen years of age;

(b) No child shall be deprived of his or her liberty unlawfully or arbitrarily. The arrest, detention or imprisonment of a child shall be in conformity with the law and shall be used only as a measure of last resort and for the shortest appropriate period of time;

(c) Every child deprived of liberty shall be treated with humanity and respect for the inherent dignity of the human person, and in a manner which takes into account the needs of persons of his or her age. In particular, every child deprived of liberty shall be separated from adults unless it is considered in the child's best interest not to do so and shall have the right to maintain contact with his or her family through correspondence and visits, save in exceptional circumstances;

(d) Every child deprived of his or her liberty shall have the right to prompt access to legal and other appropriate assistance, as well as the right to challenge the legality of the deprivation of his or her liberty before a court or other competent, independent and impartial authority, and to a prompt decision on any such action.

Article 38

1. States Parties undertake to respect and to ensure respect for rules of international humanitarian law applicable to them in armed conflicts which are relevant to the child.

2. States Parties shall take all feasible measures to ensure that persons who have not attained the age of fifteen years do not take a direct part in hostilities.

3. States Parties shall refrain from recruiting any person who has not attained the age of fifteen years into their armed forces. In recruiting among those persons who have attained the age of fifteen years but who have not attained the age of eighteen years, States Parties shall endeavour to give priority to those who are oldest.

4. In accordance with their obligations under international humanitarian law to protect the civilian population in armed conflicts, States Parties shall take all feasible measures to ensure protection and care of children who are affected by an armed conflict.

Article 39

States Parties shall take all appropriate measures to promote physical and psychological recovery and social reintegration of a child victim of: any form of neglect, exploitation, or abuse; torture or any other form of cruel, inhuman or degrading treatment or punishment; or armed conflicts. Such recovery and reintegration shall take place in an environment which fosters the health, self-respect and dignity of the child.

Article 40

1. States Parties recognize the right of every child alleged as, accused of, or recognized as having infringed the penal law to be treated in a manner consistent with the promotion of the child's sense of dignity and worth, which reinforces the child's respect for the human rights and fundamental freedoms of others and which takes into account the child's age and the desirability of promoting the child's reintegration and the child's assuming a constructive role in society.

2. To this end, and having regard to the relevant provisions of international instruments, States Parties shall, in particular, ensure that:

(a) No child shall be alleged as, be accused of, or recognized as having infringed the penal law by reason of acts or omissions that were not prohibited by national or international law at the time they were committed;

(b) Every child alleged as or accused of having infringed the penal law has at least the following guarantees:

(i) To be presumed innocent until proven guilty according to law;

(ii) To be informed promptly and directly of the charges against him or her, and, if appropriate, through his or her parents or legal guardians, and to have legal or other appropriate assistance in the preparation and presentation of his or her defence;

(iii) To have the matter determined without delay by a competent, independent and impartial authority or judicial body in a fair hearing according to law, in the presence of legal or other appropriate assistance and, unless it is considered not to be in the best interest of the child, in particular, taking into account his or her age or situation, his or her parents or legal guardians;

(iv) Not to be compelled to give testimony or to confess guilt; to examine or have examined adverse witnesses and to obtain the participation and examination of witnesses on his or her behalf under conditions of equality;

(v) If considered to have infringed the penal law, to have this decision and any measures imposed in consequence thereof reviewed by a higher competent, independent and impartial authority or judicial body according to law;

(vi) To have the free assistance of an interpreter if the child cannot understand or speak the language used;

(vii) To have his or her privacy fully respected at all stages of the proceedings.

3. States Parties shall seek to promote the establishment of laws, procedures, authorities and institutions specifically applicable to children alleged as, accused of, or recognized as having infringed the penal law, and, in particular:

(a) The establishment of a minimum age below which children shall be presumed not to have the capacity to infringe the penal law;

(b) Whenever appropriate and desirable, measures for dealing with such children without resorting to judicial proceedings, providing that human rights and legal safeguards are fully respected.

4. A variety of dispositions, such as care, guidance and supervision orders; counselling; probation; foster care; education and vocational training programmes and other alternatives to institutional care shall be available to ensure that children are dealt with in a manner appropriate to their well-being and proportionate both to their circumstances and the offence.

Article 41

Nothing in the present Convention shall affect any provisions which are more conducive to the realization of the rights of the child and which may be contained in:

(a) The law of a State party; or

(b) International law in force for that State.

PART II

Article 42

States Parties undertake to make the principles and provisions of the Convention widely known, by appropriate and active means, to adults and children alike.

Article 43

1. For the purpose of examining the progress made by States Parties in achieving the realization of the obligations undertaken in the present Convention, there shall be established a Committee on the Rights of the Child, which shall carry out the functions hereinafter provided.

2. The Committee shall consist of ten experts of high moral standing and recognized competence in the field covered by this Convention. The members of the Committee shall be elected by States Parties from among their nationals and shall serve in their personal capacity, consideration being given to equitable geographical distribution, as well as to the principal legal systems.

3. The members of the Committee shall be elected by secret ballot from a list of persons nominated by States Parties. Each State Party may nominate one person from among its own nationals.

4. The initial election to the Committee shall be held no later than six months after the date of the entry into force of the present Convention and thereafter every second year. At least four months before the date of each election, the Secretary-General of the United Nations shall address a letter to States Parties inviting them to submit their nominations within two months. The Secretary-General shall subsequently prepare a list in alphabetical order of all persons thus nominated, indicating States Parties which have nominated them, and shall submit it to the States Parties to the present Convention.

5. The elections shall be held at meetings of States Parties convened by the Secretary-General at United Nations Headquarters. At those meetings, for which two thirds of States Parties shall constitute a quorum, the persons elected to the Committee shall be those who obtain the largest number of votes and an absolute majority of the votes of the representatives of States Parties present and voting.

6. The members of the Committee shall be elected for a term of four years. They shall be eligible for re-election if renominated. The term of five of the members elected at the first election shall expire at the end of two years; immediately after the first election, the names of these five members shall be chosen by lot by the Chairman of the meeting.

7. If a member of the Committee dies or resigns or declares that for any other cause he or she can no longer perform the duties of the Committee, the State Party which nominated the member shall appoint another expert from among its nationals to serve for the remainder of the term, subject to the approval of the Committee.

8. The Committee shall establish its own rules of procedure.

9. The Committee shall elect its officers for a period of two years.

10. The meetings of the Committee shall normally be held at United Nations Headquarters or at any other convenient place as determined by the Committee. The Committee shall normally meet annually. The duration of the meetings of the Committee shall be determined, and reviewed, if necessary, by a meeting of the States Parties to the present Convention, subject to the approval of the General Assembly.

11. The Secretary-General of the United Nations shall provide the necessary staff and facilities for the effective performance of the functions of the Committee under the present Convention.

12. With the approval of the General Assembly, the members of the Committee established under the present Convention shall receive emoluments from United Nations resources on such terms and conditions as the Assembly may decide.

Article 44

1. States Parties undertake to submit to the Committee, through the Secretary-General of the United Nations, reports on the measures they have adopted which give effect to the rights recognized herein and on the progress made on the enjoyment of those rights:

(a) Within two years of the entry into force of the Convention for the State Party concerned;

(b) Thereafter every five years.

2. Reports made under the present article shall indicate factors and difficulties, if any, affecting the degree of fulfillment of the obligations under the present Convention. Reports shall also contain sufficient information to provide the Committee with a comprehensive understanding of the implementation of the Convention in the country concerned.

3. A State Party which has submitted a comprehensive initial report to the Committee need not, in its subsequent reports submitted in accordance with paragraph 1 (b) of the present article, repeat basic information previously provided.

4. The Committee may request from States Parties further information relevant to the implementation of the Convention.

5. The Committee shall submit to the General Assembly, through the Economic and Social Council, every two years, reports on its activities.

6. States Parties shall make their reports widely available to the public in their own countries.

Article 45

In order to foster the effective implementation of the Convention and to encourage international co-operation in the field covered by the Convention:

(a) The specialized agencies, the United Nations Children's Fund, and other United Nations organs shall be entitled to be represented at the consideration of the implementation of such provisions of the present Convention as fall within the scope of their mandate. The Committee may invite the specialized agencies, the United Nations Children's Fund and other competent bodies as it may consider appropriate to provide expert advice on the implementation of the Convention in areas falling within the scope of their respective mandates. The Committee may invite the specialized agencies, the United Nations Children's Fund, and other United Nations organs to submit reports on the implementation of the Convention in areas falling within the scope of their activities;

(b) The Committee shall transmit, as it may consider appropriate, to the specialized agencies, the United Nations Children's Fund and other competent bodies, any reports from States Parties that contain a request, or indicate a need, for technical advice or assistance, along with the Committee's observations and suggestions, if any, on these requests or indications;

(c) The Committee may recommend to the General Assembly to request the Secretary-General to undertake on its behalf studies on specific issues relating to the rights of the child;

(d) The Committee may make suggestions and general recommendations based on information received pursuant to articles 44 and 45 of the present Convention. Such suggestions and general recommendations shall be transmitted to any State Party concerned and reported to the General Assembly, together with comments, if any, from States Parties.

PART III

Article 46

The present Convention shall be open for signature by all States.

Article 47

The present Convention is subject to ratification. Instruments of ratification shall be deposited with the Secretary-General of the United Nations.

Article 48

The present Convention shall remain open for accession by any State. The instruments of accession shall be deposited with the Secretary-General of the United Nations.

Article 49

1. The present Convention shall enter into force on the thirtieth day following the date of deposit with the Secretary-General of the United Nations of the twentieth instrument of ratification or accession.

2. For each State ratifying or acceding to the Convention after the deposit of the twentieth instrument of ratification or accession, the Convention shall enter into force on the thirtieth day after the deposit by such State of its instrument of ratification or accession.

Article 50

1. Any State Party may propose an amendment and file it with the Secretary-General of the United Nations. The Secretary-General shall thereupon communicate the proposed amendment to States Parties, with a request that they indicate whether they favour a conference of States Parties for the purpose of considering and voting upon the proposals. In the event that, within four months from the date of such communication, at least one third of the States Parties favour such a conference, the Secretary-General shall convene the conference under the auspices of the United Nations. Any amendment adopted by a majority of States Parties present and voting at the conference shall be submitted to the General Assembly for approval.

2. An amendment adopted in accordance with paragraph 1 of the present article shall enter into

force when it has been approved by the General Assembly of the United Nations and accepted by a two-thirds majority of States Parties.

3. When an amendment enters into force, it shall be binding on those States Parties which have accepted it, other States Parties still being bound by the provisions of the present Convention and any earlier amendments which they have accepted.

Article 51

1. The Secretary-General of the United Nations shall receive and circulate to all States the text of reservations made by States at the time of ratification or accession.

2. A reservation incompatible with the object and purpose of the present Convention shall not be permitted.

3. Reservations may be withdrawn at any time by notification to that effect addressed to the Secretary-General of the United Nations, who shall then inform all States. Such notification shall take effect on the date on which it is received by the Secretary-General.

Article 52

A State Party may denounce the present Convention by written notification to the Secretary-General of the United Nations. Denunciation becomes effective one year after the date of receipt of the notification by the Secretary-General.

Article 53

The Secretary-General of the United Nations is designated as the depositary of the present Convention.

Article 54

The original of the present Convention, of which the Arabic, Chinese, English, French, Russian and Spanish texts are equally authentic, shall be deposited with the Secretary-General of the United Nations.

IN WITNESS THEREOF the undersigned plenipotentiaries, being duly authorized thereto by their respective governments, have signed the present Convention.

Protocol Additional to the Geneva Conventions of 12 August 1949, and Relating to the Protection of Victims of International Armed Conflicts (Protocol I): Children (1977)

Adopted on 8 June 1977. Entered into force 7 December 1978.
[Available at http://www.icrc.org/ihl.nsf/WebCONVFULL?OpenView]

---

* * *

Article 77
Protection of Children

1. Children shall be the object of special respect and shall be protected against any form of indecent assault. The Parties to the conflict shall provide them with the care and aid they require, whether because of their age or for any other reason.

2. The Parties to the conflict shall take all feasible measures in order that children who have not attained the age of fifteen years do not take a direct part in hostilities and, in particular, they shall re-

frain from recruiting them into their armed forces. In recruiting among those persons who have attained the age of fifteen years but who have not attained the age of eighteen years the Parties to the conflict shall endeavour to give priority to those who are oldest.

3. If, in exceptional cases, despite the provisions of paragraph 2, children who have not attained the age of fifteen years take a direct part in hostilities and fall into the power of an adverse Party, they shall continue to benefit from the special protection accorded by this Article, whether or not they are prisoners of war.

4. If arrested, detained or interned for reasons re-

lated to the armed conflict, children shall be held in quarters separate from the quarters of adults, except where families are accommodated as family units as provided in Article 75, paragraph 5.

5. The death penalty for an offence related to the armed conflict shall not be executed on persons who had not attained the age of eighteen years at the time the offence was committed.

Article 78
Evacuation of Children

1. No Party to the conflict shall arrange for the evacuation of children, other than its own nationals, to a foreign country except for a temporary evacuation where compelling reasons of the health or medical treatment of the children or, except in occupied territory, their safety, so require. Where the parents or legal guardians can be found, their written consent to such evacuation is required. If these persons cannot be found, the written consent to such evacuation of the persons who by law or custom are primarily responsible for the care of the children is required. Any such evacuation shall be supervised by the Protecting Power in agreement with the Parties concerned, namely, the Party arranging for the evacuation, the Party receiving the children and any Parties whose nationals are being evacuated. In each case, all Parties to the conflict shall take all feasible precautions to avoid endangering the evacuation.

2. Whenever an evacuation occurs pursuant to paragraph 1, each child's education, including his religious and moral education as his parents desire, shall be provided while he is away with the greatest possible continuity.

3. With a view to facilitating the return to their families and country of children evacuated pursuant to this Article, the authorities of the Party arranging for the evacuation and, as appropriate, the authorities of the receiving country shall establish for each child a card with photographs, which they shall send to the Central Tracing Agency of the International Committee of the Red Cross. Each card shall bear, whenever possible, and whenever it involves no risk of harm to the child, the following information:

(a) surname(s) of the child;
(b) the child's first name(s);
(c) the child's sex;
(d) the place and date of birth (or, if that date is not known, the approximate age);
(e) the father's full name;
(f) the mother's full name and her maiden name;
(g) the child's next-of-kin;
(h) the child's nationality;
(i) the child's native language, and any other languages he speaks;
(j) the address of the child's family;
(k) any identification number for the child;
(l) the child's state of health;
(m) the child's blood group;
(n) any distinguishing features;
(o) the date on which and the place where the child was found;
(p) the date on which and the place from which the child left the country;
(q) the child's religion, if any;
(r) the child's present address in the receiving country;
(s) should the child die before his return, the date, place and circumstances of death and place of interment.

* * *

Protocol Additional to the Geneva Conventions of 12 August 1949, and Relating to the Protection of Victims of Non-International Armed Conflicts (Protocol II): Children (1977)

Adopted on 8 June 1977. Entered into force 7 December 1978.
[Available at http://www.icrc.org/ihl.nsf/7c4d08d9b287a
42141256739003e636b/d67c3971bcff1c10c125641e0052b545?OpenDocument]

* * *

Article 4

3. Children shall be provided with the care and aid they require, and in particular:

(a) they shall receive an education, including religious and moral education, in keeping with the wishes of their parents, or in the absence of parents, of those responsible for their care;

(b) all appropriate steps shall be taken to facilitate the reunion of families temporarily separated;

(c) children who have not attained the age of fifteen years shall neither be recruited in the armed forces or groups nor allowed to take part in hostilities;

(d) the special protection provided by this Article to children who have not attained the age of fifteen years shall remain applicable to them if they take a direct part in hostilities despite the provisions of subparagraph (c) and are captured;

(e) measures shall be taken, if necessary, and whenever possible with the consent of their parents or persons who by law or custom are primarily responsible for their care, to remove children temporarily from the area in which hostilities are taking place to a safer area within the country and ensure that they are accompanied by persons responsible for their safety and well-being.

* * *

Convention Concerning the Prohibition and Immediate Action for the Elimination of the Worst Forms of Child Labour

ILO Convention C182. Adopted by the International Labor Conference at its 87th session, on 17 June 1999. Entered into force 10 November 2000. [Available at http://www.ilo.org/public/english/standards/ipec/ratification/convention/text.htm]

The General Conference of the International Labour Organization,

Having been convened at Geneva by the Governing Body of the International Labour Office, and having met in its 87th Session on 1 June 1999, and

Considering the need to adopt new instruments for the prohibition and elimination of the worst forms of child labour, as the main priority for national and international action, including international cooperation and assistance, to complement the Convention and the Recommendation concerning Minimum Age for Admission to Employment, 1973, which remain fundamental instruments on child labour, and

Considering that the effective elimination of the worst forms of child labour requires immediate and comprehensive action, taking into account the importance of free basic education and the need to remove the children concerned from all such work and to provide for their rehabilitation and social integration while addressing the needs of their families, and

Recalling the resolution concerning the elimination of child labour adopted by the International Labour Conference at its 83rd Session in 1996, and

Recognizing that child labour is to a great extent caused by poverty and that the long-term solution lies in sustained economic growth leading to social progress, in particular poverty alleviation and universal education, and

Recalling the Convention on the Rights of the Child adopted by the United Nations General Assembly on 20 November 1989, and

Recalling the ILO Declaration on Fundamental Principles and Rights at Work and its Follow-up, adopted by the International Labour Conference at its 86th Session in 1998, and

Recalling that some of the worst forms of child labour are covered by other international instruments, in particular the Forced Labour Convention, 1930, and the United Nations Supplementary Convention on the Abolition of Slavery, the Slave Trade, and Institutions and Practices Similar to Slavery, 1956, and

Having decided upon the adoption of certain proposals with regard to child labour, which is the fourth item on the agenda of the session, and

Having determined that these proposals shall take the form of an international Convention;

Adopts this seventeenth day of June of the year one thousand nine hundred and ninety-nine the following Convention, which may be cited as the Worst Forms of Child Labour Convention, 1999.

Article 1

Each Member which ratifies this Convention shall take immediate and effective measures to secure the prohibition and elimination of the worst forms of child labour as a matter of urgency.

Article 2

For the purposes of this Convention, the term child shall apply to all persons under the age of 18.

Article 3

For the purposes of this Convention, the term the worst forms of child labour comprises:

(a) all forms of slavery or practices similar to slavery, such as the sale and trafficking of children,

debt bondage and serfdom and forced or compulsory labour, including forced or compulsory recruitment of children for use in armed conflict;

(b) the use, procuring or offering of a child for prostitution, for the production of pornography or for pornographic performances;

(c) the use, procuring or offering of a child for illicit activities, in particular for the production and trafficking of drugs as defined in the relevant international treaties;

(d) work which, by its nature or the circumstances in which it is carried out, is likely to harm the health, safety or morals of children.

Article 4

1. The types of work referred to under Article 3(d) shall be determined by national laws or regulations or by the competent authority, after consultation with the organizations of employers and workers concerned, taking into consideration relevant international standards, in particular Paragraphs 3 and 4 of the Worst Forms of Child Labour Recommendation, 1999.

2. The competent authority, after consultation with the organizations of employers and workers concerned, shall identify where the types of work so determined exist.

3. The list of the types of work determined under paragraph 1 of this Article shall be periodically examined and revised as necessary, in consultation with the organizations of employers and workers concerned.

Article 5

Each Member shall, after consultation with employers' and workers' organizations, establish or designate appropriate mechanisms to monitor the implementation of the provisions giving effect to this Convention.

Article 6

1. Each Member shall design and implement programmes of action to eliminate as a priority the worst forms of child labour.

2. Such programmes of action shall be designed

and implemented in consultation with relevant government institutions and employers' and workers' organizations, taking into consideration the views of other concerned groups as appropriate.

Article 7

1. Each Member shall take all necessary measures to ensure the effective implementation and enforcement of the provisions giving effect to this Convention including the provision and application of penal sanctions or, as appropriate, other sanctions.

2. Each Member shall, taking into account the importance of education in eliminating child labour, take effective and time-bound measures to:

(a) prevent the engagement of children in the worst forms of child labour;

(b) provide the necessary and appropriate direct assistance for the removal of children from the worst forms of child labour and for their rehabilitation and social integration;

(c) ensure access to free basic education, and, wherever possible and appropriate, vocational training, for all children removed from the worst forms of child labour;

(d) identify and reach out to children at special risk; and

(e) take account of the special situation of girls.

3. Each Member shall designate the competent authority responsible for the implementation of the provisions giving effect to this Convention.

Article 8

Members shall take appropriate steps to assist one another in giving effect to the provisions of this Convention through enhanced international cooperation and/or assistance including support for social and economic development, poverty eradication programmes and universal education.

Article 9

The formal ratifications of this Convention shall be communicated to the Director-General of the International Labour Office for registration.

Article 10

1. This Convention shall be binding only upon those Members of the International Labour Organization whose ratifications have been registered with the Director-General of the International Labour Office.

2. It shall come into force 12 months after the date on which the ratifications of two Members have been registered with the Director-General.

3. Thereafter, this Convention shall come into force for any Member 12 months after the date on which its ratification has been registered.

Article 11

1. A Member which has ratified this Convention may denounce it after the expiration of ten years from the date on which the Convention first comes into force, by an act communicated to the Director-General of the International Labour Office for registration. Such denunciation shall not take effect until one year after the date on which it is registered.

2. Each Member which has ratified this Convention and which does not, within the year following the expiration of the period of ten years mentioned in the preceding paragraph, exercise the right of denunciation provided for in this Article, will be bound for another period of ten years and, thereafter, may denounce this Convention at the expiration of each period of ten years under the terms provided for in this Article.

Article 12

1. The Director-General of the International Labour Office shall notify all Members of the International Labour Organization of the registration of all ratifications and acts of denunciation communicated by the Members of the Organization.

2. When notifying the Members of the Organization of the registration of the second ratification, the Director-General shall draw the attention of the Members of the Organization to the date upon which the Convention shall come into force.

Article 13

The Director-General of the International Labour Office shall communicate to the Secretary-General of the United Nations, for registration in accordance with article 102 of the Charter of the United Nations, full particulars of all ratifications and acts of denunciation registered by the Director-General in accordance with the provisions of the preceding Articles.

Article 14

At such times as it may consider necessary, the Governing Body of the International Labour Office shall present to the General Conference a report on the working of this Convention and shall examine the desirability of placing on the agenda of the Conference the question of its revision in whole or in part.

Article 15

1. Should the Conference adopt a new Convention revising this Convention in whole or in part, then,

unless the new Convention otherwise provides —

(a) the ratification by a Member of the new revising Convention shall ipso jure involve the immediate denunciation of this Convention, notwithstanding the provisions of Article 11 above, if and when the new revising Convention shall have come into force;

(b) as from the date when the new revising Convention comes into force, this Convention shall cease to be open to ratification by the Members.

2. This Convention shall in any case remain in force in its actual form and content for those Members which have ratified it but have not ratified the revising Convention.

Article 16

The English and French versions of the text of this Convention are equally authoritative.

General Comment No. 4: Adolescent Health and Development in the Context of the Convention on the Rights of the Child (2003)

Adopted by the Committee on the Rights of the Child. [Available at
http://www.unhchr.ch/tbs/doc.nsf/(symbol)/CRC.GC.2003.4.En!OpenDocument]

[Footnotes omitted.]

INTRODUCTION

1. The Convention on the Rights of the Child defines a child as "every human being below the age of 18 years unless, under the law applicable, majority is attained earlier" (Article 1). Consequently, adolescents up to 18 years old are holders of all the rights enshrined in the Convention; they are entitled to special protection measures and, according to their evolving capacities, they can progressively exercise their rights (Article 5).

2. Adolescence is a period characterized by rapid physical, cognitive and social changes, including sexual and reproductive maturation; the gradual building up of the capacity to assume adult behaviours and roles involving new responsibilities requiring new knowledge and skills. While adoles-

cents are in general a healthy population group, adolescence also poses new challenges to health and development owing to their relative vulnerability and pressure from society, including peers, to adopt risky health behaviour. These challenges include developing an individual identity and dealing with one's sexuality. The dynamic transition period to adulthood is also generally a period of positive changes, prompted by the significant capacity of adolescents to learn rapidly, to experience new and diverse situations, to develop and use critical thinking, to familiarize themselves with freedom, to be creative and to socialize.

* * *

4. The Committee understands the concepts of "health and development" more broadly than being strictly limited to the provisions defined in Articles 6 (right to life, survival and development)

and 24 (right to health) of the Convention. One of the aims of this general comment is precisely to identify the main human rights that need to be promoted and protected in order to ensure that adolescents do enjoy the highest attainable standard of health, develop in a well-balanced manner, and are adequately prepared to enter adulthood and assume a constructive role in their communities and in society at large. This general comment should be read in conjunction with the Convention and its two Optional Protocols on the sale of children, child prostitution and child pornography, and on the involvement of children in armed conflict, as well as other relevant international human rights norms and standards.

I. FUNDAMENTAL PRINCIPLES AND OTHER OBLIGATIONS OF STATES PARTIES

* * *

The Right to Non-Discrimination
* * *

Appropriate Guidance in the Exercise of Rights
* * *

Respect for the Views of the Child

8. The right to express views freely and have them duly taken into account (Article 12) is also fundamental in realizing adolescents' right to health and development. States parties need to ensure that adolescents are given a genuine chance to express their views freely on all matters affecting them, especially within the family, in school, and in their communities. In order for adolescents to be able safely and properly exercise this right, public authorities, parents and other adults working with or for children need to create an environment based on trust, information sharing, the capacity to listen and sound guidance that is conducive for adolescents' participating equally including in decision-making processes.

Legal and Judicial Measures and Processes
* * *

Civil Rights and Freedoms
* * *

Protection from All Forms of Abuse, Neglect, Violence and Exploitation[ii]
* * *

Data Collection
* * *

II. CREATING A SAFE AND SUPPORTIVE ENVIRONMENT

14. The health and development of adolescents are strongly determined by the environments in which they live. Creating a safe and supportive environment entails addressing attitudes and actions of both the immediate environment of the adolescent — family, peers, schools and services — as well as the wider environment created by, inter alia, community and religious leaders, the media, national and local policies and legislation. The promotion and enforcement of the provisions and principles of the Convention, especially Articles 2-6, 12-17, 24, 28, 29 and 31, are key to guaranteeing adolescents' right to health and development. States parties should take measures to raise awareness and stimulate and/or regulate action through the formulation of policy or the adoption of legislation and the implementation of programmes specifically for adolescents.

15. The Committee stresses the importance of the family environment, including the members of the extended family and community or other persons legally responsible for the child or adolescent (Articles 5 and 18). While most adolescents grow up in well-functioning family environments, for some the family does not constitute a safe and supportive milieu.

* * *

20. The Committee is concerned that early marriage and pregnancy are significant factors in health problems related to sexual and reproductive health, including HIV/AIDS. Both the legal minimum age and actual age of marriage, particularly for girls, are still very low in several States parties. There are also non-health-related concerns: children who marry, especially girls, are often obliged to leave the education system and are marginalized from social activities. Further, in some States parties married children are legally

considered adults, even if they are under 18, depriving them of all the special protection measures they are entitled under the Convention. The Committee strongly recommends that States parties review and, where necessary, reform their legislation and practice to increase the minimum age for marriage with and without parental consent to 18 years, for both girls and boys. The Committee on the Elimination of Discrimination against Women has made a similar recommendation (general comment No. 21 of 1994).

* * *

22. The Committee is also very concerned about the high rate of suicide among this age group. Mental disorders and psychosocial illness are relatively common among adolescents. In many countries symptoms such as depression, eating disorders and self-destructive behaviours, sometimes leading to self-inflicted injuries and suicide, are increasing. They may be related to, inter alia, violence, ill-treatment, abuse and neglect, including sexual abuse, unrealistically high expectations, and/or bullying or hazing in and outside school. States parties should provide these adolescents with all the necessary services.

23. Violence results from a complex interplay of individual, family, community and societal factors. Vulnerable adolescents such as those who are homeless or who are living in institutions, who belong to gangs or who have been recruited as child soldiers are especially exposed to both institutional and interpersonal violence. Under Article 19 of the Convention, States parties must take all appropriate measures to prevent and eliminate: (a) institutional violence against adolescents, including through legislation and administrative measures in relation to public and private institutions for adolescents (schools, institutions for disabled adolescents, juvenile reformatories, etc.), and training and monitoring of personnel in charge of institutionalized children or who otherwise have contact with children through their work, including the police; and (b) interpersonal violence among adolescents, including by supporting adequate parenting and opportunities for social and educational development in early childhood, fostering non-violent cultural norms and values (as foreseen in Article 29 of the Convention), strictly controlling firearms and restricting access to alcohol and drugs.

24. In light of Articles 3, 6, 12, 19 and 24 (3) of the Convention, States parties should take all effective measures to eliminate all acts and activities which threaten the right to life of adolescents, including honour killings. The Committee strongly urges States parties to develop and implement awareness-raising campaigns, education programmes and legislation aimed at changing prevailing attitudes, and address gender roles and stereotypes that contribute to harmful traditional practices. Further, States parties should facilitate the establishment of multidisciplinary information and advice centres regarding the harmful aspects of some traditional practices, including early marriage and female genital mutilation.

25. The Committee is concerned about the influence exerted on adolescent health behaviours by the marketing of unhealthy products and lifestyles. In line with Article 17 of the Convention, States parties are urged to protect adolescents from information that is harmful to their health and development, while underscoring their right to information and material from diverse national and international sources. States parties are therefore urged to regulate or prohibit information on and marketing of substances such as alcohol and tobacco, particularly when it targets children and adolescents.

III. INFORMATION, SKILLS DEVELOPMENT, COUNSELLING, AND HEALTH SERVICES

26. Adolescents have the right to access adequate information essential for their health and development and for their ability to participate meaningfully in society. It is the obligation of States parties to ensure that all adolescent girls and boys, both in and out of school, are provided with, and not denied, accurate and appropriate information on how to protect their health and development and practise healthy behaviours. This should include information on the use and abuse of tobacco, alcohol and other substances, safe and respectful social and sexual behaviours, diet and physical activity.

* * *

28. In light of Articles 3, 17 and 24 of the Convention, States parties should provide adolescents with access to sexual and reproductive information, including on family planning and contraceptives, the dangers of early pregnancy, the prevention of HIV/AIDS and the prevention and treatment of sexually transmitted diseases (STDs). In addition, States parties should ensure that they have access to appropriate information, regardless of their marital status and whether their parents or guardians consent. It is essential to find proper means and methods of providing information that is adequate and sensitive to the particularities and specific rights of adolescent girls and boys. To this end, States parties are encouraged to ensure that adolescents are actively involved in the design and dissemination of information through a variety of channels beyond the school, including youth organizations, religious, community and other groups and the media.

* * *

30. Adolescents, both girls and boys, are at risk of being infected with and affected by STDs, including HIV/AIDS. States should ensure that appropriate goods, services and information for the prevention and treatment of STDs, including HIV/AIDS, are available and accessible. To this end, States parties are urged (a) to develop effective prevention programmes, including measures aimed at changing cultural views about adolescents' need for contraception and STD prevention and addressing cultural and other taboos surrounding adolescent sexuality; (b) to adopt legislation to combat practices that either increase adolescents' risk of infection or contribute to the marginalization of adolescents who are already infected with STDs, including HIV; (c) to take measures to remove all barriers hindering the access of adolescents to information, preventive measures such as condoms, and care.

31. Adolescent girls should have access to information on the harm that early marriage and early pregnancy can cause, and those who become pregnant should have access to health services that are sensitive to their rights and particular needs. States parties should take measures to reduce maternal morbidity and mortality in adolescent girls, particularly caused by early pregnancy and unsafe abortion practices, and to support adolescent parents. Young mothers, especially where support is lacking, may be prone to depression and anxiety, compromising their ability to care for their child. The Committee urges States parties (a) to develop and implement programmes that provide access to sexual and reproductive health services, including family planning, contraception and safe abortion services where abortion is not against the law, adequate and comprehensive obstetric care and counselling; (b) to foster positive and supportive attitudes towards adolescent parenthood for their mothers and fathers; and (c) to develop policies that will allow adolescent mothers to continue their education.

32. Before parents give their consent, adolescents need to have a chance to express their views freely and their views should be given due weight, in accordance with Article 12 of the Convention. However, if the adolescent is of sufficient maturity, informed consent shall be obtained from the adolescent her/himself, while informing the parents if that is in the "best interest of the child" (Article 3).

33. With regard to privacy and confidentiality, and the related issue of informed consent to treatment, States parties should (a) enact laws or regulations to ensure that confidential advice concerning treatment is provided to adolescents so that they can give their informed consent. Such laws or regulations should stipulate an age for this process, or refer to the evolving capacity of the child; and (b) provide training for health personnel on the rights of adolescents to privacy and confidentiality, to be informed about planned treatment and to give their informed consent to treatment.

IV. VULNERABILITY AND RISK

34. In ensuring respect for the right of adolescents to health and development, both individual behaviours and environmental factors which increase their vulnerability and risk should be taken into consideration. Environmental factors, such as armed conflict or social exclusion, increase the vulnerability of adolescents to abuse, other forms of violence and exploitation, thereby severely limiting adolescents' abilities to make individual, healthy behaviour choices. For example, the decision to engage in unsafe sex increases adolescents' risk of ill-health.

* * *

36. States parties have to provide special protection to homeless adolescents, including those working in the informal sector. Homeless adolescents are particularly vulnerable to violence, abuse and sexual exploitation from others, self-destructive behaviour, substance abuse and mental disorders. In this regard, States parties are required to (a) develop policies and enact and enforce legislation that protect such adolescents from violence, e.g. by law enforcement officials; (b) develop strategies for the provision of appropriate education and access to health care, and of opportunities for the development of livelihood skills.

37. Adolescents who are sexually exploited, including in prostitution and pornography, are exposed to significant health risks, including STDs, HIV/AIDS, unwanted pregnancies, unsafe abortions, violence and psychological distress. They have the right to physical and psychological recovery and social reintegration in an environment that fosters health, self-respect and dignity (Article 39). It is the obligation of States parties to enact and enforce laws to prohibit all forms of sexual exploitation and related trafficking; to collaborate with other States parties to eliminate intercountry trafficking; and to provide appropriate health and counselling services to adolescents who have been sexually exploited, making sure that they are treated as victims and not as offenders.

38. Additionally, adolescents experiencing poverty, armed conflicts, all forms of injustice, family breakdown, political, social and economic instability and all types of migration may be particularly vulnerable. These situations might seriously hamper their health and development. By investing heavily in preventive policies and measures States parties can drastically reduce levels of vulnerability and risk factors; they will also provide cost-effective ways for society to help adolescents develop harmoniously in a free society.

V. NATURE OF STATES' OBLIGATIONS

39. In exercising their obligations in relation to the health and development of adolescents, States parties shall always take fully into account the four general principles of the Convention. It is the view of the Committee that States parties must take all appropriate legislative, administrative and other measures for the realization and monitoring of the rights of adolescents to health and development as recognized in the Convention. To this end, States parties must notably fulfil the following obligations:

(a) To create a safe and supportive environment for adolescents, including within their family, in schools, in all types of institutions in which they may live, within their workplace and/or in the society at large;

(b) To ensure that adolescents have access to the information that is essential for their health and development and that they have opportunities to participate in decisions affecting their health (notably through informed consent and the right of confidentiality), to acquire life skills, to obtain adequate and age-appropriate information, and to make appropriate health behaviour choice;

(c) To ensure that health facilities, goods and services, including counselling and health services for mental and sexual and reproductive health, of appropriate quality and sensitive to adolescents' concerns are available to all adolescents;

(d) To ensure that adolescent girls and boys have the opportunity to participate actively in planning and programming for their own health and development;

(e) To protect adolescents from all forms of labour which may jeopardize the enjoyment of their rights, notably by abolishing all forms of child labour and by regulating the working environment and conditions in accordance with international standards;

(f) To protect adolescents from all forms of intentional and unintentional injuries, including those resulting from violence and road traffic accidents;

(g) To protect adolescents from all harmful traditional practices, such as early marriages, honour killings and female genital mutilation;

(h) To ensure that adolescents belonging to especially vulnerable groups are fully taken into account in the fulfilment of all aforementioned obligations;

(i) To implement measures for the prevention of mental disorders and the promotion of mental health of adolescents.

* * *

41. In accordance with Articles 24, 39 and other related provisions of the Convention, States parties should provide health services that are sensitive to the particular needs and human rights of all adolescents, paying attention to the following characteristics:

(a) Availability. Primary health care should include services sensitive to the needs of adolescents, with special attention given to sexual and reproductive health and mental health;

(b) Accessibility. Health facilities, goods and services should be known and easily accessible (economically, physically and socially) to all adolescents, without discrimination. Confidentiality should be guaranteed, when necessary;

(c) Acceptability. While fully respecting the provisions and principles of the Convention, all health facilities, goods and services should respect cultural values, be gender sensitive, be respectful of medical ethics and be acceptable to both adolescents and the communities in which they live;

(d) Quality. Health services and goods should be scientifically and medically appropriate, which requires personnel trained to care for adolescents, adequate facilities and scientifically accepted methods.

* * *

C. Disabilities

General Comment 5: Persons with Disabilities (1994)
*Adopted by the Committee on Economic, Social and Cultural Rights
on 9 December 1994. UN document E/1995/22.
[Available at http://www.unhchr.ch/tbs/doc.nsf/(Symbol)/
4b0c449a9ab4ff72c12563ed0054f17d?Opendocument*

[Footnotes omitted.]

1. The central importance of the International Covenant on Economic, Social and Cultural Rights in relation to the human rights of persons with disabilities has frequently been underlined by the international community. Thus a 1992 review by the Secretary-General of the implementation of the World Programme of Action concerning Disabled Persons and the United Nations Decade of Disabled Persons concluded that "disability is closely linked to economic and social factors" and that "conditions of living in large parts of the world are so desperate that the provision of basic needs for all — food, water, shelter, health protection and education — must form the cornerstone of national programmes". Even in countries which have a relatively high standard of living, persons with disabilities are very often denied the opportunity to enjoy the full range of economic, social and cultural rights recognized in the Covenant.

* * *

3. There is still no internationally accepted definition of the term "disability". For present purposes, however, it is sufficient to rely on the approach adopted in the Standard Rules of 1993, which state:

"The term 'disability' summarizes a great number of different functional limitations occurring in any population ... People may be disabled by physical, intellectual or sensory impairment, medical conditions or mental illness. Such impairments, conditions or illnesses may be permanent or transitory in nature".

* * *

I. GENERAL OBLIGATIONS OF STATES PARTIES

* * *

8. The United Nations has estimated that there are more than 500 million persons with disabilities in the world today. Of that number, 80 per cent live in rural areas in developing countries. Seventy per cent of the total are estimated to have either limited or no access to the services they need. The challenge of improving the situation of persons with disabilities is thus of direct relevance to every State party to the Covenant. While the means chosen to promote the full realization of the economic, social and cultural rights of this group will inevitably differ significantly from one country to another, there is no country in which a major policy and programme effort is not required.

9. The obligation of States parties to the Covenant to promote progressive realization of the relevant rights to the maximum of their available resources clearly requires Governments to do much more than merely abstain from taking measures which might have a negative impact on persons with disabilities. The obligation in the case of such a vulnerable and disadvantaged group is to take positive action to reduce structural disadvantages and to give appropriate preferential treatment to people with disabilities in order to achieve the objectives of full participation and equality within society for all persons with disabilities. This almost invariably means that additional resources will need to be made available for this purpose and that a wide range of specially tailored measures will be required.

* * *

11. Given the increasing commitment of Governments around the world to market-based policies, it is appropriate in that context to emphasize certain aspects of States parties' obligations. One is the need to ensure that not only the public sphere, but also the private sphere, are, within appropriate limits, subject to regulation to ensure the equitable treatment of persons with disabilities. In a context in which arrangements for the provision of public services are increasingly being privatized and in which the free market is being relied on to an ever greater extent, it is essential that private employers, private suppliers of goods and services, and other non-public entities be subject to both non-discrimination and equality norms in relation to persons with disabilities.

* * *

12. In the absence of government intervention there will always be instances in which the operation of the free market will produce unsatisfactory results for persons with disabilities, either individually or as a group, and in such circumstances it is incumbent on Governments to step in and take appropriate measures to temper, complement, compensate for, or override the results produced by market forces. Similarly, while it is appropriate for Governments to rely on private, voluntary groups to assist persons with disabilities in various ways, such arrangements can never absolve Governments from their duty to ensure full compliance with their obligations under the Covenant. As the World Programme of Action concerning Disabled Persons states, "the ultimate responsibility for remedying the conditions that lead to impairment and for dealing with the consequences of disability rests with Governments". World Programme of Action concerning Disabled Persons (see note 3 above), paragraph. 3.

II. MEANS OF IMPLEMENTATION

* * *

III. THE OBLIGATION TO ELIMINATE DISCRIMINATION ON THE GROUNDS OF DISABILITY

15. Both de jure and de facto discrimination against persons with disabilities have a long history and take various forms. They range from invidious discrimination, such as the denial of educational opportunities, to more "subtle" forms of discrimination such as segregation and isolation achieved through the imposition of physical and social barriers. For the purposes of the Covenant, "disability-based discrimination" may be defined as including any distinction, exclusion, restriction or preference, or denial of reasonable accommodation based on disability which has the effect of nullifying or impairing the recognition, enjoyment or exercise of economic, social or cultural rights. Through neglect, ignorance, prejudice and false assumptions, as well as through exclusion, distinction or separation, persons with disabilities have very often been prevented from exercising their economic, social or cultural rights on an equal basis with persons without disabilities. The effects of disability-based discrimination have been particularly severe in the fields of education, employment, housing, transport, cultural life, and access to public places and services.

16. Despite some progress in terms of legislation over the past decade, the legal situation of persons with disabilities remains precarious. In order to remedy past and present discrimination, and to deter future discrimination, comprehensive anti-discrimination legislation in relation to disability would seem to be indispensable in virtually all States parties. Such legislation should not only provide persons with disabilities with judicial remedies as far as possible and appropriate, but also provide for social-policy programmes which enable persons with disabilities to live an integrated, self-determined and independent life.

17. Anti-discrimination measures should be based on the principle of equal rights for persons with disabilities and the non-disabled, which, in the words of the World Programme of Action concerning Disabled Persons, "implies that the needs of each and every individual are of equal importance, that these needs must be made the basis for the planning of societies, and that all resources must be employed in such a way as to ensure, for every individual, equal opportunity for participation. Disability policies should ensure the access of [persons with disabilities] to all community services".

18. Because appropriate measures need to be taken to undo existing discrimination and to estab-

lish equitable opportunities for persons with disabilities, such actions should not be considered discriminatory in the sense of article 2 (2) of the International Covenant on Economic, Social and Cultural Rights as long as they are based on the principle of equality and are employed only to the extent necessary to achieve that objective.

IV. SPECIFIC PROVISIONS OF THE COVENANT

A. Article 3 — Equal rights for Men and Women
* * *

B. Articles 6-8 — Rights Relating to Work
* * *

C. Article 9 — Social Security
* * *

D. Article 10 — Protection of the Family and of Mothers and Children
* * *

E. Article 11 — The Right to an Adequate Standard of Living
* * *

F. Article 12 — The Right to Physical and Mental Health

34. According to the Standard Rules, "States should ensure that persons with disabilities, par-

ticularly infants and children, are provided with the same level of medical care within the same system as other members of society". The right to physical and mental health also implies the right to have access to, and to benefit from, those medical and social services — including orthopaedic devices — which enable persons with disabilities to become independent, prevent further disabilities and support their social integration. Similarly, such persons should be provided with rehabilitation services which would enable them "to reach and sustain their optimum level of independence and functioning". All such services should be provided in such a way that the persons concerned are able to maintain full respect for their rights and dignity.

G. Articles 13 and 14 — The Right to Education
* * *

H. Article 15 — The Right to Take Part in Cultural Life and Enjoy the Benefits of Scientific Progress

Principles for the Protection of Persons with Mental Illness and the Improvement of Mental Health Care (1991)

Adopted by General Assembly Resolution 46/119 of 17 December 1991.
[Available at: http://www.unhchr.ch/html/menu3/b/68.htm]

APPLICATION

These Principles shall be applied without discrimination of any kind such as on grounds of disability, race, colour, sex, language, religion, political or other opinion, national, ethnic or social origin, legal or social status, age, property or birth.

DEFINITIONS

In these Principles:

"Counsel" means a legal or other qualified representative;

"Independent authority" means a competent and independent authority prescribed by domestic law;

"Mental health care" includes analysis and diagnosis of a person's mental condition, and treatment, care and rehabilitation for a mental illness or suspected mental illness;

"Mental health facility" means any establishment, or any unit of an establishment, which as its primary function provides mental health care;

"Mental health practitioner" means a medical doctor, clinical psychologist, nurse, social worker or other appropriately trained and qualified person with specific skills relevant to mental health care;

"Patient" means a person receiving mental health care and includes all persons who are admitted to a mental health facility;

"Personal representative" means a person charged by law with the duty of representing a patient's interests in any specified respect or of exercising specified rights on the patient's behalf, and includes the parent or legal guardian of a minor unless otherwise provided by domestic law;

"The review body" means the body established in accordance with Principle 17 to review the involuntary admission or retention of a patient in a mental health facility.

General Limitation Clause

The exercise of the rights set forth in these Principles may be subject only to such limitations as are prescribed by law and are necessary to protect the health or safety of the person concerned or of others, or otherwise to protect public safety, order, health or morals or the fundamental rights and freedoms of others.

Principle 1

Fundamental Freedoms and Basic Rights

1. All persons have the right to the best available mental health care, which shall be part of the health and social care system.

2. All persons with a mental illness, or who are being treated as such persons, shall be treated with humanity and respect for the inherent dignity of the human person.

3. All persons with a mental illness, or who are being treated as such persons, have the right to protection from economic, sexual and other forms of exploitation, physical or other abuse and degrading treatment.

4. There shall be no discrimination on the grounds of mental illness. "Discrimination" means any distinction, exclusion or preference that has the effect of nullifying or impairing equal enjoyment of rights. Special measures solely to protect the rights, or secure the advancement, of persons with mental illness shall not be deemed to be discriminatory. Discrimination does not include any distinction, exclusion or preference undertaken in accordance with the provisions of these Principles and necessary to protect the human rights of a person with a mental illness or of other individuals.

5. Every person with a mental illness shall have the right to exercise all civil, political, economic, social and cultural rights as recognized in the Universal Declaration of Human Rights, the International Covenant on Economic, Social and Cultural Rights, the International Covenant on Civil and Political Rights, and in other relevant instruments, such as the Declaration on the Rights of Disabled Persons and the Body of Principles for the Protection of All Persons under Any Form of Detention or Imprisonment.

6. Any decision that, by reason of his or her mental illness, a person lacks legal capacity, and any decision that, in consequence of such incapacity, a personal representative shall be appointed, shall be made only after a fair hearing by an independent and impartial tribunal established by domestic law. The person whose capacity is at issue shall be entitled to be represented by a counsel. If the person whose capacity is at issue does not himself or herself secure such representation, it shall be made available without payment by that person to the extent that he or she does not have sufficient means to pay for it. The counsel shall not in the same proceedings represent a mental health facility or its personnel and shall not also represent a member of the family of the person whose capacity is at issue unless the tribunal is satisfied that there is no conflict of interest. Decisions regarding capacity and the need for a personal representative shall be reviewed at reasonable intervals prescribed by domestic law. The person whose capacity is at issue, his or her personal representative, if any, and any other interested person shall have the right to appeal to a higher court against any such decision.

7. Where a court or other competent tribunal finds that a person with mental illness is unable to manage his or her own affairs, measures shall be taken, so far as is necessary and appropriate to that person's condition, to ensure the protection of his or her interest.

Principle 2

Protection of Minors
Special care should be given within the purposes of these Principles and within the context of domestic law relating to the protection of minors to protect the rights of minors, including, if necessary, the appointment of a personal representative other than a family member.

Principle 3

Life in the Community
Every person with a mental illness shall have the right to live and work, as far as possible, in the community.

Principle 4

Determination of Mental Illness
1. A determination that a person has a mental illness shall be made in accordance with internationally accepted medical standards.

2. A determination of mental illness shall never be made on the basis of political, economic or social status, or membership of a cultural, racial or religious group, or any other reason not directly relevant to mental health status.

3. Family or professional conflict, or non-conformity with moral, social, cultural or political values or religious beliefs prevailing in a person's community, shall never be a determining factor in diagnosing mental illness.

4. A background of past treatment or hospitalization as a patient shall not of itself justify any present or future determination of mental illness.

5. No person or authority shall classify a person as having, or otherwise indicate that a person has, a mental illness except for purposes directly relating to mental illness or the consequences of mental illness.

Principle 5

Medical Examination
No person shall be compelled to undergo medical examination with a view to determining whether or not he or she has a mental illness except in accordance with a procedure authorized by domestic law.

Principle 6

Confidentiality
The right of confidentiality of information concerning all persons to whom these Principles apply shall be respected.

Principle 7

Role of Community and Culture
1. Every patient shall have the right to be treated and cared for, as far as possible, in the community in which he or she lives.

2. Where treatment takes place in a mental health facility, a patient shall have the right, whenever possible, to be treated near his or her home or the home of his or her relatives or friends and shall have the right to return to the community as soon as possible.

3. Every patient shall have the right to treatment suited to his or her cultural background.

Principle 8

Standards of Care
1. Every patient shall have the right to receive such health and social care as is appropriate to his or her health needs, and is entitled to care and treatment in accordance with the same standards as other ill persons.

2. Every patient shall be protected from harm, including unjustified medication, abuse by other patients, staff or others or other acts causing mental distress or physical discomfort.

Principle 9

Treatment
1. Every patient shall have the right to be treated in the least restrictive environment and with the least restrictive or intrusive treatment appropriate to the patient's health needs and the need to protect the physical safety of others.

2. The treatment and care of every patient shall be based on an individually prescribed plan, discussed with the patient, reviewed regularly, revised as necessary and provided by qualified professional staff.

3. Mental health care shall always be provided in accordance with applicable standards of ethics for mental health practitioners, including internationally accepted standards such as the Principles of Medical Ethics adopted by the United Nations General Assembly. Mental health knowledge and skills shall never be abused.

4. The treatment of every patient shall be directed towards preserving and enhancing personal autonomy.

Principle 10

Medication
1. Medication shall meet the best health needs of the patient, shall be given to a patient only for therapeutic or diagnostic purposes and shall never be administered as a punishment or for the convenience of others. Subject to the provisions of paragraph 15 of Principle 11, mental health practitioners shall only administer medication of known or demonstrated efficacy.

2. All medication shall be prescribed by a mental health practitioner authorized by law and shall be recorded in the patient's records.

Principle 11

Consent to Treatment
1. No treatment shall be given to a patient without his or her informed consent, except as provided for in paragraphs 6, 7, 8, 13 and 15 below.

2. Informed consent is consent obtained freely, without threats or improper inducements, after appropriate disclosure to the patient of adequate and understandable information in a form and language understood by the patient on:

(a) The diagnostic assessment;

(b) The purpose, method, likely duration and expected benefit of the proposed treatment;

(c) Alternative modes of treatment, including those less intrusive; and

(d) Possible pain or discomfort, risks and side-effects of the proposed treatment.

3. A patient may request the presence of a person or persons of the patient's choosing during the procedure for granting consent.

4. A patient has the right to refuse or stop treatment, except as provided for in paragraphs 6, 7, 8, 13 and 15 below. The consequences of refusing or stopping treatment must be explained to the patient.

5. A patient shall never be invited or induced to waive the right to informed consent. If the patient should seek to do so, it shall be explained to the patient that the treatment cannot be given without informed consent.

6. Except as provided in paragraphs 7, 8, 12, 13, 14 and 15 below, a proposed plan of treatment may be

given to a patient without a patient's informed consent if the following conditions are satisfied:

(a) The patient is, at the relevant time, held as an involuntary patient;

(b) An independent authority, having in its possession all relevant information, including the information specified in paragraph 2 above, is satisfied that, at the relevant time, the patient lacks the capacity to give or withhold informed consent to the proposed plan of treatment or, if domestic legislation so provides, that, having regard to the patient's own safety or the safety of others, the patient unreasonably withholds such consent; and

(c) The independent authority is satisfied that the proposed plan of treatment is in the best interest of the patient's health needs.

7. Paragraph 6 above does not apply to a patient with a personal representative empowered by law to consent to treatment for the patient; but, except as provided in paragraphs 12, 13, 14 and 15 below, treatment may be given to such a patient without his or her informed consent if the personal representative, having been given the information described in paragraph 2 above, consents on the patient's behalf.

8. Except as provided in paragraphs 12, 13, 14 and 15 below, treatment may also be given to any patient without the patient's informed consent if a qualified mental health practitioner authorized by law determines that it is urgently necessary in order to prevent immediate or imminent harm to the patient or to other persons. Such treatment shall not be prolonged beyond the period that is strictly necessary for this purpose.

9. Where any treatment is authorized without the patient's informed consent, every effort shall nevertheless be made to inform the patient about the nature of the treatment and any possible alternatives and to involve the patient as far as practicable in the development of the treatment plan.

10. All treatment shall be immediately recorded in the patient's medical records, with an indication of whether involuntary or voluntary.

11. Physical restraint or involuntary seclusion of a patient shall not be employed except in accordance with the officially approved procedures of the mental health facility and only when it is the only means available to prevent immediate or imminent harm to the patient or others. It shall not be prolonged beyond the period which is strictly necessary for this purpose. All instances of physical restraint or involuntary seclusion, the reasons for them and their nature and extent shall be recorded in the patient's medical record. A patient who is restrained or secluded shall be kept under humane conditions and be under the care and close and regular supervision of qualified members of the staff. A personal representative, if any and if relevant, shall be given prompt notice of any physical restraint or involuntary seclusion of the patient.

12. Sterilization shall never be carried out as a treatment for mental illness.

13. A major medical or surgical procedure may be carried out on a person with mental illness only where it is permitted by domestic law, where it is considered that it would best serve the health needs of the patient and where the patient gives informed consent, except that, where the patient is unable to give informed consent, the procedure shall be authorized only after independent review.

14. Psychosurgery and other intrusive and irreversible treatments for mental illness shall never be carried out on a patient who is an involuntary patient in a mental health facility and, to the extent that domestic law permits them to be carried out, they may be carried out on any other patient only where the patient has given informed consent and an independent external body has satisfied itself that there is genuine informed consent and that the treatment best serves the health needs of the patient.

15. Clinical trials and experimental treatment shall never be carried out on any patient without informed consent, except that a patient who is unable to give informed consent may be admitted to a clinical trial or given experimental treatment, but only with the approval of a competent, independent review body specifically constituted for this purpose.

16. In the cases specified in paragraphs 6, 7, 8, 13, 14 and 15 above, the patient or his or her personal representative, or any interested person, shall have the right to appeal to a judicial or other independent authority concerning any treatment given to him or her.

Principle 12

Notice of Rights

1. A patient in a mental health facility shall be informed as soon as possible after admission, in a form and a language which the patient understands, of all his or her rights in accordance with these Principles and under domestic law, which information shall include an explanation of those rights and how to exercise them.

2. If and for so long as a patient is unable to understand such information, the rights of the patient shall be communicated to the personal representative, if any and if appropriate, and to the person or persons best able to represent the patient's interests and willing to do so.

3. A patient who has the necessary capacity has the right to nominate a person who should be informed on his or her behalf, as well as a person to represent his or her interests to the authorities of the facility.

Principle 13

Rights and Conditions in Mental Health Facilities

1. Every patient in a mental health facility shall, in particular, have the right to full respect for his or her:

(a) Recognition everywhere as a person before the law;

(b) Privacy;

(c) Freedom of communication, which includes freedom to communicate with other persons in the facility; freedom to send and receive uncensored private communications; freedom to receive, in private, visits from a counsel or personal representative and, at all reasonable times, from other visitors; and freedom of access to postal and telephone services and to newspapers, radio and television;

(d) Freedom of religion or belief.

2. The environment and living conditions in mental health facilities shall be as close as possible to those of the normal life of persons of similar age and in particular shall include:

(a) Facilities for recreational and leisure activities;

(b) Facilities for education;

(c) Facilities to purchase or receive items for daily living, recreation and communication;

(d) Facilities, and encouragement to use such facilities, for a patient's engagement in active occupation suited to his or her social and cultural background, and for appropriate vocational rehabilitation measures to promote reintegration in the community. These measures should include vocational guidance, vocational training and placement services to enable patients to secure or retain employment in the community.

3. In no circumstances shall a patient be subject to forced labour. Within the limits compatible with the needs of the patient and with the requirements of institutional administration, a patient shall be able to choose the type of work he or she wishes to perform.

4. The labour of a patient in a mental health facility shall not be exploited. Every such patient shall have the right to receive the same remuneration for any work which he or she does as would, according to domestic law or custom, be paid for such work to a non-patient. Every such patient shall, in any event, have the right to receive a fair share of any remuneration which is paid to the mental health facility for his or her work.

Principle 14

Resources for Mental Health Facilities

1. A mental health facility shall have access to the same level of resources as any other health establishment, and in particular:

(a) Qualified medical and other appropriate professional staff in sufficient numbers and with adequate space to provide each patient with privacy and a programme of appropriate and active therapy;

(b) Diagnostic and therapeutic equipment for the patient;

(c) Appropriate professional care; and

(d) Adequate, regular and comprehensive treatment, including supplies of medication.

2. Every mental health facility shall be inspected by the competent authorities with sufficient frequency to ensure that the conditions, treatment and care of patients comply with these Principles.

Principle 15
Admission Principles

1. Where a person needs treatment in a mental health facility, every effort shall be made to avoid involuntary admission.

2. Access to a mental health facility shall be administered in the same way as access to any other facility for any other illness.

3. Every patient not admitted involuntarily shall have the right to leave the mental health facility at any time unless the criteria for his or her retention as an involuntary patient, as set forth in Principle 16, apply, and he or she shall be informed of that right.

Principle 16
Involuntary Admission

1. A person may (a) be admitted involuntarily to a mental health facility as a patient; or (b) having already been admitted voluntarily as a patient, be retained as an involuntary patient in the mental health facility if, and only if, a qualified mental health practitioner authorized by law for that purpose determines, in accordance with Principle 4, that person has a mental illness and considers:

(a) That, because of that mental illness, there is a serious likelihood of immediate or imminent harm to that person or to other persons; or

(b) That, in the case of a person whose mental illness is severe and whose judgement is impaired, failure to admit or retain that person is likely to lead to a serious deterioration in his or her condition or will prevent the giving of appropriate treatment that can only be given by admission to a mental health facility in accordance with the principle of the least restrictive alternative.

In the case referred to in subparagraph (b), a second such mental health practitioner, independent of the first, should be consulted where possible. If such consultation takes place, the involuntary admission or retention may not take place unless the second mental health practitioner concurs.

2. Involuntary admission or retention shall initially be for a short period as specified by domestic law for observation and preliminary treatment pending review of the admission or retention by the review body. The grounds of the admission shall be communicated to the patient without delay and the fact of the admission and the grounds for it shall also be communicated promptly and in detail to the review body, to the patient's personal representative, if any, and, unless the patient objects, to the patient's family.

3. A mental health facility may receive involuntarily admitted patients only if the facility has been designated to do so by a competent authority prescribed by domestic law.

Principle 17
Review Body

1. The review body shall be a judicial or other independent and impartial body established by domestic law and functioning in accordance with procedures laid down by domestic law. It shall, in formulating its decisions, have the assistance of one or more qualified and independent mental health practitioners and take their advice into account.

2. The review body's initial review, as required by paragraph 2 of Principle 16, of a decision to admit or retain a person as an involuntary patient shall take place as soon as possible after that decision and shall be conducted in accordance with simple and expeditious procedures as specified by domestic law.

3. The review body shall periodically review the cases of involuntary patients at reasonable intervals as specified by domestic law.

4. An involuntary patient may apply to the review body for release or voluntary status, at reasonable intervals as specified by domestic law.

5. At each review, the review body shall consider whether the criteria for involuntary admission set out in paragraph 1 of Principle 16 are still satisfied, and, if not, the patient shall be discharged as an involuntary patient.

6. If at any time the mental health practitioner responsible for the case is satisfied that the conditions for the retention of a person as an involuntary

patient are no longer satisfied, he or she shall order the discharge of that person as such a patient.

7. A patient or his personal representative or any interested person shall have the right to appeal to a higher court against a decision that the patient be admitted to, or be retained in, a mental health facility.

Principle 18
Procedural Safeguards

1. The patient shall be entitled to choose and appoint a counsel to represent the patient as such, including representation in any complaint procedure or appeal. If the patient does not secure such services, a counsel shall be made available without payment by the patient to the extent that the patient lacks sufficient means to pay.

2. The patient shall also be entitled to the assistance, if necessary, of the services of an interpreter. Where such services are necessary and the patient does not secure them, they shall be made available without payment by the patient to the extent that the patient lacks sufficient means to pay.

3. The patient and the patient's counsel may request and produce at any hearing an independent mental health report and any other reports and oral, written and other evidence that are relevant and admissible.

4. Copies of the patient's records and any reports and documents to be submitted shall be given to the patient and to the patient's counsel, except in special cases where it is determined that a specific disclosure to the patient would cause serious harm to the patient's health or put at risk the safety of others. As domestic law may provide, any document not given to the patient should, when this can be done in confidence, be given to the patient's personal representative and counsel. When any part of a document is withheld from a patient, the patient or the patient's counsel, if any, shall receive notice of the withholding and the reasons for it and shall be subject to judicial review.

5. The patient and the patient's personal representative and counsel shall be entitled to attend, participate and be heard personally in any hearing.

6. If the patient or the patient's personal representative or counsel requests that a particular person be present at a hearing, that person shall be admitted unless it is determined that the person's presence could cause serious harm to the patient's health or put at risk the safety of others.

7. Any decision whether the hearing or any part of it shall be in public or in private and may be publicly reported shall give full consideration to the patient's own wishes, to the need to respect the privacy of the patient and of other persons and to the need to prevent serious harm to the patient's health or to avoid putting at risk the safety of others.

8. The decision arising out of the hearing and the reasons for it shall be expressed in writing. Copies shall be given to the patient and his or her personal representative and counsel. In deciding whether the decision shall be published in whole or in part, full consideration shall be given to the patient's own wishes, to the need to respect his or her privacy and that of other persons, to the public interest in the open administration of justice and to the need to prevent serious harm to the patient's health or to avoid putting at risk the safety of others.

Principle 19
Access to Information

1. A patient (which term in this Principle includes a former patient) shall be entitled to have access to the information concerning the patient in his or her health and personal records maintained by a mental health facility. This right may be subject to restrictions in order to prevent serious harm to the patient's health and avoid putting at risk the safety of others. As domestic law may provide, any such information not given to the patient should, when this can be done in confidence, be given to the patient's personal representative and counsel. When any of the information is withheld from a patient, the patient or the patient's counsel, if any, shall receive notice of the withholding and the reasons for it and it shall be subject to judicial review.

2. Any written comments by the patient or the patient's personal representative or counsel shall, on request, be inserted in the patient's file.

Principle 20

Criminal Offenders

1. This Principle applies to persons serving sentences of imprisonment for criminal offences, or who are otherwise detained in the course of criminal proceedings or investigations against them, and who are determined to have a mental illness or who it is believed may have such an illness.

2. All such persons should receive the best available mental health care as provided in Principle 1. These Principles shall apply to them to the fullest extent possible, with only such limited modifications and exceptions as are necessary in the circumstances. No such modifications and exceptions shall prejudice the persons' rights under the instruments noted in paragraph 5 of Principle 1.

3. Domestic law may authorize a court or other competent authority, acting on the basis of competent and independent medical advice, to order that such persons be admitted to a mental health facility.

4. Treatment of persons determined to have a mental illness shall in all circumstances be consistent with Principle 11.

Principle 21

Complaints

Every patient and former patient shall have the right to make a complaint through procedures as specified by domestic law.

Principle 22

Monitoring and Remedies

States shall ensure that appropriate mechanisms are in force to promote compliance with these Principles, for the inspection of mental health facilities, for the submission, investigation and resolution of complaints and for the institution of appropriate disciplinary or judicial proceedings for professional misconduct or violation of the rights of a patient.

Principle 23

Implementation

1. States should implement these Principles through appropriate legislative, judicial, administrative, educational and other measures, which they shall review periodically.

2. States shall make these Principles widely known by appropriate and active means.

Principle 24

Scope of Principles Relating to Mental Health Facilities

These Principles apply to all persons who are admitted to a mental health facility.

Principle 25

Saving of Existing Rights

There shall be no restriction upon or derogation from any existing rights of patients, including rights recognized in applicable international or domestic law, on the pretext that these Principles do not recognize such rights or that they recognize them to a lesser extent.

Draft Comprehensive and Integral International Convention on the Protection and Promotion of the Rights and Dignity of Persons with Disabilities (2004)

Draft text as presented to the Working Group to the Ad Hoc Committee at its session on 5-16 January 2004. UN document A/AC.265/2004/WG/1.
[Available at http://www.un.org/esa/socdev/enable/rights/ahcwgreportax1.htm]

The States Parties to this Convention,

* * *

(e) Recognizing the importance of the principles and policy guidelines contained in the Standard Rules on the Equalization of Opportunities for Persons with Disabilities in influencing the promotion, formulation and evaluation of the policies, plans, programmes and actions at the national, regional and international levels to further equalize opportunities for persons with disabilities,

(f) Recognizing also that discrimination against any person on the basis of disability is a violation of the inherent dignity of the human person,

(g) Recognizing further the diversity of persons with disabilities,

(h) Concerned that, despite the efforts and actions undertaken by Governments, bodies and relevant organizations, persons with disabilities continue to face barriers in their participation as equal members of society and violations to their human rights in all parts of the world,

(i) Emphasizing the importance of international cooperation to promote the full enjoyment of human rights and fundamental freedoms of persons with disabilities,

(j) Emphasizing also the existing and potential contributions made by persons with disabilities to the overall well-being and diversity of their communities, and that the promotion of the full enjoyment by persons with disabilities of their human rights and fundamental freedoms and of full participation by persons with disabilities will result in significant advances in the human, social and economic development of their societies and the eradication of poverty,

(k) Recognizing the importance for persons with disabilities of their individual autonomy and independence, including the freedom to make their own choices,

(l) Considering that persons with disabilities should have the opportunity to be actively involved in decision-making processes about policies and programmes, especially those directly concerning them,

(m) Concerned about the difficult conditions faced by persons with severe or multiple disabilities and of persons with disabilities who are subject to multiple or aggravated forms of discrimination on the basis of race, colour, sex, language, religion, political or other opinion, national or social origin, property, birth or other status,

(n) Emphasizing the need to incorporate a gender perspective in all efforts to promote the full enjoyment of human rights and fundamental freedoms by persons with disabilities,

(o) Mindful of the need to alleviate the negative impact of poverty on the conditions of persons with disabilities,

(p) Concerned that situations of armed conflict have especially devastating consequences for the human rights of persons with disabilities,

(q) Recognizing the importance of accessibility to the physical, social and economic environment and to information and communication, including information and communication technologies, in enabling persons with disabilities to fully enjoy all human rights and fundamental freedoms,

(r) Convinced that a convention dealing specifically with the human rights of persons with disabilities will make a significant contribution to redressing the profound social disadvantage of persons with disabilities and promote their participation in the civil, political, economic, social and cultural spheres with equal opportunities, in both developing and developed countries,

Hereby agree as follows:

Article 1
Purpose

The purpose of this Convention shall be to ensure the full, effective and equal enjoyment of all human rights and fundamental freedoms by persons with disabilities.

Article 2
General Principles

The fundamental principles of this Convention shall be:

(a) Dignity, individual autonomy including the freedom to make one's own choices, and independence of persons;

(b) Non-discrimination;

(c) Full inclusion of persons with disabilities as equal citizens and participants in all aspects of life;

(d) Respect for difference and acceptance of disability as part of human diversity and humanity;

(e) Equality of opportunity.

Article 3
Definitions
* * *

Article 4
General Obligations

1. States Parties undertake to ensure the full realization of all human rights and fundamental freedoms for all individuals within their jurisdiction without discrimination of any kind on the basis of disability. To this end, States Parties undertake:

(a) To adopt legislative, administrative and other measures to give effect to this Convention, and to amend, repeal or nullify any laws and regulations and to discourage customs or practices that are inconsistent with this Convention;

(b) To embody the rights of equality and non-discrimination on the ground of disability in their national constitutions or other appropriate legislation, if not yet incorporated therein, and to ensure, through law and other appropriate means, the practical realization of these rights;

(c) To mainstream disability issues into all economic and social development policies and programmes;

(d) To refrain from engaging in any act or practice that is inconsistent with this Convention and to ensure that public authorities and institutions act in conformity with this Convention;

(e) To take all appropriate measures to eliminate discrimination on the ground of disability by any person, organization or private enterprise;

(f) To promote the development, availability and use of universally designed goods, services, equipment and facilities. Such goods, services, equipment and facilities should require the minimum possible adaptation and the least cost to meet the specific needs of a person with disabilities.

2. In the development and implementation of policies and legislation to implement this Convention, States Parties shall do so in close consultation with, and include the active involvement of, persons with disabilities and their representative organizations.

Article 5. Promotion of Positive Attitudes to Persons with Disabilities
* * *

Article 6. Statistics and Data Collection
* * *

Article 7
Equality and Non-Discrimination

1. States Parties recognize that all persons are equal before the law and are entitled without any discrimination to the equal protection of the law. States Parties shall prohibit any discrimination on the basis of disability, and guarantee to all persons with disabilities equal and effective protection against discrimination. States Parties shall also prohibit any discrimination and guarantee to all persons with disabilities equal and effective pro-

tection against discrimination on any ground such as race, colour, sex, language, religion, political or other opinion, national or social origin, property, birth, source or type of disability, age or any other status.

2. (a) Discrimination shall mean any distinction, exclusion or restriction which has the purpose or effect of impairing or nullifying the recognition, enjoyment or exercise by persons with disabilities, on an equal footing, of all human rights and fundamental freedoms.

(b) Discrimination shall include all forms of discrimination, including direct, indirect and systemic, and shall also include discrimination based on an actual or perceived disability.

3. Discrimination does not include a provision, criterion or practice that is objectively and demonstrably justified by the State Party by a legitimate aim and where the means of achieving that aim are reasonable and necessary.

4. In order to secure the right to equality for persons with disabilities, States Parties undertake to take all appropriate steps, including by legislation, to provide reasonable accommodation, defined as necessary and appropriate modification and adjustments to guarantee to persons with disabilities the enjoyment or exercise on an equal footing of all human rights and fundamental freedoms, unless such measures would impose a disproportionate burden.

5. Special measures aimed at accelerating de facto equality of persons with disabilities shall not be considered discrimination as defined in the present Convention, but shall in no way entail as a consequence the maintenance of unequal or separate standards; those measures shall be discontinued when the objectives of equality of opportunity and treatment have been achieved.

Article 8. Right to Life
* * *

Article 9. Equal Recognition as a Person Before the Law
* * *

Article 10. Liberty and Security of the Person
* * *

Article 11. Freedom from Torture or Cruel,

Inhuman or Degrading Treatment or Punishment
* * *

Article 12. Freedom from Violence and Abuse
* * *

Article 13. Freedom of Expression and Opinion and Access to Information
* * *

Article 14. Respect for Privacy, the Home and the Family
* * *

Article 15. Living Independently and Being Included in the Community
* * *

Article 16. Children with Disabilities
* * *

Article 17. Education
* * *

Article 18. Participation in Political and Public Life
* * *

Article 19. Accessibility
* * *

Article 20. Personal Mobility
* * *

Article 21
Right to Health and Rehabilitation

States Parties recognize that all persons with disabilities have the right to the enjoyment of the highest attainable standard of health without discrimination on the basis of disability. States Parties shall strive to ensure no person with a disability is deprived of that right, and shall take all appropriate measures to ensure access for persons with disabilities to health and rehabilitation services. In particular, States Parties shall:

(a) Provide persons with disabilities with the same range and standard of health and rehabilitation services as provided other citizens, including sexual and reproductive health services;

(b) Strive to provide those health and rehabilitation services needed by persons with disabilities specifically because of their disabilities;

(c) Endeavour to provide these health and rehabilitation services as close as possible to people's own communities;

(d) Ensure that health and rehabilitation services include the provision of safe respite places, to use on a voluntary basis, and counselling and support groups, including those provided by persons with disabilities;

(e) Provide programmes and services to prevent and protect against secondary disabilities, including among children and the elderly;

(f) Encourage research and the development, dissemination and application of new knowledge and technologies that benefit persons with disabilities;

(g) Encourage the development of sufficient numbers of health and rehabilitation professionals, including persons who have disabilities, covering all disciplines needed to meet the health and rehabilitation needs of persons with disabilities, and ensure that they have adequate specialized training;

(h) Provide to all health and rehabilitation professionals an appropriate education and training to increase their disability-sensitive awareness and respect for the rights, dignity and needs of persons with disabilities, in line with the principles of this Convention;

(i) Ensure that a code of ethics for public and private health care, which promotes quality care, openness and respect for the human rights, dignity and autonomy of persons with disabilities, is put in place nationally, and ensure that the services and conditions of public and private health care and rehabilitation facilities and institutions are well monitored;

(j) Ensure that health and rehabilitation services provided to persons with disabilities, and the sharing of their personal health or rehabilitation information, occur only after the person concerned has given their free and informed consent, and that health and rehabilitation professionals inform persons with disabilities of their relevant rights;

(k) Prevent unwanted medical and related interventions and corrective surgeries from being imposed on persons with disabilities;

(l) Protect the privacy of health and rehabilitation information of persons with disabilities on an equal basis;

(m) Promote the involvement of persons with disabilities and their organizations in the formulation of health and rehabilitation legislation and policy as well as in the planning, delivery and evaluation of health and rehabilitation services.

Article 22. Right to Work
* * *
Article 23. Social Security and an Adequate Standard of Living
* * *
Article 24. Participation in Cultural Life, Recreation, Leisure and Sport
* * *
Article 25. Monitoring
* * *
National Implementation Framework
* * *

D. Rights of Older Persons

World Medical Association Declaration on the Abuse of the Elderly (1989, 1990)

Adopted by the 41st World Medical Assembly, Hong Kong, September 1989 and editorially revised at the 126th Council Session, Jerusalem, Israel, May 1990.
[Available at http://www.wma.net/e/policy/a4.htm]

Elderly people may suffer pathological problems such as motor disturbances and psychic and orientation disorders. As a result of such problems, elderly patients may require assistance with their daily activities which, in turn can lead to a state of dependence. Such a situation may cause their families and the community to consider them to be a burden and to limit care and services to a minimum. It is against this background that the subject of abuse of the elderly must be considered.

Abuse of the elderly can be manifested in a variety of ways, such as physical, psychological, and financial and/or material, medical abuse or self-neglect. Variations in the definition of elder abuse present difficulties in comparing findings on the nature and causes of the problem. A number of preliminary hypotheses have been proposed on the etiology of elder abuse, including: dependency on others to provide services; lack of close family ties; family violence; lack of financial resources; psychopathology of the abuser; lack of community support, and institutional factors such as low pay and poor working conditions that contribute to pessimistic attitudes of caretakers, resulting in neglect of the elderly.

The phenomenon of elder abuse is becoming increasingly recognized by both medical facilities and social agencies. Physicians played a prominent role in the child abuse movement by defining and publicizing the problem and in shaping public policy. Elder abuse, however, has just recently attracted the attention of the medical profession. The first step in preventing elder abuse and neglect is to increase levels of awareness and knowledge among physicians and other health professionals. Once high-risk individuals and families have been identified, physicians can participate in the primary prevention of maltreatment by making referrals to appropriate community and social service centers. Physicians may also participate by providing support and information on high risk situations directly to patients and their families.

The World Medical Association therefore adopts the following General Principles relating to abuse of the elderly.

GENERAL PRINCIPLES

The elderly have the same rights to care, welfare and respect as other human beings.

The World Medical Association recognizes that it is the physicians' responsibility to help prevent the physical and psychological abuse of elderly patients.

Physicians whether consulted by an aged person directly, the nursing home or the family will see that the patient receives the best possible care.

If in terms of this statement physicians verify or suspect ill treatment, they will discuss the situation with those in charge, be it the nursing home or the family. If ill treatment is confirmed, or death is considered to be suspicious, they will report to the relevant authorities.

To guarantee protection of the elderly in any environment there should be no restrictions on their right of free choice of physician. National member associations will strive to make certain that such free choice is preserved within the socio-medical system.

The World Medical Association also makes the following recommendations to physicians involved in treating the elderly, and urges all National Medical Associations to publicize this Declaration to their members and the public.

RECOMMENDATIONS

Physicians involved in treating the elderly should:

• identify the elder who may have been abused and/or neglected

• identify the elder who may have been abused and/or neglected

• remain objective and nonjudgmental

• attempt to establish or maintain a therapeutic alliance with the family (often the physician is the only professional who maintains long-term contact with the patient and the family)

• report all suspected cases of elder abuse and/or neglect in accordance with local statutes

• encourage the development and utilization of supportive community resources that provide in-home services, respite care, and stress reduction with high-risk families.

General Comment 6: The Economic, Social and Cultural Rights of Older Persons (1995)
Adopted by the Committee on Economic, Social and Cultural Rights on 8 December 1995. UN document E/1996/22.
[Available at http://www.unhchr.ch/tbs/doc.nsf/099b725fe87555ec8025670c004 fc803/482a0aced8049067c12563ed005acf9e?OpenDocument#*%20Contained]

[Footnotes omitted.]

1. INTRODUCTION

1. The world population is ageing at a steady, quite spectacular rate. The total number of persons aged 60 and above rose from 200 million in 1950 to 400 million in 1982 and is projected to reach 600 million in the year 2001 and 1.2 billion by the year 2025, at which time over 70 per cent of them will be living in what are today's developing countries. The number of people aged 80 and above has grown and continues to grow even more dramatically, going from 13 million in 1950 to over 50 million today and projected to increase to 137 million in 2025. This is the fastest growing population group in the world, projected to increase by a factor of 10 between 1950 and 2025, compared with a factor of six for the group aged 60 and above and a factor of little more than three for the total population.

2. These figures are illustrations of a quiet revolution, but one which has far-reaching and unpredictable consequences and which is now affecting the social and economic structures of societies both at the world level and at the country level, and will affect them even more in future.

3. Most of the States parties to the Covenant, and the industrialized countries in particular, are faced with the task of adapting their social and economic policies to the ageing of their populations, especially as regards social security. In the developing countries, the absence or deficiencies of social security coverage are being aggravated by the emigration of the younger members of the population and the consequent weakening of the traditional role of the family, the main support of older people.

2. INTERNATIONALLY ENDORSED POLICIES IN RELATION TO OLDER PERSONS

4. In 1982 the World Assembly on Ageing adopted the Vienna International Plan of Action on Ageing. This important document was endorsed by the General Assembly and is a very useful guide, for it details the measures that should be taken by Member States to safeguard the rights of older persons within the context of the rights proclaimed by the International Covenants on Human Rights. It contains 62 recommendations, many of which are of direct relevance to the Covenant.

5. In 1991 the General Assembly adopted the United Nations Principles for Older Persons which, because of their programmatic nature, is

also an important document in the present context. It is divided into five sections which correlate closely to the rights recognized in the Covenant. "Independence" includes access to adequate food, water, shelter, clothing and health care. To these basic rights are added the opportunity to remunerated work and access to education and training. By "participation" is meant that older persons should participate actively in the formulation and implementation of policies that affect their well-being and share their knowledge and skills with younger generations, and should be able to form movements and associations. The section headed "care" proclaims that older persons should benefit from family care, health care and be able to enjoy human rights and fundamental freedoms when residing in a shelter, care or treatment facility. With regard to "self-fulfilment", the Principles that older persons should pursue opportunities for the full development of their potential through access to the educational, cultural, spiritual and recreational resources of their societies. Lastly, the section entitled "dignity" states that older persons should be able to live in dignity and security and be free of exploitation and physical or mental abuse, should be treated fairly, regardless of age, gender, racial or ethnic background, disability, financial situation or any other status, and be valued independently of their economic contribution.

6. In 1992, the General Assembly adopted eight global targets on ageing for the year 2001 and a brief guide for setting national targets. In a number of important respects, these global targets serve to reinforce the obligations of States parties to the Covenant.

7. Also in 1992, and in commemoration of the tenth anniversary of the adoption of the Vienna International Plan of Action by the Conference on Ageing, the General Assembly adopted the Proclamation on Ageing in which it urged support of national initiatives on ageing so that older women are given adequate support for their largely unrecognized contributions to society and older men are encouraged to develop social, cultural and emotional capacities which they may have been prevented from developing during breadwinning years; families are supported in providing care and all family members encouraged to cooperate in caregiving; and that international co-operation is expanded in the context of the strategies for reaching the global targets on ageing for the year 2001. It also proclaimed the year 1999 as the International Year of Older Persons in recognition of humanity's demographic "coming of age".

8. The United Nations specialized agencies, especially the International Labour Organization, have also given attention to the problem of ageing in their respective fields of competence.

3. THE RIGHTS OF OLDER PERSONS IN RELATION TO THE INTERNATIONAL COVENANT ON ECONOMIC, SOCIAL AND CULTURAL RIGHTS

9. The terminology used to describe older persons varies considerably, even in international documents. It includes: "older persons", "the aged", "the elderly", "the third age", "the ageing", and, to denote persons more than 80 years of age, "the fourth age". The Committee opted for "older persons" (in French, personnes âgées; in Spanish, personas mayores), the term employed in General Assembly resolutions 47/5 and 48/98. According to the practice in the United Nations statistical services, these terms cover persons aged 60 and above (Eurostat, the statistical service of the European Union, considers "older persons" to mean persons aged 65 or above, since 65 is the most common age of retirement and the trend is towards later retirement still).

10. The International Covenant on Economic, Social and Cultural Rights does not contain any explicit reference to the rights of older persons, although article 9 dealing with "the right of everyone to social security, including social insurance", implicitly recognizes the right to old-age benefits. Nevertheless, in view of the fact that the Covenant's provisions apply fully to all members of society, it is clear that older persons are entitled to enjoy the full range of rights recognized in the Covenant. This approach is also fully reflected in the Vienna International Plan of Action on Ageing. Moreover, in so far as respect for the rights of older persons requires special measures to be taken, States parties are required by the Covenant to do so to the maximum of their available resources.

11. Another important issue is whether discrimination on the basis of age is Prohibited by the Covenant. Neither the Covenant nor the Universal Declaration of Human Rights refers explicitly to age as one of the prohibited grounds. Rather than being seen as an intentional exclusion, this omission is probably best explained by the fact that, when these instruments were adopted, the problem of demographic ageing was not as evident or as pressing as it is now.

12. This is not determinative of the matter, however, since the prohibition of discrimination on the grounds of "other status" could be interpreted as applying to age. The Committee notes that while it may not yet be possible to conclude that discrimination on the grounds of age is comprehensively prohibited by the Covenant, the range of matters in relation to which such discrimination can be accepted is very limited. Moreover, it must be emphasized that the unacceptableness of discrimination against older persons is underlined in many international policy documents and is confirmed in the legislation of the vast majority of States. In the few areas in which discrimination continues to be tolerated, such as in relation to mandatory retirement ages or access to tertiary education, there is a clear trend towards the elimination of such barriers. The Committee is of the view that States parties should seek to expedite this trend to the greatest extent possible.

13. Accordingly, the Committee on Economic, Social and Cultural Rights is of the view that States parties to the Covenant are obligated to pay particular attention to promoting and protecting the economic, social and cultural rights of older persons. The Committee's own role in this regard is rendered all the more important by the fact that, unlike the case of other population groups such as women and children, no comprehensive international convention yet exists in relation to the rights of older persons and no binding supervisory arrangements attach to the various sets of United Nations principles in this area.

14. By the end of its thirteenth session, the Committee and, before that, its predecessor, the Sessional Working Group of Governmental Experts, had examined 144 initial reports, 70 second periodic reports and 20 initial and periodic global reports on articles 1 to 15. This examination made it possible to identify many of the problems that may be encountered in implementing the Covenant in a considerable number of States parties that represent all the regions of the world and have different political, socio-economic and cultural systems. The reports examined to date have not provided any information in a systematic way on the situation of older persons with regard to compliance with the Covenant, apart from information, of varying completeness, on the implementation of article 9 relating to the right to social security.

15. In 1993, the Committee devoted a day of general discussion to this issue in order to plan its future activity in this area. Moreover, it has, at recent sessions, begun to attach substantially more importance to information on the rights of older persons and its questioning has elicited some very valuable information in some instances. Nevertheless, the Committee notes that the great majority of States parties reports continue to make little reference to this important issue. It therefore wishes to indicate that, in future, it will insist that the situation of older persons in relation to each of the rights recognized in the Covenant should be adequately addressed in all reports. The remainder of this General Comment identifies the specific issues which are relevant in this regard.

4. GENERAL OBLIGATIONS OF STATES PARTIES

16. Older persons as a group are as heterogeneous and varied as the rest of the population and their situation depends on a country's economic and social situation, on demographic, environmental cultural and employment factors and, at the individual level, on the family situation, the level of education, the urban or rural environment and the occupation of workers and retirees.

17. Side by side with older persons who are in good health and whose financial situation is acceptable, there are many who do not have adequate means of support, even in developed countries, and who feature prominently among the most vulnerable, marginal and unprotected groups. In times of recession and of restructuring of the economy, older persons are particularly at risk. As the Committee has previously stressed (General Comment No. 3 (1990), para. 12), even in times of severe resource constraints, States parties have the duty to protect the vulnerable members of society.

18. The methods that States parties use to fulfil the obligations they have assumed under the Covenant in respect of older persons will be basically the same as those for the fulfilment of other obligations (see General Comment No. 1 (1989)). They include the need to determine the nature and scope of problems within a State through regular monitoring, the need to adopt properly designed policies and programmes to meet requirements, the need to enact legislation when necessary and to eliminate any discriminatory legislation and the need to ensure the relevant budget support or, as appropriate, to request international cooperation. In the latter connection, international cooperation in accordance with articles 22 and 23 of the Covenant may be a particularly important way of enabling some developing countries to fulfil their obligations under the Covenant.

19. In this context, attention may be drawn to Global target No. 1, adopted by the General Assembly in 1992, which calls for the establishment of national support infrastructures to promote policies and programmes on ageing in national and international development plans and programmes. In this regard, the Committee notes that one of the United Nations Principles for Older Persons which Governments were encouraged to incorporate into their national programmes is that older persons should be able to form movements or associations of older persons.

5. SPECIFIC PROVISIONS OF THE COVENANT

Article 3: Equal Rights of Men and Women
* * *

Articles 6 to 8: Rights Relating to Work
* * *

Article 9: Right to Social Security
* * *

Article 10: Protection of the Family
* * *

Article 11: Right to an Adequate Standard of Living
* * *

Article 12
Right to Physical and Mental Health

34. With a view to the realization of the right of elderly persons to the enjoyment of a satisfactory standard of physical and mental health, in accordance with article 12, paragraph 1, of the Covenant, States parties should take account of the content of recommendations 1 to 17 of the Vienna International Plan of Action on Ageing, which focus entirely on providing guidelines on health policy to preserve the health of the elderly and take a comprehensive view, ranging from prevention and rehabilitation to the care of the terminally ill.

35. Clearly, the growing number of chronic, degenerative diseases and the high hospitalization costs they involve cannot be dealt with only by curative treatment. In this regard, States parties should bear in mind that maintaining health into old age requires investments during the entire life span, basically through the adoption of healthy lifestyles (food, exercise, elimination of tobacco and alcohol, etc.). Prevention, through regular checks suited to the needs of the elderly, plays a decisive role, as does rehabilitation, by maintaining the functional capacities of elderly persons, with a resulting decrease in the cost of investments in health care and social services.

Articles 13 to 15: Right to Education and Culture

* * *

E. Refugees and Displaced Persons

Convention Relating to the Status of Refugees (1951)
Adopted on 28 July 1951 by the United Nations Conference of Plenipotentiaries on the Status of Refugees and Stateless Persons. Entered into force 22 April 1954
[Available at http://www.unhchr.ch/html/menu3/b/o_c_ref.htm]

PREAMBLE

The High Contracting Parties,

Considering that the Charter of the United Nations and the Universal Declaration of Human Rights approved on 10 December 1948 by the General Assembly have affirmed the principle that human beings shall enjoy fundamental rights and freedoms without discrimination,

Considering that the United Nations has, on various occasions, manifested its profound concern for refugees and endeavoured to assure refugees the widest possible exercise of these fundamental rights and freedoms,

* * *

Have agreed as follows:

CHAPTER I: GENERAL PROVISIONS

Article 1
Definition of the Term "Refugee"

A. For the purposes of the present Convention, the term "refugee" shall apply to any person who:

(1) Has been considered a refugee under the Arrangements of 12 May 1926 and 30 June 1928 or under the Conventions of 28 October 1933 and 10 February 1938, the Protocol of 14 September 1939 or the Constitution of the International Refugee Organization;

Decisions of non-eligibility taken by the International Refugee Organization during the period of its activities shall not prevent the status of refugee being accorded to persons who fulfil the conditions of paragraph 2 of this section;

(2) As a result of events occurring before 1 January 1951 and owing to well-founded fear of being persecuted for reasons of race, religion, nationality, membership of a particular social group or political opinion, is outside the country of his nationality and is unable, or owing to such fear, is unwilling to avail himself of the protection of that country; or who, not having a nationality and being outside the country of his former habitual residence as a result of such events, is unable or, owing to such fear, is unwilling to return to it.

In the case of a person who has more than one nationality, the term "the country of his nationality" shall mean each of the countries of which he is a national, and a person shall not be deemed to be lacking the protection of the country of his nationality if, without any valid reason based on well-founded fear, he has not availed himself of the protection of one of the countries of which he is a national.

B. (1) For the purposes of this Convention, the words "events occurring before 1 January 1951" in article 1, section A, shall be understood to mean either (a) "events occurring in Europe before 1 January 1951"; or (b) "events occurring in Europe or elsewhere before 1 January 1951"; and each Contracting State shall make a declaration at the time of signature, ratification or accession, specifying which of these meanings it applies for the purpose of its obligations under this Convention.

(2) Any Contracting State which has adopted alternative (a) may at any time extend its obligations by adopting alternative (b) by means of a notification addressed to the Secretary-General of the United Nations.

C. This Convention shall cease to apply to any person falling under the terms of section A if:

(1) He has voluntarily re-availed himself of the protection of the country of his nationality; or

(2) Having lost his nationality, he has voluntarily re-acquired it; or

(3) He has acquired a new nationality, and enjoys the protection of the country of his new nationality; or

(4) He has voluntarily re-established himself in the country which he left or outside which he remained owing to fear of persecution; or

(5) He can no longer, because the circumstances in connection with which he has been recognized as a refugee have ceased to exist, continue to refuse to avail himself of the protection of the country of his nationality;

Provided that this paragraph shall not apply to a refugee falling under section A (1) of this article who is able to invoke compelling reasons arising out of previous persecution for refusing to avail himself of the protection of the country of nationality;

(6) Being a person who has no nationality he is, because the circumstances in connection with which he has been recognized as a refugee have ceased to exist, able to return to the country of his former habitual residence;

Provided that this paragraph shall not apply to a refugee falling under section A (1) of this article who is able to invoke compelling reasons arising out of previous persecution for refusing to return to the country of his former habitual residence.

D. This Convention shall not apply to persons who are at present receiving from organs or agencies of the United Nations other than the United Nations High Commissioner for Refugees protection or assistance.

When such protection or assistance has ceased for any reason, without the position of such persons being definitively settled in accordance with the relevant resolutions adopted by the General Assembly of the United Nations, these persons shall ipso facto be entitled to the benefits of this Convention.

E. This Convention shall not apply to a person who is recognized by the competent authorities of the country in which he has taken residence as having the rights and obligations which are attached to the possession of the nationality of that country.

F. The provisions of this Convention shall not apply to any person with respect to whom there are serious reasons for considering that.

(a) He has committed a crime against peace, a war crime, or a crime against humanity, as defined in the international instruments drawn up to make provision in respect of such crimes;

(b) He has committed a serious non-political crime outside the country of refuge prior to his admission to that country as a refugee;

(c) He has been guilty of acts contrary to the purposes and principles of the United Nations.

Article 2
General Obligations

Every refugee has duties to the country in which he finds himself, which require in particular that he conform to its laws and regulations as well as to measures taken for the maintenance of public order.

Article 3
Non-Discrimination

The Contracting States shall apply the provisions of this Convention to refugees without discrimination as to race, religion or country of origin.

Article 4
Religion

The Contracting States shall accord to refugees within their territories treatment at least as favourable as that accorded to their nationals with respect to freedom to practise their religion and freedom as regards the religious education of their children.

Article 5
Rights Granted Apart from
This Convention

Nothing in this Convention shall be deemed to impair any rights and benefits granted by a Contracting State to refugees apart from this Convention.

Article 6
The Term "in the same circumstances"

For the purposes of this Convention, the term "in the same circumstances," implies that any requirements (including requirements as to length and conditions of sojourn or residence) which the particular individual would have to fulfil for the enjoyment of the right in question, if he were not a refugee, must be fulfilled by him, with the exception of requirements which by their nature a refugee is incapable of fulfilling.

Article 7
Exemption from Reciprocity

* * *

Article 8
Exemption from Exceptional Measures

* * *

Article 9
Provisional Measures

Nothing in this Convention shall prevent a Contracting State, in time of war or other grave and exceptional circumstances, from taking provisionally measures which it considers to be essential to the national security in the case of a particular person, pending a determination by the Contracting State that that person is in fact a refugee and that the continuance of such measures is necessary in his case in the interests of national security.

Article 10
Continuity of Residence

* * *

Article 11
Refugee Seamen

* * *

CHAPTER II: JURIDICAL STATUS
Article 12
Personal Status

1. The personal status of a refugee shall be governed by the law of the country of his domicile or, if he has no domicile, by the law of the country of his residence.

2. Rights previously acquired by a refugee and dependent on personal status, more particularly rights attaching to marriage, shall be respected by a Contracting State, subject to compliance, if this be necessary, with the formalities required by the law of that State, provided that the right in question is one which would have been recognized by the law of that State had he not become a refugee.

Article 13
Movable and Immovable Property

The Contracting States shall accord to a refugee treatment as favourable as possible and, in any event, not less favourable than that accorded to aliens generally in the same circumstances, as regards the acquisition of movable and immovable property and other rights pertaining thereto, and to leases and other contracts relating to movable and immovable property.

Article 14
Artistic Rights and Industrial Property

In respect of the protection of industrial property, such as inventions, designs or models, trade marks, trade names, and of rights in literary, artistic and scientific works, a refugee shall be accorded in the country in which he has his habitual residence the same protection as is accorded to nationals of that country. In the territory of any other Contracting States, he shall be accorded the same protection as is accorded in that territory to nationals of the country in which he has his habitual residence.

Article 15
Right of Association

As regards non-political and non-profit-making associations and trade unions the Contracting States shall accord to refugees lawfully staying in their territory the most favourable treatment accorded to nationals of a foreign country, in the same circumstances.

Article 16
Access to Courts

1. A refugee shall have free access to the courts of law on the territory of all Contracting States.

2. A refugee shall enjoy in the Contracting State in which he has his habitual residence the same treatment as a national in matters pertaining to access to the courts, including legal assistance and exemption from cautio judicatum solvi.

3. A refugee shall be accorded in the matters referred to in paragraph 2 in countries other than that in which he has his habitual residence the treatment granted to a national of the country of his habitual residence.

CHAPTER III:
GAINFUL EMPLOYMENT

Article 17
Wage-Earning Employment

1. The Contracting States shall accord to refugees lawfully staying in their territory the most favourable treatment accorded to nationals of a foreign country in the same circumstances, as regards the right to engage in wage-earning employment.

2. In any case, restrictive measures imposed on aliens or the employment of aliens for the protection of the national labour market shall not be applied to a refugee who was already exempt from them at the date of entry into force of this Convention for the Contracting State concerned, or who fulfils one of the following conditions:

(a) He has completed three years' residence in the country;

(b) He has a spouse possessing the nationality of the country of residence. A refugee may not invoke the benefit of this provision if he has abandoned his spouse;

(c) He has one or more children possessing the nationality of the country of residence.

3. The Contracting States shall give sympathetic consideration to assimilating the rights of all refugees with regard to wage-earning employment to those of nationals, and in particular of those refugees who have entered their territory pursuant to programmes of labour recruitment or under immigration schemes.

Article 18
Self-Employment

The Contracting States shall accord to a refugee lawfully in their territory treatment as favourable as possible and, in any event, not less favourable than that accorded to aliens generally in the same circumstances, as regards the right to engage on his own account in agriculture, industry, handi-crafts and commerce and to establish commercial and industrial companies.

Article 19
Liberal Professions

1. Each Contracting State shall accord to refugees lawfully staying in their territory who hold diplomas recognized by the competent authorities of that State, and who are desirous of practising a liberal profession, treatment as favourable as possible and, in any event, not less favourable than that accorded to aliens generally in the same circumstances.

2. The Contracting States shall use their best endeavours consistently with their laws and constitutions to secure the settlement of such refugees in the territories, other than the metropolitan territory, for whose international relations they are responsible.

CHAPTER IV: WELFARE

Article 20
Rationing

Where a rationing system exists, which applies to the population at large and regulates the general distribution of products in short supply, refugees shall be accorded the same treatment as nationals.

Article 21
Housing

As regards housing, the Contracting States, in so far as the matter is regulated by laws or regulations or is subject to the control of public authorities, shall accord to refugees lawfully staying in their territory treatment as favourable as possible and, in any event, not less favourable than that accorded to aliens generally in the same circumstances.

Article 22
Public Education

1. The Contracting States shall accord to refugees the same treatment as is accorded to nationals with respect to elementary education.

2. The Contracting States shall accord to refugees treatment as favourable as possible, and, in any event, not less favourable than that accorded to aliens generally in the same circumstances, with respect to education other than elementary educa-

tion and, in particular, as regards access to studies, the recognition of foreign school certificates, diplomas and degrees, the remission of fees and charges and the award of scholarships.

Article 23
Public Relief

The Contracting States shall accord to refugees lawfully staying in their territory the same treatment with respect to public relief and assistance as is accorded to their nationals.

Article 24
Labour Legislation and Social Security

1. The Contracting States shall accord to refugees lawfully staying in their territory the same treatment as is accorded to nationals in respect of the following matters;

(a) In so far as such matters are governed by laws or regulations or are subject to the control of administrative authorities: remuneration, including family allowances where these form part of remuneration, hours of work, overtime arrangements, holidays with pay, restrictions on home work, minimum age of employment, apprenticeship and training, women's work and the work of young persons, and the enjoyment of the benefits of collective bargaining;

(b) Social security (legal provisions in respect of employment injury, occupational diseases, maternity, sickness, disability, old age, death, unemployment, family responsibilities and any other contingency which, according to national laws or regulations, is covered by a social security scheme), subject to the following limitations:

(i) There may be appropriate arrangements for the maintenance of acquired rights and rights in course of acquisition;

(ii) National laws or regulations of the country of residence may prescribe special arrangements concerning benefits or portions of benefits which are payable wholly out of public funds, and concerning allowances paid to persons who do not fulfil the contribution conditions prescribed for the award of a normal pension.

2. The right to compensation for the death of a refugee resulting from employment injury or from occupational disease shall not be affected by the fact that the residence of the beneficiary is outside the territory of the Contracting State.

3. The Contracting States shall extend to refugees the benefits of agreements concluded between them, or which may be concluded between them in the future, concerning the maintenance of acquired rights and rights in the process of acquisition in regard to social security, subject only to the conditions which apply to nationals of the States signatory to the agreements in question.

4. The Contracting States will give sympathetic consideration to extending to refugees so far as possible the benefits of similar agreements which may at any time be in force between such Contracting States and non-contracting States.

CHAPTER V: ADMINISTRATIVE MEASURES
Article 25
Administrative Assistance

* * *

Article 26
Freedom of Movement

Each Contracting State shall accord to refugees lawfully in its territory the right to choose their place of residence and to move freely within its territory subject to any regulations applicable to aliens generally in the same circumstances.

Article 27
Identity Papers

The Contracting States shall issue identity papers to any refugee in their territory who does not possess a valid travel document.

Article 28
Travel Documents

1. The Contracting States shall issue to refugees lawfully staying in their territory travel documents for the purpose of travel outside their territory, unless compelling reasons of national security or public order otherwise require, and the provisions of the Schedule to this Convention shall apply with respect to such documents. The Contracting States may issue such a travel document to any other refugee in their territory; they shall in particular give sympathetic consideration to the issue of

such a travel document to refugees in their territory who are unable to obtain a travel document from the country of their lawful residence.

2. Travel documents issued to refugees under previous international agreements by Parties thereto shall be recognized and treated by the Contracting States in the same way as if they had been issued pursuant to this article.

Article 29
Fiscal Charges

1. The Contracting States shall not impose upon refugees duties, charges or taxes, of any description whatsoever, other or higher than those which are or may be levied on their nationals in similar situations.

2. Nothing in the above paragraph shall prevent the application to refugees of the laws and regulations concerning charges in respect of the issue to aliens of administrative documents including identity papers.

Article 30
Transfer of Assets

* * *

Article 31
Refugees Unlawfully in the Country of Refuge

1. The Contracting States shall not impose penalties, on account of their illegal entry or presence, on refugees who, coming directly from a territory where their life or freedom was threatened in the sense of article 1, enter or are present in their territory without authorization, provided they present themselves without delay to the authorities and show good cause for their illegal entry or presence.

2. The Contracting States shall not apply to the movements of such refugees restrictions other than those which are necessary and such restrictions shall only be applied until their status in the country is regularized or they obtain admission into another country. The Contracting States shall allow such refugees a reasonable period and all the necessary facilities to obtain admission into another country.

Article 32
Expulsion

1. The Contracting States shall not expel a refugee lawfully in their territory save on grounds of national security or public order.

2. The expulsion of such a refugee shall be only in pursuance of a decision reached in accordance with due process of law. Except where compelling reasons of national security otherwise require, the refugee shall be allowed to submit evidence to clear himself, and to appeal to and be represented for the purpose before competent authority or a person or persons specially designated by the competent authority.

3. The Contracting States shall allow such a refugee a reasonable period within which to seek legal admission into another country. The Contracting States reserve the right to apply during that period such internal measures as they may deem necessary.

Article 33
Prohibition of Expulsion
or Return ("Refoulement")

1. No Contracting State shall expel or return ("refouler") a refugee in any manner whatsoever to the frontiers of territories where his life or freedom would be threatened on account of his race, religion, nationality, membership in a particular social group or political opinion.

2. The benefit of the present provision may not, however, be claimed by a refugee whom there are reasonable grounds for regarding as a danger to the security of the country in which he is, or who, having been convicted by a final judgement of a particularly serious crime, constitutes a danger to the community of that country.

Article 34
Naturalization

The Contracting States shall as far as possible facilitate the assimilation and naturalization of refugees. They shall in particular make every effort to expedite naturalization proceedings and to reduce as far as possible the charges and costs of such proceedings.

CHAPTER VI: EXECUTORY AND TRANSITORY PROVISIONS

Article 35
Co-Operation of the National Authorities with the United Nations

* * *

Article 36
Information on National Legislation

* * *

Article 37
Relation to Previous Conventions

* * *

CHAPTER VII: FINAL CLAUSES

Article 38
Settlement of Disputes

Any dispute between Parties to this Convention relating to its interpretation or application, which cannot be settled by other means, shall be referred to the International Court of Justice at the request of any one of the parties to the dispute.

Article 39
Signature, Ratification and Accession

* * *

Article 40
Territorial Application Clause

* * *

Article 41
Federal Clause

* * *

Article 42
Reservations

1. At the time of signature, ratification or accession, any State may make reservations to articles of the Convention other than to articles 1, 3, 4, 16 (1), 33, 36-46 inclusive.

2. Any State making a reservation in accordance with paragraph 1 of this article may at any time withdraw the reservation by a communication to that effect addressed to the Secretary-General of the United Nations.

Article 43
Entry into Force

* * *

Article 44
Denunciation

* * *

Article 46
Notifications by the Secretary-General of the United Nations

* * *

IN FAITH WHEREOF the undersigned, duly authorized, have signed this Convention on behalf of their respective Governments.

DONE at Geneva, this twenty-eighth day of July, one thousand nine hundred and fifty-one, in a single copy, of which the English and French texts are equally authentic and which shall remain deposited in the archives of the United Nations, and certified true copies of which shall be delivered to all Members of the United Nations and to the non-member States referred to in article 39.

Guiding Principles on Internal Displacement (1998)

Prepared at the request of the Commission on Human Rights and the General Assembly by the Representative of the Secretary General on internally displaced and contained in UN Doc. No. E/CN.4/1998/53/Add.2 of 11 February 1998.
[Available at http://www.reliefweb.int/ocha_ol/pub/idp_gp/idp.html]

A. INTRODUCTION: SCOPE AND PURPOSE

1. These Guiding Principles address the specific needs of internally displaced persons worldwide. They identify rights and guarantees relevant to the protection of persons from forced displacement and to their protection and assistance during displacement as well as during return or resettlement and reintegration.

2. For the purposes of these Principles, internally displaced persons are persons or groups of persons who have been forced or obliged to flee or to leave their homes or places of habitual residence, in particular as a result of or in order to avoid the effects of armed conflict, situations of generalized violence, violations of human rights or natural or human-made disasters, and who have not crossed an internationally recognized State border.

3. These Principles reflect and are consistent with international human rights law and international humanitarian law. They provide guidance to:

(a) The Representative of the Secretary-General on internally displaced persons in carrying out his mandate;

(b) States when faced with the phenomenon of internal displacement;

(c) All other authorities, groups and persons in their relations with internally displaced persons; and

(d) Intergovernmental and non-governmental organizations when addressing internal displacement.

4. These Guiding Principles should be disseminated and applied as widely as possible.

SECTION I
GENERAL PRINCIPLES

Principle 1

1. Internally displaced persons shall enjoy, in full equality, the same rights and freedoms under international and domestic law as do other persons in their country. They shall not be discriminated against in the enjoyment of any rights and freedoms on the ground that they are internally displaced.

2. These Principles are without prejudice to individual criminal responsibility under international law, in particular relating to genocide, crimes against humanity and war crimes.

Principle 2

1. These Principles shall be observed by all authorities, groups and persons irrespective of their legal status and applied without any adverse distinction. The observance of these Principles shall not affect the legal status of any authorities, groups or persons involved.

2. These Principles shall not be interpreted as restricting, modifying or impairing the provisions of any international human rights or international humanitarian law instrument or rights granted to persons under domestic law. In particular, these Principles are without prejudice to the right to seek and enjoy asylum in other countries.

Principle 3

1. National authorities have the primary duty and responsibility to provide protection and humanitarian assistance to internally displaced persons within their jurisdiction.

2. Internally displaced persons have the right to request and to receive protection and humanitarian assistance from these authorities. They shall not be persecuted or punished for making such a request.

Principle 4

1. These Principles shall be applied without discrimination of any kind, such as race, colour, sex, language, religion or belief, political or other opinion, national, ethnic or social origin, legal or social status, age, disability, property, birth, or on any other similar criteria.

2. Certain internally displaced persons, such as children, especially unaccompanied minors, expectant mothers, mothers with young children, female heads of household, persons with disabilities and elderly persons, shall be entitled to protection and assistance required by their condition and to treatment which takes into account their special needs.

SECTION II: PRINCIPLES RELATING TO PROTECTION FROM DISPLACEMENT

Principle 5

All authorities and international actors shall respect and ensure respect for their obligations under international law, including human rights and humanitarian law, in all circumstances, so as to prevent and avoid conditions that might lead to displacement of persons.

Principle 6

1. Every human being shall have the right to be protected against being arbitrarily displaced from his or her home or place of habitual residence.

2. The prohibition of arbitrary displacement includes displacement:

(a) When it is based on policies of apartheid, "ethnic cleansing" or similar practices aimed at/or resulting in altering the ethnic, religious or racial composition of the affected population;

(b) In situations of armed conflict, unless the security of the civilians involved or imperative military reasons so demand;

(c) In cases of large-scale development projects, which are not justified by compelling and overriding public interests;

(d) In cases of disasters, unless the safety and health of those affected requires their evacuation; and

(e) When it is used as a collective punishment.

3. Displacement shall last no longer than required by the circumstances.

Principle 7

1. Prior to any decision requiring the displacement of persons, the authorities concerned shall ensure that all feasible alternatives are explored in order to avoid displacement altogether. Where no alternatives exist, all measures shall be taken to minimize displacement and its adverse effects.

2. The authorities undertaking such displacement shall ensure, to the greatest practicable extent, that proper accommodation is provided to the displaced persons, that such displacements are effected in satisfactory conditions of safety, nutrition, health and hygiene, and that members of the same family are not separated.

3. If displacement occurs in situations other than during the emergency stages of armed conflicts and disasters, the following guarantees shall be complied with:

(a) A specific decision shall be taken by a State authority empowered by law to order such measures;

(b) Adequate measures shall be taken to guarantee to those to be displaced full information on the reasons and procedures for their displacement and, where applicable, on compensation and relocation;

(c) The free and informed consent of those to be displaced shall be sought;

(d) The authorities concerned shall endeavour to involve those affected, particularly women, in the planning and management of their relocation;

(e) Law enforcement measures, where required, shall be carried out by competent legal authorities; and

(f) The right to an effective remedy, including the review of such decisions by appropriate judicial authorities, shall be respected.

Principle 8

Displacement shall not be carried out in a manner

that violates the rights to life, dignity, liberty and security of those affected.

Principle 9

States are under a particular obligation to protect against the displacement of indigenous peoples, minorities, peasants, pastoralists and other groups with a special dependency on and attachment to their lands.

SECTION III: PRINCIPLES RELATING TO PROTECTION DURING DISPLACEMENT

Principle 10

1. Every human being has the inherent right to life which shall be protected by law. No one shall be arbitrarily deprived of his or her life. Internally displaced persons shall be protected in particular against:

(a) Genocide;

(b) Murder;

(c) Summary or arbitrary executions; and

(d) Enforced disappearances, including abduction or unacknowledged detention, threatening or resulting in death.

Threats and incitement to commit any of the foregoing acts shall be prohibited.

2. Attacks or other acts of violence against internally displaced persons who do not or no longer participate in hostilities are prohibited in all circumstances. Internally displaced persons shall be protected, in particular, against:

(a) Direct or indiscriminate attacks or other acts of violence, including the creation of areas wherein attacks on civilians are permitted;

(b) Starvation as a method of combat;

(c) Their use to shield military objectives from attack or to shield, favour or impede military operations;

(d) Attacks against their camps or settlements; and

(e) The use of anti-personnel landmines.

Principle 11

1. Every human being has the right to dignity and physical, mental and moral integrity.

2. Internally displaced persons, whether or not their liberty has been restricted, shall be protected in particular against:

(a) Rape, mutilation, torture, cruel, inhuman or degrading treatment or punishment, and other outrages upon personal dignity, such as acts of gender-specific violence, forced prostitution and any form of indecent assault;

(b) Slavery or any contemporary form of slavery, such as sale into marriage, sexual exploitation, or forced labour of children; and

(c) Acts of violence intended to spread terror among internally displaced persons. Threats and incitement to commit any of the foregoing acts shall be prohibited.

Principle 12

1. Every human being has the right to liberty and security of person. No one shall be subjected to arbitrary arrest or detention.

2. To give effect to this right for internally displaced persons, they shall not be interned in or confined to a camp. If in exceptional circumstances such internment or confinement is absolutely necessary, it shall not last longer than required by the circumstances.

3. Internally displaced persons shall be protected from discriminatory arrest and detention as a result of their displacement.

4. In no case shall internally displaced persons be taken hostage.

Principle 13

1. In no circumstances shall displaced children be recruited nor be required or permitted to take part in hostilities.

2. Internally displaced persons shall be protected against discriminatory practices of recruitment into any armed forces or groups as a result of their displacement. In particular any cruel, inhuman or

degrading practices that compel compliance or punish non-compliance with recruitment are prohibited in all circumstances.

Principle 14

1. Every internally displaced person has the right to liberty of movement and freedom to choose his or her residence.

2. In particular, internally displaced persons have the right to move freely in and out of camps or other settlements.

Principle 15

Internally displaced persons have:

(a) The right to seek safety in another part of the country;

(b) The right to leave their country;

(c) The right to seek asylum in another country; and

(d) The right to be protected against forcible return to or resettlement in any place where their life, safety, liberty and/or health would be at risk.

Principle 16

1. All internally displaced persons have the right to know the fate and whereabouts of missing relatives.

2. The authorities concerned shall endeavour to establish the fate and whereabouts of internally displaced persons reported missing, and cooperate with relevant international organizations engaged in this task. They shall inform the next of kin on the progress of the investigation and notify them of any result.

3. The authorities concerned shall endeavour to collect and identify the mortal remains of those deceased, prevent their despoliation or mutilation, and facilitate the return of those remains to the next of kin or dispose of them respectfully.

4. Grave sites of internally displaced persons should be protected and respected in all circumstances. Internally displaced persons should have the right of access to the grave sites of their deceased relatives.

Principle 17

1. Every human being has the right to respect of his or her family life.

2. To give effect to this right for internally displaced persons, family members who wish to remain together shall be allowed to do so.

3. Families which are separated by displacement should be reunited as quickly as possible. All appropriate steps shall be taken to expedite the reunion of such families, particularly when children are involved. The responsible authorities shall facilitate inquiries made by family members and encourage and cooperate with the work of humanitarian organizations engaged in the task of family reunification.

4. Members of internally displaced families whose personal liberty has been restricted by internment or confinement in camps shall have the right to remain together.

Principle 18

1. All internally displaced persons have the right to an adequate standard of living.

2. At the minimum, regardless of the circumstances, and without discrimination, competent authorities shall provide internally displaced persons with and ensure safe access to:

(a) Essential food and potable water;

(b) Basic shelter and housing;

(c) Appropriate clothing; and

(d) Essential medical services and sanitation.

3. Special efforts should be made to ensure the full participation of women in the planning and distribution of these basic supplies.

Principle 19

1. All wounded and sick internally displaced persons as well as those with disabilities shall receive to the fullest extent practicable and with the least possible delay, the medical care and attention they require, without distinction on any grounds other than medical ones. When necessary, internally dis-

placed persons shall have access to psychological and social services.

2. Special attention should be paid to the health needs of women, including access to female health care providers and services, such as reproductive health care, as well as appropriate counselling for victims of sexual and other abuses.

3. Special attention should also be given to the prevention of contagious and infectious diseases, including AIDS, among internally displaced persons.

Principle 20

1. Every human being has the right to recognition everywhere as a person before the law.

2. To give effect to this right for internally displaced persons, the authorities concerned shall issue to them all documents necessary for the enjoyment and exercise of their legal rights, such as passports, personal identification documents, birth certificates and marriage certificates. In particular, the authorities shall facilitate the issuance of new documents or the replacement of documents lost in the course of displacement, without imposing unreasonable conditions, such as requiring the return to one's area of habitual residence in order to obtain these or other required documents.

3. Women and men shall have equal rights to obtain such necessary documents and shall have the right to have such documentation issued in their own names.

Principle 21

1. No one shall be arbitrarily deprived of property and possessions.

2. The property and possessions of internally displaced persons shall in all circumstances be protected, in particular, against the following acts:

(a) Pillage;

(b) Direct or indiscriminate attacks or other acts of violence;

(c) Being used to shield military operations or objectives;

(d) Being made the object of reprisal; and

(e) Being destroyed or appropriated as a form of collective punishment.

3. Property and possessions left behind by internally displaced persons should be protected against destruction and arbitrary and illegal appropriation, occupation or use.

Principle 22

1. Internally displaced persons, whether or not they are living in camps, shall not be discriminated against as a result of their displacement in the enjoyment of the following rights:

(a) The rights to freedom of thought, conscience, religion or belief, opinion and expression;

(b) The right to seek freely opportunities for employment and to participate in economic activities;

(c) The right to associate freely and participate equally in community affairs;

(d) The right to vote and to participate in governmental and public affairs, including the right to have access to the means necessary to exercise this right; and

(e) The right to communicate in a language they understand.

Principle 23

1. Every human being has the right to education.

2. To give effect to this right for internally displaced persons, the authorities concerned shall ensure that such persons, in particular displaced children, receive education which shall be free and compulsory at the primary level. Education should respect their cultural identity, language and religion.

3. Special efforts should be made to ensure the full and equal participation of women and girls in educational programmes.

4. Education and training facilities shall be made available to internally displaced persons, in particular adolescents and women, whether or not living in camps, as soon as conditions permit.

SECTION IV: PRINCIPLES RELATING TO HUMANITARIAN ASSISTANCE

Principle 24

1. All humanitarian assistance shall be carried out in accordance with the principles of humanity and impartiality and without discrimination.

2. Humanitarian assistance to internally displaced persons shall not be diverted, in particular for political or military reasons.

Principle 25

1. The primary duty and responsibility for providing humanitarian assistance to internally displaced persons lies with national authorities.

2. International humanitarian organizations and other appropriate actors have the right to offer their services in support of the internally displaced. Such an offer shall not be regarded as an unfriendly act or an interference in a State's internal affairs and shall be considered in good faith. Consent thereto shall not be arbitrarily withheld, particularly when authorities concerned are unable or unwilling to provide the required humanitarian assistance.

3. All authorities concerned shall grant and facilitate the free passage of humanitarian assistance and grant persons engaged in the provision of such assistance rapid and unimpeded access to the internally displaced.

Principle 26

Persons engaged in humanitarian assistance, their transport and supplies shall be respected and protected. They shall not be the object of attack or other acts of violence.

Principle 27

1. International humanitarian organizations and other appropriate actors when providing assistance should give due regard to the protection needs and human rights of internally displaced persons and take appropriate measures in this regard. In so doing, these organizations and actors should respect relevant international standards and codes of conduct.

2. The preceding paragraph is without prejudice to the protection responsibilities of international organizations mandated for this purpose, whose services may be offered or requested by States.

SECTION V: PRINCIPLES RELATING TO RETURN, RESETTLEMENT AND REINTEGRATION

Principle 28

1. Competent authorities have the primary duty and responsibility to establish conditions, as well as provide the means, which allow internally displaced persons to return voluntarily, in safety and with dignity, to their homes or places of habitual residence, or to resettle voluntarily in another part of the country. Such authorities shall endeavour to facilitate the reintegration of returned or resettled internally displaced persons.

2. Special efforts should be made to ensure the full participation of internally displaced persons in the planning and management of their return or resettlement and reintegration.

Principle 29

1. Internally displaced persons who have returned to their homes or places of habitual residence or who have resettled in another part of the country shall not be discriminated against as a result of their having been displaced. They shall have the right to participate fully and equally in public affairs at all levels and have equal access to public services.

2. Competent authorities have the duty and responsibility to assist returned and/or resettled internally displaced persons to recover, to the extent possible, their property and possessions which they left behind or were dispossessed of upon their displacement. When recovery of such property and possessions is not possible, competent authorities shall provide or assist these persons in obtaining appropriate compensation or another form of just reparation.

Principle 30

All authorities concerned shall grant and facilitate for international humanitarian organizations and other appropriate actors, in the exercise of their respective mandates, rapid and unimpeded access to internally displaced persons to assist in their return or resettlement and reintegration.

VI. HUMAN RIGHTS ASPECTS OF HEALTH POLICY
A. Infectious Diseases

International Guidelines on HIV/AIDS and Human Rights (with revised Guideline 6) (1998, 2002)

Issued by the Office of the High Commissioner for Human Rights and the Joint United Nations Programme on HIV/AIDS (UNAIDS) in 1998, updated in 2002.
[Available at http://www.unhchr.ch/hiv/g6.pdf]

[Footnotes omitted.]

INTRODUCTION

1. The Commission on Human Rights, at its fifty-second session, in its resolution 1996/43 of 19 April 1996, requested that the United Nations High Commissioner for Human Rights, inter alia, continue the efforts, in cooperation with UNAIDS and nongovernmental organizations, as well as groups of people living with HIV/AIDS, towards the elaboration of guidelines on promoting and protecting respect for human rights in the context of HIV/AIDS. At the same time, the Commission requested that the Secretary-General of the United Nations prepare for the consideration of the Commission at its fifty-third session a report on the abovementioned guidelines, including the outcome of the second expert consultation on human rights and HIV/AIDS, and on their international dissemination.

2. The call for guidelines on human rights and HIV/AIDS was based on a recommendation contained in an earlier report of the Secretary-General to the Commission at its fifty-first session (E/CN.4/1995/45, para. 135), which stated that "the development of such guidelines or principles could provide an international framework for discussion of human rights considerations at the national, regional and international levels in order to arrive at a more comprehensive understanding of the complex relationship between the public health rationale and the human rights rationale of HIV/AIDS. In particular, governments could benefit from guidelines that outline clearly how human rights standards apply in the area of HIV/AIDS and indicate concrete and specific measures, both in terms of legislation and practice, that should be undertaken".

3. In response to the above requests, the United Nations Centre for Human Rights and the Joint United Nations Programme on HIV/AIDS (UNAIDS) convened the Second International Consultation on HIV/AIDS and Human Rights in Geneva, from 23 to 25 September 1996. The first International Consultation on AIDS and Human Rights was organized by the United Nations Centre for Human Rights, in cooperation with the World Health Organization, in Geneva, from 26 to 28 July 1989. In the report of the first consultation (HR/PUB/90/2), the elaboration of guidelines to assist policymakers and others in complying with international human rights standards regarding law, administrative practice and policy had already been proposed.

4. The Second International Consultation on HIV/AIDS and Human Rights brought together 35 experts in the field of HIV/AIDS and human rights, comprising government officials and staff of national AIDS programmes, 10 people living with HIV/AIDS (PLWHA), human rights activists, academics, representatives of regional and national networks on ethics, law, human rights and HIV/AIDS, and representatives of United Nations bodies and agencies, nongovernmental organizations and AIDS service organizations (ASOs).

5. The Second International Consultation on HIV/AIDS and Human Rights had before it five background papers that had been commissioned for the purpose of eliciting specific regional and thematic experiences and concerns regarding HIV/AIDS and human rights, prepared by the following nongovernmental organizations and networks of people living with HIV/AIDS: the Alternative Law Research and Development

Center (ALTERLAW) (Philippines); the Network of African People Living with HIV/AIDS (NAP+) (Zambia); Colectivo Sol (Mexico); the International Community of Women Living with HIV/AIDS (ICW+) (global); and the Global Network of People Living with HIV/AIDS (GNP+). The groups were asked, each within its specific context, to identify the most important human rights principles and concerns in the context of HIV/AIDS, as well as concrete measures that States could take to protect HIV/AIDS-related human rights.

6. The full text of the International Guidelines on HIV/AIDS and Human Rights, as adopted by the Second International Consultation, is contained in Annex I to the report of the Secretary-General to the Commission on Human Rights in document E/CN.4/1997/37. The summary of the 12 guidelines is provided below:

Guideline 1

States should establish an effective national framework for their response to HIV/AIDS, which ensures a coordinated, participatory, transparent and accountable approach, integrating HIV/AIDS policy and programme responsibilities across all branches of government.

Guideline 2

States should ensure, through political and financial support, that community consultation occurs in all phases of HIV/AIDS policy design, programme implementation and evaluation and that community organizations are enabled to carry out their activities, including in the field of ethics, law and human rights, effectively.

Guideline 3

States should review and reform public health laws to ensure that they adequately address public health issues raised by HIV/AIDS, that their provisions applicable to casually transmitted diseases are not inappropriately applied to HIV/AIDS and that they are consistent with international human rights obligations.

Guideline 4

States should review and reform criminal laws and correctional systems to ensure that they are consistent with international human rights obliga-

tions and are not misused in the context of HIV/AIDS or targeted against vulnerable groups.

Guideline 5

States should enact or strengthen anti-discrimination and other protective laws that protect vulnerable groups, people living with HIV/AIDS and people with disabilities from discrimination in both the public and private sectors, ensure privacy and confidentiality and ethics in research involving human subjects, emphasize education and conciliation, and provide for speedy and effective administrative and civil remedies.

Guideline 6

States should enact legislation to provide for the regulation of HIV-related goods, services and information, so as to ensure widespread availability of qualitative prevention measures and services, adequate HIV prevention and care information, and safe and effective medication at an affordable price.

Guideline 7

States should implement and support legal support services that will educate people affected by HIV/AIDS about their rights, provide free legal services to enforce those rights, develop expertise on HIV-related legal issues and utilize means of protection in addition to the courts, such as offices of ministries of justice, ombudspersons, health complaint units and human rights commissions.

Guideline 8

States, in collaboration with and through the community, should promote a supportive and enabling environment for women, children and other vulnerable groups by addressing underlying prejudices and inequalities through community dialogue, specially designed social and health services and support to community groups.

Guideline 9

States should promote the wide and ongoing distribution of creative education, training and media programmes explicitly designed to change attitudes of discrimination and stigmatization associated with HIV/AIDS to understanding and acceptance.

Guideline 10

States should ensure that government and the private sector develop codes of conduct regarding HIV/AIDS issues that translate human rights principles into codes of professional responsibility and practice, with accompanying mechanisms to implement and enforce these codes.

Guideline 11

States should ensure monitoring and enforcement mechanisms to guarantee the protection of HIV-related human rights, including those of people living with HIV/AIDS, their families and communities.

Guideline 12

States should cooperate through all relevant programmes and agencies of the United Nations system, including UNAIDS, to share knowledge and experience concerning HIV-related human rights issues and should ensure effective mechanisms to protect human rights in the context of HIV/AIDS at international level.

7. The International Guidelines on HIV/AIDS and Human Rights were also subsequently issued in 1998 by OHCHR and UNAIDS as a joint policy paper.

8. Since their publication in 1998, the International Guidelines on HIV/AIDS and Human Rights have provided policy guidance to governments, international organizations, non-governmental organizations and civil society groups on the development and implementation of effective national strategies for combating HIV/AIDS. The Commission on Human Rights has asked States to take all necessary steps to ensure the respect, protection and fulfilment of HIV-related human rights as contained in the guidelines, and has urged States to ensure that their laws, policies and practices comply with the guidelines1. The Secretary-General has submitted reports to the Commission on steps taken by governments and United Nations organs, programmes and specialized agencies to promote and implement the guidelines.

9. Significant developments have taken place with regard to the right to health and access to HIV/AIDS-related prevention, treatment, care and support, including advances in the availability of diagnostic tests and HIV/AIDS related treatments,

including antiretroviral therapies. There have been increased commitments at the international, regional and domestic levels towards the full realization of all human rights related to HIV/AIDS, including improved access to health services for people living with HIV/AIDS. Key among these are the Declaration of Commitment on HIV/AIDS; the Millennium Development Goals; General Comment 14 of the Committee on Economic, Social and Cultural Rights; and Commission on Human Rights resolutions on the right to the highest attainable standard of health and access to medication.

10. In light of these developments, the High Commissioner for Human Rights and the Executive Director of UNAIDS decided to convene a Third International Consultation on HIV/AIDS and Human Rights in order to update Guideline 6. The third consultation reviewed advances in HIV/AIDS-related treatment and antiretroviral medication, the current global disparity in access to treatment, as well as political and legal developments since the elaboration of the guidelines in 1996. The mandate of the third consultation was limited to a consideration of changes relevant to Guideline 6 that had occurred since the second consultation in 1996.

11. The revised Guideline 6 provides relevant and up-to-date policy guidance based on the current state of international law and on best practice experiences at the country level. It is based upon the following key premises:

• access to HIV/AIDS-related treatment is fundamental to realizing the right to health;

• prevention, treatment, care and support are a continuum;

• access to medication is one element of comprehensive treatment, care and support;

• ensuring sustainable access to medication requires action on numerous fronts; and

• international cooperation is vital in realizing equitable access to care, treatment and support to all in need. The revised Guideline 6, its related commentary and recommendations for implementation are contained in this document. The revised guideline replaces the original Guideline 6 of the International Guidelines on HIV/AIDS and Human Rights.

Revised Guideline 6: Access to Prevention, Treatment, Care and Support

States should enact legislation to provide for the regulation of HIV-related goods, services and information, so as to ensure widespread availability of quality prevention measures and services, adequate HIV prevention and care information, and safe and effective medication at an affordable price.

States should also take measures necessary to ensure for all persons, on a sustained and equal basis, the availability and accessibility of quality goods, services and information for HIV/AIDS prevention, treatment, care and support, including antiretroviral and other safe and effective medicines, diagnostics and related technologies for preventive, curative and palliative care of HIV/AIDS and related opportunistic infections and conditions.

States should take such measures at both the domestic and international levels, with particular attention to vulnerable individuals and populations.

Commentary on Guideline 6

Prevention, treatment, care and support are mutually reinforcing elements and a continuum of an effective response to HIV/AIDS. They must be integrated into a comprehensive approach, and a multifaceted response is needed. Comprehensive treatment, care and support include antiretroviral and other medicines, diagnostics and related technologies for the care of HIV/AIDS, related opportunistic infections and other conditions, good nutrition, and social, spiritual and psychological support, as well as family, community and home-based care. HIV-prevention technologies include condoms, lubricants, sterile injection equipment, antiretroviral medicines (e.g. to prevent mother-to-child transmission or as post-exposure prophylaxis) and, once developed, safe and effective microbicides and vaccines. Based on human rights principles, universal access requires that these goods, services and information not only be available, acceptable and of good quality, but also within physical reach and affordable for all.

Recommendations for Implementation of Guideline 6

a) States should develop and implement national plans to progressively realize universal access to comprehensive treatment, care and support for all persons living with HIV/AIDS, as well as universal access to a full range of goods, services and information for HIV prevention. National plans should be developed in consultation with nongovernmental organizations to ensure the active participation of people living with HIV/AIDS and vulnerable groups.

b) Universal access to HIV/AIDS prevention, treatment, care and support is necessary to respect, protect and fulfil human rights related to health, including the right to enjoy the highest attainable standard of health. Universal access will be achieved progressively over time. However, States have an immediate obligation to take steps, and to move as quickly and effectively as possible, towards realizing access for all to HIV/AIDS prevention, treatment, care and support at both the domestic and global levels. This requires, among other things, setting benchmarks and targets for measuring progress.

c) Access to HIV/AIDS-related information, goods and services is affected by a range of social, economic, cultural, political and legal factors. States should review and, where necessary, amend or adopt laws, policies, programmes and plans to realize universal and equal access to medicines, diagnostics and related technologies, taking these factors into account. As one example, duties, customs laws and valueadded taxes may hinder access to medicines, diagnostics and related technologies at affordable prices. Such laws should be revised so as to maximize access. States should ensure that national laws, policies, programmes and plans affecting access to HIV/AIDS-related goods, services or information are consistent with international human rights norms, principles and standards. States should consider the experience and expertise of other States, and consult with people living with HIV/ AIDS, nongovernmental organizations, and domestic and international health organizations with relevant expertise.

d) States should also ensure that their laws, policies, programmes and practices do not exclude, stigmatize or discriminate against people living with HIV/AIDS or their families, either on the basis of their HIV status or on other grounds contrary to international or domestic human rights norms, with respect to their entitlement or access to health-care goods, services and information.

e) States' legislation, policies, programmes, plans and practices should include positive measures to address factors that hinder the equal access of vulnerable individuals and populations to prevention, treatment, care and support, such as poverty, migration, rural location or discrimination of various kinds. These factors may have a cumulative effect. For example, children (particularly girls) and women may be the last to receive access even if treatment is otherwise available in their communities.

f) States should recognize, affirm and strengthen the involvement of communities as part of comprehensive HIV/AIDS prevention, treatment, care and support, while also complying with their own obligations to take steps in the public sector to respect, protect and fulfil human rights related to health. Mechanisms should be developed to enable affected communities to access resources to assist families who have lost income earners to AIDS. Particular attention must be paid to gender inequalities, with respect to access to care in the community for women and girls, as well as the burdens that delivering care at the community level may impose on them.

g) To assist caregivers and, where relevant, employers and insurers, States should ensure the availability, use and implementation of sound, scientifically up-to-date guidelines for prevention, treatment, care and support to people living with HIV/AIDS in respect of available health-care goods, services and information. States should develop mechanisms to monitor and improve, as necessary, the availability, use and implementation of these guidelines.

h) Legislation, policies and programmes should take into account the fact that persons living with HIV/AIDS may recurrently and progressively experience ill-health and greater health-care needs, which should be accommodated accordingly within benefit schemes in both the public and private sectors. States should work with employers, and employers' and workers' organizations, to adopt or adapt benefit schemes, where necessary,

to ensure universal and equal access to benefits for workers living with HIV/AIDS. Particular attention must also be paid to ensuring access to health care for individuals outside the formal employment sector, who lack work-related health-care benefits.

i) States should ensure that domestic legislation provides for prompt and effective remedies in cases in which a person living with HIV/AIDS is denied or not provided access to treatment, care and support. States should also ensure due process of law so that the merits of such complaints can be independently and impartially assessed. At the international level, States should strengthen existing mechanisms, and develop new mechanisms where they do not currently exist, enabling persons living with HIV/AIDS to seek prompt, effective redress for breaches of States' international legal obligations to respect, protect and fulfil rights related to health.

j) States should ensure the quality assurance and control of HIV/AIDS-elated products. States should ensure, through legislative and other measures (e.g. functional systems for pre-marketing approval and post-marketing surveillance), that medicines, diagnostics and related technologies are safe and effective.

k) States should take legislative and other measures to ensure that medicines are supplied in adequate quantities and in a timely fashion, and with accurate, current and accessible information regarding their use. For example, consumer protection laws or other relevant legislation should be enacted or strengthened to prevent fraudulent claims regarding the safety and efficacy of drugs, vaccines and medical devices, including those relating to HIV/AIDS.

l) Laws and/or regulations should be enacted to ensure the quality and availability of HIV tests and counselling. If home tests and/or rapid HIV test kits are permitted on the market, they should be strictly regulated to ensure quality and accuracy. The consequences of loss of epidemiological information, the lack of accompanying counselling and the risk of unauthorized use, such as for employment or immigration, should also be addressed. Legal and social support services should be established to protect individuals from any abuses arising from HIV testing. States should also ensure supervision of the quality of delivery of voluntary counselling and testing (VCT) services.

m) Legal quality control of condoms should be enforced, and compliance with the International Condom Standard should be monitored in practice. Restrictions on the availability of preventive measures, such as condoms, bleach, clean needles and syringes, should be repealed.

Widespread provision of these preventive measures through various means, including vending machines in appropriate locations, should be considered, in light of the greater effectiveness provided by the increased accessibility and anonymity afforded by this method of distribution. Condom promotion initiatives should be coupled with HIV/AIDS information campaigns for optimal impact.

n) Laws and/or regulations should be enacted to enable widespread provision of information about HIV/AIDS through the mass media. This information should be aimed at the general public, as well as at various vulnerable groups that may have difficulty in accessing information. HIV/AIDS information should be effective for its designated audience and not be inappropriately subject to censorship or other broadcasting standards, particularly as this will have the effect of damaging access to information vital to life, health and human dignity.

o) In order to improve prevention and therapeutic options related to HIV/AIDS, States should increase funds allocated to the public sector for researching, developing and promoting therapies and technologies for the prevention, treatment, care and support of HIV/AIDS and related infections and conditions. The private sector should also be encouraged to undertake such research and development and to make the resulting options widely and promptly available at prices affordable to those who need them.

p) States and the private sector should pay special attention to supporting research and development that address the health needs of developing countries. In recognition of the human right to share in scientific advancement and its benefits, States should adopt laws and policies, at the domestic and international levels, ensuring that the out-

comes of research and development are of national and global benefit, with particular attention to the needs of people in developing countries and people who are poor or otherwise marginalized.

q) States should integrate HIV/AIDS prevention, treatment, care and support into all aspects of their planning for development, including in poverty eradication strategies, national budget allocations and sectoral development plans. In so doing, States should have particular regard, at a minimum, for internationally agreed targets in addressing HIV/AIDS.

r) States should increase their national budget allocations for measures promoting secure and sustainable access to affordable HIV/AIDS prevention, treatment, care and support, at both the domestic and international levels. States should, among other steps, make contributions, in proportion to their resources, to mechanisms such as the Global Fund to Fight AIDS, Tuberculosis and Malaria. Developed countries should make concrete commitments of increased official development assistance that will move them without delay towards meeting international targets to which they have agreed, paying particular attention to assistance in realizing access to health-care goods, services and information.

s) States should ensure that international and bilateral mechanisms for financing responses to HIV/AIDS provide funds for prevention, treatment, care and support, including the purchase of antiretroviral and other medicines, diagnostics and related technologies. States should support and implement policies maximizing the benefit of donor assistance, including policies ensuring that such resources are used to purchase generic medicines, diagnostics and related technologies, where these are more economical.

t) States' international and bilateral financing mechanisms should also provide funding for strengthening health-care systems, for improving the capacity and working conditions of health-care personnel and the effectiveness of supply systems, for financing plans and referral mechanisms to provide access to prevention, treatment, care and support, and for family, community and home-based care.

u) States should collaborate with nongovernmental organizations, intergovernmental organizations, and United Nations bodies, agencies and programmes in creating, maintaining and expanding international, publicly-accessible sources of information on the sources, quality and worldwide prices of medicines, diagnostics and related technologies for the preventive, curative and palliative care of HIV/AIDS and related opportunistic infections and conditions.

v) Creditor countries and international financing institutions should implement debt relief for developing countries more quickly and extensively, and should ensure that resources provided for this purpose do not detract from those made available for official development assistance. Developing countries should use the resources freed up by debt relief (as well as other sources of development finance) in a manner that fully takes into account their obligations to respect, protect and fulfil rights related to health. States should, among other things, dedicate an appropriate proportion of such resources, in the light of domestic conditions, priorities and internationally agreed commitments, to HIV/AIDS prevention, treatment, care and support.

w) States should support and cooperate with international mechanisms for monitoring and reporting on the measures they have taken for progressively realizing access to comprehensive HIV/AIDS prevention, treatment, care and support, including anti-retroviral and other medicines, diagnostics and related technologies. States should include relevant information in their reports to bodies monitoring their progress in complying with their international legal obligations. The data in these reports should be disaggregated in a manner that helps identify and remedy possible disparities in access to prevention, treatment, care and support, and should use existing, or develop new, evaluation tools such as indicators or audits to measure implementation. States should actively involve nongovernmental organizations, including those representing people living with HIV/AIDS and vulnerable groups, in preparing such reports and in acting on the observations and recommendations received from such monitoring bodies.

x) States should pursue and implement international and regional cooperation aimed at transferring to developing countries technologies and expertise for HIV/AIDS prevention, treatment, care and support. States should support cooperation between developing countries in this regard, and should join international organizations in providing and supporting technical assistance aimed at realizing access to HIV/AIDS prevention, treatment, care and support.

y) In their conduct in international forums and negotiations, States should take due account of international norms, principles and standards relating to human rights. In particular, they should take account of their obligations to respect, protect and fulfil rights related to health, as well as of their commitments to provide international assistance and cooperation. States should also avoid taking measures that would undermine access to HIV/AIDS prevention, treatment, care and support, including access to antiretroviral and other medicines, diagnostics and related technologies, either domestically or in other countries, and should ensure that medicine is never used as a tool for political pressure. Particular attention must be paid by all States to the needs and situations of developing countries.

z) States should, in light of their human rights obligations, ensure that bilateral, regional and international agreements, such as those dealing with intellectual property, do not impede access to HIV/AIDS prevention, treatment, care and support, including access to antiretroviral and other medicines, diagnostics and related technologies. States should ensure that, in interpreting and implementing international agreements, domestic legislation incorporates to the fullest extent any safeguards and flexibilities therein that may be used to promote and ensure access to HIV/AIDS prevention, treat-ment, care and support for all, including access to medicines, diagnostics and related technologies. States should make use of these safeguards to the extent necessary to satisfy their domestic and international obligations in relation to human rights. States should review their international agreements (including on trade and investment) to ensure that these are consistent with treaties, legislation and policies designed to promote and protect all human rights and, where those agreements impede access to prevention, treatment, care and support, should amend them as necessary.

General Comment No. 3:
HIV/AIDS and the Rights of the Child (2003)

Adopted by the Committee on the Rights of the Child in January 2003. [Available at
http://www.unhchr.ch/html/menu2/6/crc/doc/comment/hiv.pdf]

[Footnotes omitted.]

I. INTRODUCTION

1. The HIV/AIDS epidemic has drastically changed the world in which children live. Millions of children have been infected and have died and many more are gravely affected as HIV spreads through their families and communities. The epidemic impacts on the daily life of younger children, and increases the victimization and marginalization of children, especially those living in particularly difficult circumstances. HIV/AIDS is not a problem of some countries but of the entire world. To truly bring its impact on children under control will require concerted and well-targeted efforts from all countries at all stages of development.

2. Initially children were considered to be only marginally affected by the epidemic. However, the international community has discovered that, unfortunately, children are at the heart of the problem. According to the Joint United Nations Programme on HIV/AIDS (UNAIDS), the most recent trends are alarming: in most parts of the world the majority of new infections are among young people between the ages of 15 and 24, sometimes younger. Women, including young girls, are also increasingly becoming infected. In most regions of the world, the vast majority of infected women do not know that they are infected and may unknowingly infect their children. Consequently, many States have recently registered an increase in their infant and child mortality rates. Adolescents are also vulnerable to HIV/AIDS because their first sexual experience may take place in an environment in which they have no access to proper information and guidance. Children who use drugs are at high risk.

3. Yet, all children can be rendered vulnerable by the particular circumstances of their lives, especially (a) children who are themselves HIV-infected; (b) children who are affected by the epidemic because of the loss of a parental caregiver or teacher and/or because their families or communities are severely strained by its consequences; and (c) children who are most prone to be infected or affected.

II. THE OBJECTIVES OF THE PRESENT GENERAL COMMENT

4. The objectives of the present General Comment are:

(a) To identify further and strengthen understanding of all the human rights of children in the context of HIV/AIDS;

(b) To promote the realization of the human rights of children in the context of HIV/AIDS, as guaranteed under the Convention on the Rights of the Child (hereafter "the Convention");

(c) To identify measures and good practices to increase the level of implementation by States of the rights related to the prevention of HIV/AIDS and the support, care and protection of children infected with or affected by this pandemic;

(d) To contribute to the formulation and promotion of child-oriented plans of action, strategies, laws, polices and programmes to combat the spread and mitigate the impact of HIV/AIDS at the national and international levels.

III. THE CONVENTION'S PERSPECTIVES ON HIV/AIDS: THE HOLISTIC CHILD RIGHTS-BASED APPROACH

5. The issue of children and HIV/AIDS is perceived as mainly a medical or health problem, although in reality it involves a much wider range of issues. In this regard, the right to health (article 24 of the Convention) is, however, central. But HIV/AIDS impacts so heavily on the lives of all children that it affects all their rights-civil, polit-

ical, economic, social and cultural. The rights embodied in the general principles of the Convention-the right to nondiscrimination (article 2), the right of the child to have his/her interest as a primary consideration (article 3), the right to life, survival and development (article 6) and the right to have his/her views respected (article 12)-should therefore be the guiding themes in the consideration of HIV/AIDS at all levels of prevention, treatment, care and support.

6. Adequate measures to address HIV/AIDS can be undertaken only if the rights of children and adolescents are fully respected. The most relevant rights in this regard, in addition to those enumerated in paragraph 5 above, are the following: the right to access information and material aimed at the promotion of their social, spiritual and moral well being and physical and mental health (article 17); the right to preventive health care, sex education and family planning education and services (article 24 (f)); the right to an appropriate standard of living (article 27); the right to privacy (article 16); the right not to be separated from parents (article 9); the right to be protected from violence (article 19); the right to special protection and assistance by the State (article 20); the rights of children with disabilities (article 23); the right to health (article 24); the right to social security, including social insurance (article 26); the right to education and leisure (arts. 28 and 31); the right to be protected from economic and sexual exploitation and abuse, and from illicit use of narcotic drugs (articles. 32, 33, 34 and 36); the right to be protected from abduction, sale and trafficking as well as torture or other cruel, inhuman or degrading treatment or punishment (arts. 35 and 37); and the right to physical and psychological recovery and social reintegration (article 39). Children are confronted with serious challenges to the above-mentioned rights as a result of the epidemic. The Convention, and in particular the four general principles with their comprehensive approach, provide a powerful framework for efforts to reduce the negative impact of the pandemic on the lives of children. The holistic rights-based approach required to implement the Convention is the optimal tool for addressing the broader range of issues that relate to prevention, treatment and care efforts.

A. The Right to Non-Discrimination (Article 2)

7. Discrimination is responsible for heightening the vulnerability of children to HIV and AIDS, as well as seriously impacting the lives of children who are affected by HIV/AIDS, or are themselves HIV infected. Girls and boys of parents living with HIV/AIDS are often victims of stigma and discrimination as they too are often assumed to be infected. As a result of discrimination, children are denied access to information, education (see the Committee's General Comment No. 1 on the aims of education), health or social care services or community life. At its extreme, discrimination against HIIV infected children has resulted in their abandonment by their family, community and/or society. Discrimination also fuels the epidemic by making children in particular those belonging to certain groups like children living in remote or rural areas where services are less accessible, more vulnerable to infection. These children are thus doubly victimized.

8. Of particular concern is gender-based discrimination combined with taboos or negative or judgmental attitudes to sexual activity of girls, often limiting their access to preventive measures and other services. Of concern also is discrimination based on sexual orientation. In the design of HIV/AIDS-related strategies, and in keeping with their obligations under the Convention, States parties must give careful consideration to prescribed gender norms within their societies with a view to eliminating gender-based discrimination as these norms impact on the vulnerability of both girls and boys to HIV/AIDS. States parties should, in particular, recognize that discrimination in the context of HIV/AIDS often impacts girls more severely than boys.

9. All the above-mentioned discriminatory practices are violations of children's rights under the Convention. Article 2 of the Convention obliges States parties to ensure all the rights set forth in the Convention without discrimination of any kind, "irrespective of the child's or his or her parent's or legal guardian's race, colour, sex, language, religion, political or other opinion, national, ethnic or social origin, property, disability, birth or other status". The Committee interprets "other status" under article 2 of the Convention to

include HIV/AIDS status of the child or his/her parent(s). Laws, policies, strategies and practices should address all forms of discrimination that contribute to increasing the impact of the epidemic. Strategies should also promote education and training programmes explicitly designed to change attitudes of discrimination and stigmatization associated with HIV/AIDS.

B. Best Interests of the Child (Article 3)

10. Policies and programmes for the prevention, care and treatment of HIV/AIDS have generally been designed for adults with scarce attention to the principle of the best interests of the child as a primary consideration. Article 3, paragraph 1, of the Convention states "In all actions concerning children, whether undertaken by public or private social welfare institutions, courts of law, administrative authorities or legislative bodies, the best interests of the child shall be a primary consideration". The obligations attached to this right are fundamental to guiding the action of States in relation to HIV/AIDS. The child should be placed at the centre of the response to the pandemic, and strategies should be adapted to children's rights and needs.

C. The Right to Life, Survival and Development (Article 6)

11. Children have the right not to have their lives arbitrarily taken, as well as to benefit from economic and social policies that will allow them to survive into adulthood and develop in the broadest sense of the word. State obligation to realize the right to life, survival and development also highlights the need to give careful attention to sexuality as well as to the behaviors and lifestyles of children, even if they do not conform with what society determines to be acceptable under prevailing cultural norms for a particular age group. In this regard, the female child is often subject to harmful traditional practices, such as early and/or forced marriage, which violate her rights and make her more vulnerable to HIV infection, including because such practices often interrupt access to education and information. Effective prevention programmes are only those that acknowledge the realities of the lives of adolescents, while addressing sexuality by ensuring equal access to appropriate information, life skills, and to preventive measures.

D. The Right to Express Views and Have Them Taken into Account (Article 12)

12. Children are rights holders and have a right to participate, in accordance with their evolving capacities, in raising awareness by speaking out about the impact of HIV/AIDS on their lives and in the development of HIV/AIDS policies and programmes. Interventions have been found to benefit children most when they are actively involved in assessing needs, devising solutions, shaping strategies and carrying them out rather than being seen as objects for whom decisions are made. In this regard, the participation of children as peer educators, both within and outside schools, should be actively promoted. States, international agencies and non-governmental organizations must provide children with a supportive and enabling environment to carry out their own initiatives, and to fully participate at both community and national levels in HIV policy and programme conceptualization, design, implementation, coordination, monitoring and review. A variety of approaches are likely to be necessary to ensure the participation of children from all sectors of society, including mechanisms which encourage children, consistent with their evolving capacities, to express their views, have them heard, and given due weight in accordance with their age and maturity (article 12, para. 1). Where appropriate, the involvement of children living with HIV/AIDS in raising awareness, by sharing their experiences with their peers and others, is critical both to effective prevention and to reducing stigmatization and discrimination. States parties must ensure that children who participate in these awareness-raising efforts do so voluntarily, after being counselled, and that they receive both the social support and legal protection to allow them to lead normal lives during and after their involvement.

E. Obstacles

13. Experience has shown that many obstacles hinder effective prevention, delivery of care services and support for community initiatives on HIV/AIDS. These are mainly cultural, structural and financial. Denying that a problem exists, cultural practices and attitudes, including taboos and stigmatization, poverty and patronizing attitudes towards children are just some of the obstacles that may block the political and individual commitment needed for effective programmes.

14. With regard to financial, technical and human resources, the Committee is aware that such resources may not be immediately available. However, concerning this obstacle, the Committee wishes to remind States parties of their obligations under article 4. It further notes that resource constraints should not be used by States parties to justify their failure to take any or enough of the technical or financial measures required. Finally, the Committee wishes to emphasize in this regard the essential role of international cooperation.

IV. PREVENTION, CARE, TREATMENT AND SUPPORT

15. The Committee wishes to stress that prevention, care, treatment and support are mutually reinforcing elements and provide a continuum within an effective response to HIV/AIDS.

A. Information on HIV Prevention and Awareness-Raising

16. Consistent with the obligations of States parties in relation to the rights to health and information (arts. 24, 13 and 17), children should have the right to access adequate information related to HIV/AIDS prevention and care, through formal channels (e.g. through educational opportunities and child-targeted media) as well as informal channels (e.g. those targeting street children, institutionalized children or children living in difficult circumstances). States parties are reminded that children require relevant, appropriate and timely information which recognizes the differences in levels of understanding among them, is tailored appropriately to age level and capacity and enables them to deal positively and responsibly with their sexuality in order to protect themselves from HIV infection. The Committee wishes to emphasize that effective HIV/AIDS prevention requires States to refrain from censoring, withholding or intentionally misrepresenting health-related information, including sexual education and information, and that, consistent with their obligations to ensure the right to life, survival and development of the child (article 6), States parties must ensure that children have the ability to acquire the knowledge and skills to protect themselves and others as they begin to express their sexuality.

17. Dialogue with community, family and peer counsellors, and the provision of "life skills" edu-
cation within schools, including skills in communicating on sexuality and healthy living, have been found to be useful approaches to delivering HIV prevention messages to both girls and boys, but different approaches may be necessary to reach different groups of children. States parties must make efforts to address gender differences as they may impact on the access children have to prevention messages, and ensure that children are reached with appropriate prevention messages even if they face constraints due to language, religion, disability or other factors of discrimination. Particular attention must be paid to raising awareness among hard to reach populations. In this respect, the role of the mass media and/or oral tradition in ensuring that children have access to information and material, as recognized in article 17 of the Convention, is crucial both to providing appropriate information and to reducing stigmatization and discrimination. States parties should support the regular monitoring and evaluation of HIV/AIDS awareness campaigns to ascertain their effectiveness in providing information, reducing ignorance, stigmatization and discrimination, as well as addressing fear and misperceptions concerning HIV and its transmission among children, including adolescents.

B. The Role of Education

18. Education plays a critical role in providing children with relevant and appropriate information on HIV/AIDS, which can contribute to increased awareness and better understanding of this pandemic and prevent negative attitudes towards victims of HIV/AIDS (see also the Committee's General Comment No. 1 on the aims of education). Furthermore, education can and should empower children to protect themselves from the risk of HIV infection. In this regard, the Committee wishes to remind States parties of their obligation to ensure that primary education is available to all children, whether infected, orphaned or otherwise affected by HIV/AIDS. In many communities where HIV has spread widely, children from affected families, in particular girls, are facing serious difficulties staying in school and the number of teachers and other school employees lost to AIDS is limiting and threatening to destroy the ability of children to access education. States parties must make adequate provision to ensure that children affected by HIV/AIDS can stay in school and ensure the qualified replace-

ment of sick teachers so that children's regular attendance at schools is not affected, and that the right to education (article 28) of all children living within these communities is fully protected.

19. States parties must make every effort to ensure that schools are safe places for children, which offer them security and do not contribute to their vulnerability to HIV infection. In accordance with article 34 of the Convention, States parties are under obligation to take all appropriate measures to prevent, inter alia, the inducement or coercion of a child to engage in any unlawful sexual activity.

C. Child and Adolescent Sensitive Health Services

20.The Committee is concerned that health services are generally still insufficiently responsive to the needs of children under 18 years of age, in particular adolescents. As the Committee has noted on numerous occasions, children are more likely to use services that are friendly and supportive, provide a wide range of services and information, are geared to their needs, give them the opportunity to participate in decisions affecting their health, are accessible, affordable, confidential and non-judgmental, do not require parental consent and are not discriminatory. In the context of HIV/AIDS and taking into account the evolving capacities of the child, States parties are encouraged to ensure that health services employ trained personnel who fully respect the rights of children to privacy (article 16) and non-discrimination in offering them access to HIV-related information, voluntary counselling and testing, knowledge of their HIV status, confidential sexual and reproductive health services, and free or low cost contraceptive, methods and services, as well as HIV-related care and treatment if and when needed, including for the prevention and treatment of health problems related to HIV/AIDS, e.g. tuberculosis and opportunistic infections.

21. In some countries, even when child- and adolescent-friendly HIV-related services are available, they are not sufficiently accessible to children with disabilities, indigenous children, children belonging to minorities, children living in rural areas, children living in extreme poverty or children who are otherwise marginalized within the society. In others, where the health system's overall capacity is already strained, children with

HIV have been routinely denied access to basic health care. States parties must ensure that services are provided to the maximum extent possible to all children living within their borders, without discrimination, and that they sufficiently take into account differences in gender, age and the social, economic, cultural and political context in which children live.

D. HIV Counselling and Testing

22. The accessibility of voluntary, confidential HIV counselling and testing services, with due attention to the evolving capacities of the child, is fundamental to the rights and health of children. Such services are critical to children's ability to reduce the risk of contracting or transmitting HIV, to access HIV-specific care, treatment and support, and to better plan for their futures. Consistent with their obligation under article 24 of the Convention to ensure that no child is deprived of his or her right of access to necessary health services, States parties should ensure access to voluntary, confidential HIV counselling and testing for all children.

23. The Committee wishes to stress that, as the duty of States parties is first and foremost to ensure that the rights of the child are protected, States parties must refrain from imposing mandatory HIV/AIDS testing of children in all circumstances and ensure protection against it. While the evolving capacities of the child will determine whether consent is required from him or her directly or from his or her parent or guardian, in all cases, consistent with the child's right to receive information under articles 13 and 17 of the Convention, States parties must ensure that, prior to any HIV testing, whether by health-care providers in relation to children who are accessing health services for another medical condition or otherwise, the risks and benefits of such testing are sufficiently conveyed so that an informed decision can be made.

24. States parties must protect the confidentiality of HIV test results, consistent with the obligation to protect the right to privacy of children (article 16), including within health and social welfare settings, and information on the HIV status of children may not be disclosed to third parties, including parents, without the child's consent.

E. Mother-to-Child Transmission

25. Mother-to-child transmission (MTCT) is responsible for the majority of HIV infections in infants and young children. Infants and young children can be infected with HIV during pregnancy, labour and delivery, and through breastfeeding. States parties are requested to ensure implementation of the strategies recommended by the United Nations agencies to prevent HIV infection in infants and young children. These include: (a) the primary prevention of HIV infection among parents-to-be; (b) the prevention of unintended pregnancies in HIV-infected women, (c) the prevention of HIV transmission from HIV-infected women to their infants; and (d) the provision of care, treatment and support to HIV-infected women, their infants and families.

26. To prevent MTCT of HIV, States parties must take steps, including the provision of essential drugs, e.g. anti-retroviral drugs, appropriate antenatal, delivery and post-partum care, and making HIV voluntary counselling and testing services available to pregnant women and their partners. The Committee recognizes that anti-retroviral drugs administered to a woman during pregnancy and/or labour and, in some regimens, to her infant, have been shown to significantly reduce the risk of transmission from mother to child. However, in addition, States parties should provide support for mothers and children, including counselling on infant feeding options. States parties are reminded that counselling of HIV-positive mothers should include information about the risks and benefits of different infant feeding options, and guidance on selecting the option most likely to be suitable for their situation. Follow-up support is also required in order for women to be able to implement their selected option as safely as possible.

27. Even in populations with high HIV prevalence, the majority of infants are born to women who are not HIV-infected. For the infants of HIV-negative women and women who do not know their HIV status, the Committee wishes to emphasize, consistent with articles 6 and 24 of the Convention, that breastfeeding remains the best feeding choice. For the infants of HIV-positive mothers, available evidence indicates that breastfeeding can add to the risk of HIV transmission by 10-20 per cent, but that lack of breastfeeding can expose children to an increased risk of malnutrition or infectious diseases other than HIV. United Nations agencies have recommended that, where replacement feeding is affordable, feasible, acceptable, sustainable and safe, avoidance of all breastfeeding by HIV-infected mothers is recommended; otherwise, exclusive breastfeeding is recommended during the first months of life and should then be discontinued as soon as it is feasible.

F. Treatment and Care

28. The obligations of States parties under the Convention extend to ensuring that children have sustained and equal access to comprehensive treatment and care, including necessary HIV-related drugs, goods and services on a basis of non-discrimination. It is now widely recognized that comprehensive treatment and care includes anti-retroviral and other drugs, diagnostics and related technologies for the care of HIV/AIDS, related opportunistic infections and other conditions, good nutrition, and social, spiritual and psychological support, as well as family, community and home-based care. In this regard, States parties should negotiate with the pharmaceutical industry in order to make the necessary medicines locally available at the lowest costs possible. Furthermore, States parties are requested to affirm, support and facilitate the involvement of communities in the provision of comprehensive HIV/AIDS treatment, care and support, while at the same time complying with their own obligations under the Convention. States parties are called upon to pay special attention to addressing those factors within their societies that hinder equal access to treatment, care and support for all children.

G. Involvement of Children in Research

29. Consistent with article 24 of the Convention, States parties must ensure that HIV/AIDS research programmes include specific studies that contribute to effective prevention, care, treatment and impact reduction for children. States parties must, nonetheless, ensure that children do not serve as research subjects until an intervention has already been thoroughly tested on adults. Rights and ethical concerns have arisen in relation to HIV/AIDS biomedical research, HIV/ADS operations, and social, cultural and behavioural research. Children have been subjected to unnecessary or inappropriately designed research with little or no voice to either refuse or consent to par-

ticipation. In line with the child's evolving capacities, consent of the child should be sought and consent may be sought from parents or guardians if necessary, but in all cases consent must be based on full disclosure of the risks and benefits of research to the child. States parties are further reminded to ensure that the privacy rights of children, in line with their obligations under article 16 of the Convention, are not inadvertently violated through the research process and that personal information about children, which is accessed through research, is, under no circumstances, used for purposes other than that for which consent was given. States parties must make every effort to ensure that children and, according to their evolving capacities, their parents and/or their guardians participate in decisions on research priorities and that a supportive environment is created for children who participate in such research.

V. VULNERABILITY AND CHILDREN NEEDING SPECIAL PROTECTION

30. The vulnerability of children to HIV/AIDS resulting from political, economic, social, cultural and other factors determines the likelihood of their being left with insufficient support to cope with the impact of HIV/AIDS on their families and communities, exposed to the risk of infection, subjected to inappropriate research, or deprived of access to treatment, care and support if and when HIV infection sets in. Vulnerability to HIV/AIDS is most acute for children living in refugee and internally displaced persons camps, children in detention, children living in institutions, as well as children living in extreme poverty, children living in situations of armed conflict, child soldiers, economically and sexually exploited children, and disabled, migrant, minority, indigenous, and street children. However, all children can be rendered vulnerable by the particular circumstances of their lives. Even in times of severe resource constraints, the Committee wishes to note that the rights of vulnerable members of society must be protected and that many measures can be pursued with minimum resource implications. Reducing vulnerability to HIV/AIDS requires first and foremost that children, their families and communities be empowered to make informed choices about decisions, practices or policies affecting them in relation to HIV/AIDS.

A. Children Affected and Orphaned by HIV/AIDS

31. Special attention must be given to children orphaned by AIDS and to children from affected families, including child-headed households, as these impact on vulnerability to HIV infection. For children from families affected by HIV/AIDS, the stigmatization and social isolation they experience may be accentuated by the neglect or violation of their rights, in particular discrimination resulting in a decrease or loss of access to education, health and social services. The Committee wishes to underline the necessity of providing legal, economic and social protection to affected children to ensure their access to education, inheritance, shelter and health and social services, as well as to make them feel secure in disclosing their HIV status and that of their family members when the children deem it appropriate. In this respect, States parties are reminded that these measures are critical to the realization of the rights of children and to giving them the skills and support necessary to reduce their vulnerability and risk of becoming infected.

32. The Committee wishes to emphasize the critical implications of proof of identity for children affected by HIV/AIDS, as it relates to securing recognition as a person before the law, safeguarding the protection of rights, in particular to inheritance, education, health and other social services, as well as to making children less vulnerable to abuse and exploitation, particularly if separated from their families due to illness or death. In this respect, birth registration is critical to ensuring the rights of the child and is also necessary to minimize the impact of HIV/AIDS on the lives of affected children. States parties are, therefore, reminded of their obligation under article 7 of the Convention to ensure that systems are in place for the registration of every child at or immediately after birth.

33. The trauma HIV/AIDS brings to the lives of orphans often begins with the illness and death of one of their parents, and is frequently compounded by the effects of stigmatization and discrimination. In this respect, States parties are particularly reminded to ensure that both law and practice support the inheritance and property rights of orphans, with particular attention to the underlying gender-based discrimination which

may interfere with the fulfilment of these rights. Consistent with their obligations under article 27 of the Convention, States parties must also support and strengthen the capacity of families and communities of children orphaned by AIDS to provide them with a standard of living adequate for their physical, mental, spiritual, moral, economic and social development, including access to psychosocial care, as needed.

34. Orphans are best protected and cared for when efforts are made to enable siblings to remain together, and in the care of relatives or family members. The extended family, with the support of the surrounding community, may be the least traumatic and therefore the best way to care for orphans when there are no other feasible alternatives. Assistance must be provided so that, to the maximum extent possible, children can remain within existing family structures. This option may not be available due to the impact HIV/AIDS has on the extended family. In that case, States parties should provide, as far as possible, for family-type alternative care (e.g. foster care). States parties are encouraged to provide support, financial and otherwise, when necessary, to child-headed households. States parties must ensure that their strategies recognize that communities are at the front line of the response to HIV/AIDS and that these strategies are designed to assist communities in determining how best to provide support to the orphans living there.

35. Although institutionalized care may have detrimental effects on child development, States parties may, nonetheless, determine that it has an interim role to play in caring for children orphaned by HIV/AIDS when family-based care within their own communities is not a possibility. It is the opinion of the Committee that any form of institutionalized care for children should only serve as a measure of last resort, and that measures must be fully in place to protect the rights of the child and guard against all forms of abuse and exploitation. In keeping with the right of children to special protection and assistance when within these environments, and consistent with articles 3, 20 and 25 of the Convention, strict measures are needed to ensure that such institutions meet specific standards of care and comply with legal protection safeguards. States parties are reminded that limits must be placed on the length of time

children spend in these institutions, and programmes must be developed to support any children who stay in these institutions, whether infected or affected by HIV/AIDS, to successfully reintegrate them into their communities.

B. Victims of Sexual and Economic Exploitation

36. Girls and boys who are deprived of the means of survival and development, particularly children orphaned by AIDS, may be subjected to sexual and economic exploitation in a variety of ways, including the exchange of sexual services or hazardous work for money to survive, support their sick or dying parents and younger siblings, or to pay for school fees. Children who are infected or directly affected by HIV/AIDS may find themselves at a double disadvantage-experiencing discrimination on the basis of both their social and economic marginalization and their, or their parents', HIV status. Consistent with the right of children under articles 32, 34, 35 and 36 of the Convention, and in order to reduce children's vulnerability to HIV/AIDS, States parties are under obligation to protect children from all forms of economic and sexual exploitation, including ensuring they do not fall prey to prostitution networks, and that they are protected from performing any work likely to be prejudicial to, or to interfere with, their education, health, or physical, mental, spiritual, moral or social development. States parties must take bold action to protect children from sexual and economic exploitation, trafficking and sale and, consistent with the rights under article 39, create opportunities for those who have been subjected to such treatment to benefit from the support and caring services of the State and non-governmental entities engaged in these issues.

C. Victims of Violence and Abuse

37. Children may be exposed to various forms of violence and abuse which may increase the risk of their becoming HIV-infected, and may also be subjected to violence as a result of their being infected or affected by HIV/AIDS. Violence, including rape and other forms of sexual abuse, can occur in the family or foster setting or may be perpetrated by those with specific responsibilities towards children, including teachers and employees of institutions working with children, such as

prisons and institutions concerned with mental health and other disabilities. In keeping with the rights of the child set forth in article 19 of the Convention, States parties have the obligation to protect children from all forms of violence and abuse, whether at home, in school or other institutions, or in the community.

38. Programmes must be specifically adapted to the environment in which children live, to their ability to recognize and report abuses and to their individual capacity and autonomy. The Committee considers that the relationship between HIV/AIDS and the violence or abuse suffered by children in the context of war and armed conflict requires specific attention. Measures to prevent violence and abuse in these situations are critical, and States parties must ensure the incorporation of HIV/AIDS and child rights issues in addressing and supporting children-girls and boys-who were used by military or other uniformed personnel to provide domestic help or sexual services, or who are internally displaced or living in refugee camps. In keeping with States parties' obligations, including under articles 38 and 39 of the Convention, active information campaigns, combined with the counselling of children and mechanisms for the prevention and early detection of violence and abuse, must be put in place within conflict- and disaster-affected regions, and must form part of national and community responses to HIV/AIDS.

Substance Abuse

39. The use of substances, including alcohol and drugs, may reduce the ability of children to exert control over their sexual conduct and, as a result, may increase their vulnerability to HIV infection. Injecting practices using unsterilized instruments further increase the risk of HIV transmission. The Committee notes that greater understanding of substance use behaviors among children is needed, including the impact that neglect and violation of the rights of the child has on these behaviors. In most countries, children have not benefited from pragmatic HIV prevention programmes related to substance use, which even when they do exist have largely targeted adults. The Committee wishes to emphasize that policies and programmes aimed at reducing substance use and HIV transmission must recognize the particular sensitivities and lifestyles of children, including adolescents, in the context of HIV/AIDS prevention. Consistent with the rights of children under articles 33 and 24 of the Convention, States parties are obligated to ensure the implementation of programmes which aim to reduce the factors that expose children to the use of substances, as well as those that provide treatment and support to children who are abusing substances.

VI. RECOMMENDATIONS

40. The Committee hereby reaffirms the recommendations, which emerged at the day of general discussion on children living in a world with HIV/AIDS (CRC/C/80), and calls upon States parties:

(a) To adopt and implement national and local HIV/AIDS-related policies, including effective plans of action, strategies, and programmes that are child-centred, rights-based and incorporate the rights of the child under the Convention, including by taking into account the recommendations made in the previous paragraphs of the present General Comment and those adopted at the United Nations General Assembly special session on children (2002);

(b) To allocate financial, technical and human resources, to the maximum extent possible, to supporting national and community-based action (article 4), and, where appropriate, within the context of international cooperation (see paragraph 41 below).

(c) To review existing laws or enact new legislation with a view to implementing fully article 2 of the Convention, and in particular to expressly prohibiting discrimination based on real or perceived HIV/AIDS status so as to guarantee equal access for of all children to all relevant services, with particular attention to the child's right to privacy and confidentiality and to other recommendations made by the Committee in the previous paragraphs relevant to legislation;

(d) To include HIV/AIDS plans of action, strategies, policies and programmes in the work of national mechanisms responsible for monitoring and coordinating children's rights and to consider the establishment of a review procedure, which responds specifically to complaints of neglect or violation of the rights of the child in relation to HIV/AIDS, whether this entails the creation of a new legislative or administrative body or is entrusted to an existing national institution;

(e) To reassess their HIV-related data collection and evaluation to ensure that they adequately cover children as defined under the Convention, are disaggregated by age and gender ideally in five-year age groups, and include, as far as possible, children belonging to vulnerable groups and those in need of special protection;

(f) To include, in their reporting process under article 44 of the Convention, information on national HIV/AIDS policies and programmes and, to the extent possible, budgeting and resource allocations at the national, regional and local levels, as well as within these breakdowns the proportions allocated to prevention, care, research and impact reduction. Specific attention must be given to the extent to which these programmes and policies explicitly recognize children (in the light of their evolving capacities) and their rights, and the extent to which HIV-related rights of children are dealt with in laws, policies and practices, with specific attention to discrimination against children on the basis of their HIV status, as well as because they are orphans or the children of parents living with HIV/AIDS. The Committee requests States parties to provide a detailed indication in their reports of what they consider to be the most important priorities within their jurisdiction in relation to children and HIV/AIDS, and to outline the programme of activities they intend to pursue over the coming five years in order to address the problems identified. This would allow activities to be progressively assessed over time.

41. In order to promote international cooperation, the Committee calls upon UNICEF, World Health Organization, United Nations Population Fund, UNAIDS and other relevant international bodies, organizations and agencies to contribute systematically, at the national level, to efforts to ensure the rights of children in the context of HIV/AIDS, and also to continue to work with the Committee to improve the rights of the child in the context of HIV/AIDS. Further, the Committee urges States providing development cooperation to ensure that HIV/AIDS strategies are so designed as to take fully into account the rights of the child.

42. Non-governmental organizations, as well as community-based groups and other civil society actors, such as youth groups, faith-based organizations, women's organizations and traditional leaders, including religious and cultural leaders, all have a vital role to play in the response to the HIV/AIDS pandemic. States parties are called upon to ensure an enabling environment for participation by civil society groups, which includes facilitating collaboration and coordination among the various players, and that these groups are given the support needed to enable them to operate effectively without impediment (in this regard, States parties are specifically encouraged to support the full involvement of people living with HIV/AIDS, with particular attention to the inclusion of children, in the provision of HIV/AIDS prevention, care, treatment and support services).

Commission on Human Rights Resolution 2004/26:
Access to Medication in the Context of Pandemics Such as HIV/AIDS, Tuberculosis and Malaria (2004)

Adopted by the UN Commission on Human Rights without a vote on 16 April 2004.
[Available at http://www.ohchr.org/english/issues/hiv/documeent.htm]

The Commission on Human Rights,

* * *

Welcoming the decision on the implementation of paragraph 6 of the Doha Declaration on the TRIPS Agreement and public health, adopted by the General Council of the World Trade Organization on 30 August 2003,

Recognizing the existing efforts and the desirability of further promoting the transfer of technology and capacity building in the pharmaceutical sector to countries with insufficient or no manufacturing capacities in the pharmaceutical sector, in accordance with applicable international law, including international agreements acceded to,

Stressing the importance of fully implementing the Declaration of Commitment on HIV/AIDS, "Global Crisis Global Action", adopted by the General Assembly in its resolution S26/2 of 27 June 2001 at its special session on HIV/AIDS, and taking note of the report of the Secretary General on progress towards implementation of the Declaration of Commitment on HIV/AIDS (A/58/184),

Expressing its support for the work of the Global Fund to Fight AIDS, Tuberculosis and Malaria and of other international bodies combating such pandemics, and encouraging the Global Fund to develop further effective and appropriate processes for the disbursement of funds,

* * *

Recognizing that the spread of HIV/AIDS can have a uniquely devastating impact on all sectors and levels of society and stressing that the HIV/AIDS pandemic, if unchecked, may pose a risk to stability and security, as stated in Security Council resolution 1308 (2000) of 17 July 2000,

Emphasizing, in view of the increasing challenges presented by pandemics such as HIV/AIDS, tuberculosis and malaria, the need for intensified efforts to ensure universal respect for and observance of human rights and fundamental freedoms for all, including by reducing vulnerability to pandemics such as HIV/AIDS, tuberculosis and malaria and by preventing related discrimination and stigma,

1. Recognizes that access to medication in the context of pandemics such as HIV/AIDS, tuberculosis and malaria is one fundamental element for achieving progressively the full realization of the right of everyone to the enjoyment of the highest attainable standard of physical and mental health;

2. Calls upon States to consider taking into account the guidelines elaborated at the Second International Consultation on HIV/AIDS and Human Rights held in Geneva from 23 to 25 September 1996 (E/CN.4/1997/37, annex I), as well as the revision of guideline 6 at the Third International Consultation, held on 25 and 26 July 2002;

3. Also calls upon States to develop and implement national strategies, in accordance with applicable international law, including international agreements acceded to, in order progressively to realize access for all to prevention related goods, services and information as well as access to comprehensive treatment, care and support for all individuals infected and affected by pandemics such as HIV/AIDS, tuberculosis and malaria;

4. Further calls upon States to establish or strengthen national health and social infrastructures and health care systems, with the assistance of the international community as necessary, for the effective delivery of prevention, treatment, care and support to respond to pandemics such as HIV/AIDS, tuberculosis and malaria;

5. Affirms the importance of public health interests in both pharmaceutical and health policies;

6. Calls upon States to pursue policies, in accordance with applicable international law, including international agreements acceded to, which would promote:

(a) The availability, in sufficient quantities, of pharmaceutical products and medical technologies used to treat pandemics such as HIV/AIDS, tuberculosis and malaria or the most common opportunistic infections that accompany them;

(b) The accessibility and affordability for all without discrimination, including the most vulnerable or socially disadvantaged groups of the population, of pharmaceutical products or medical technologies used to treat pandemics such as HIV/AIDS, tuberculosis, malaria or the most common opportunistic infections that accompany them;

(c) The assurance that pharmaceutical products or medical technologies used to treat pandemics such as HIV/AIDS, tuberculosis, malaria or the most common opportunistic infections that accompany them, irrespective of their sources and countries of origin, are scientifically and medically appropriate and of good quality;

7. Calls upon States, at the national level, on a non discriminatory basis, in accordance with applicable international law, including international agreements acceded to:

(a) To refrain from taking measures which would deny or limit equal access for all persons to preventive, curative or palliative pharmaceutical products or medical technologies used to treat pandemics such as HIV/AIDS, tuberculosis, malaria or the most common opportunistic infections that accompany them;

(b) To adopt and implement legislation or other measures, in accordance with applicable international law, including international agreements acceded to, to safeguard access to such preventive, curative or palliative pharmaceutical products or medical technologies from any limitations by third parties;

(c) To adopt all appropriate positive measures, to the maximum of the resources allocated for this purpose, to promote effective access to such preventive, curative or palliative pharmaceutical products or medical technologies;

8. Also calls upon States, in furtherance of the Declaration of Commitment on HIV/AIDS, to address factors affecting the provision of drugs related to the treatment of pandemics such as HIV/AIDS and the most common opportunistic infections that accompany them, as well as to develop integrated strategies to strengthen health care systems, including voluntary counselling and testing, laboratory capacities and the training of health care providers and technicians, in order to provide treatment and monitor the use of medications, diagnostics and related technologies;

9. Further calls upon States to take all appropriate measures, nationally and through cooperation, to promote research and development of new and more effective preventive, curative or palliative pharmaceutical products and diagnostic tools, in accordance with applicable international law, including international agreements acceded to;

10. Calls upon States, at the international level, to take steps, individually and/or through international cooperation, in accordance with applicable international law, including international agreements acceded to, such as:

(a) To facilitate, wherever possible, access in other countries to essential preventive, curative or palliative pharmaceutical products or medical technologies used to treat pandemics such as HIV/AIDS, tuberculosis and malaria or the most common opportunistic infections that accompany them, as well as to extend the necessary cooperation, wherever possible, especially in times of emergency;

(b) To ensure that their actions as members of international organizations take due account of the right of everyone to the enjoyment of the highest attainable standard of physical and mental health and that the application of international agreements is supportive of public health policies that promote broad access to safe, effective and affordable preventive, curative or palliative pharmaceutical products and medical technologies;

11. Urges States to consider, whenever necessary, adapting national legislation in order to use to the full the flexibilities contained in the TRIPS Agreement;

12. Welcomes the financial contributions made to date to the Global Fund to Fight AIDS, Tuberculosis and Malaria, urges that further contributions be made by States and other donors, and also calls upon all States to encourage the private sector to contribute to the Fund as a matter of urgency;

13. Calls upon all States and other donors to cooperate in supporting the "3 by 5" Initiative launched jointly by the World Health Organization and UN-AIDS with the aim of providing antiretroviral therapy to 3 million people in the developing world by 2005;

14. Calls upon UNAIDS to mobilize further resources to combat the HIV/AIDS pandemic and upon all Governments to take measures to ensure that the necessary resources are made available to UNAIDS, in line with the Declaration of Commitment on HIV/AIDS;

15. Calls upon States to ensure that those at risk of contracting malaria, in particular pregnant women and children under five years of age, benefit from the most suitable combination of personal and community protective measures, such as insecticide treated bed nets and other interventions that are accessible and affordable, to prevent infection and suffering;

16. Also calls upon States to provide the necessary support for the World Health Organization "Roll Back Malaria" and "Stop TB" partnerships in ongoing measures to combat malaria and tuberculosis;

17. Calls upon the international community, the developed countries in particular, to continue to assist the developing countries in the fight against pandemics such as HIV/AIDS, tuberculosis and malaria through financial and technical support, as well as through the training of personnel;

* * *

B. Business, Trade, and Intellectual Property

Doha Declaration on the TRIPS Agreement and Public Health
Adopted by the Fourth Ministerial Conference of the World Trade Organization in Doha, Qatar, on 14 November 2001.
[Available in WTO doc. WT/MIN (01)/DEC/2 of 20 November 2001 and at http://www.wto.org/english/thewto_e/minist_e/min01_e/mindecl_trips_e.htm

1. We recognize the gravity of the public health problems afflicting many developing and least-developed countries, especially those resulting from HIV/AIDS, tuberculosis, malaria and other epidemics.

2. We stress the need for the World Trade Organization (WTO) Agreement on Trade-Related Aspects of Intellectual Property Rights (TRIPS Agreement) to be part of the wider national and international action to address these problems.

3. We recognize that intellectual property protection is important for the development of new medicines. We also recognize the concerns about its effects on prices.

4. We agree that the TRIPS Agreement does not and should not prevent members from taking measures to protect public health. Accordingly, while reiterating our commitment to the TRIPS Agreement, we affirm that the Agreement can and should be interpreted and implemented in a manner supportive of WTO members' right to protect public health and, in particular, to promote access to medicines for all.

In this connection, we reaffirm the right of WTO members to use, to the full, the provisions in the TRIPS Agreement, which provide flexibility for this purpose.

5. Accordingly and in the light of paragraph 4 above, while maintaining our commitments in the TRIPS Agreement, we recognize that these flexibilities include:

a. In applying the customary rules of interpretation of public international law, each provision of the TRIPS Agreement shall be read in the light of the object and purpose of the Agreement as expressed, in particular, in its objectives and principles.

b. Each member has the right to grant compulsory licences and the freedom to determine the grounds upon which such licences are granted.

c. Each member has the right to determine what constitutes a national emergency or other circumstances of extreme urgency, it being understood that public health crises, including those relating to HIV/AIDS, tuberculosis, malaria and other epidemics, can represent a national emergency or other circumstances of extreme urgency.

d. The effect of the provisions in the TRIPS Agreement that are relevant to the exhaustion of intellectual property rights is to leave each member free to establish its own regime for such exhaustion without challenge, subject to the MFN and national treatment provisions of Articles 3 and 4.

6. We recognize that WTO members with insufficient or no manufacturing capacities in the pharmaceutical sector could face difficulties in making effective use of compulsory licensing under the TRIPS Agreement. We instruct the Council for TRIPS to find an expeditious solution to this problem and to report to the General Council before the end of 2002.

7. We reaffirm the commitment of developed-country members to provide incentives to their enterprises and institutions to promote and encourage technology transfer to least-developed country members pursuant to Article 66.2. We also agree that the least-developed country members will not be obliged, with respect to pharmaceutical products, to implement or apply Sections 5 and 7 of Part II of the TRIPS Agreement or to

enforce rights provided for under these Sections until 1 January 2016, without prejudice to the right of least-developed country members to seek other extensions of the transition periods as provided for in Article 66.1 of the TRIPS Agreement.

We instruct the Council for TRIPS to take the necessary action to give effect to this pursuant to Article 66.1 of the TRIPS Agreement.

Implementation of Paragraph 6 of the Doha Declaration on the TRIPS Agreement and Public Health
Decision of the General Council of 30 August 2003.
[Available in WTO doc. WT/GC/M/82 and at
http://www.wto.org/english/tratop_e/trips_e/implem_para6_e.htm]

[Footnotes omitted.]

The General Council,

Having regard to paragraphs 1, 3 and 4 of Article IX of the Marrakesh Agreement Establishing the World Trade Organization ("the WTO Agreement");

Conducting the functions of the Ministerial Conference in the interval between meetings pursuant to paragraph 2 of Article IV of the WTO Agreement;

Noting the Declaration on the TRIPS Agreement and Public Health (WT/MIN(01)/DEC/2) (the "Declaration") and, in particular, the instruction of the Ministerial Conference to the Council for TRIPS contained in paragraph 6 of the Declaration to find an expeditious solution to the problem of the difficulties that WTO Members with insufficient or no manufacturing capacities in the pharmaceutical sector could face in making effective use of compulsory licensing under the TRIPS Agreement and to report to the General Council before the end of 2002;

Recognizing, where eligible importing Members seek to obtain supplies under the system set out in this Decision, the importance of a rapid response to those needs consistent with the provisions of this Decision;

Noting that, in the light of the foregoing, exceptional circumstances exist justifying waivers from the obligations set out in paragraphs (f) and (h) of Article 31 of the TRIPS Agreement with respect to pharmaceutical products;

Decides as follows:

·1. For the purposes of this Decision:

(a) "pharmaceutical product" means any patented product, or product manufactured through a patented process, of the pharmaceutical sector needed to address the public health problems as recognized in paragraph 1 of the Declaration. It is understood that active ingredients necessary for its manufacture and diagnostic kits needed for its use would be included;

(b) "eligible importing Member" means any least-developed country Member, and any other Member that has made a notification to the Council for TRIPS of its intention to use the system as an importer, it being understood that a Member may notify at any time that it will use the system in whole or in a limited way, for example only in the case of a national emergency or other circumstances of extreme urgency or in cases of public non-commercial use. It is noted that some Members will not use the system set out in this Decision as importing Members and that some other Members have stated that, if they use the system, it would be in no more than situations of national emergency or other circumstances of extreme urgency;

(c) "exporting Member" means a Member using the system set out in this Decision to produce pharmaceutical products for, and export them to, an eligible importing Member.

2. The obligations of an exporting Member under Article 31(f) of the TRIPS Agreement shall be waived with respect to the grant by it of a compul-

sory licence to the extent necessary for the purposes of production of a pharmaceutical product(s) and its export to an eligible importing Member(s) in accordance with the terms set out below in this paragraph:

(a) the eligible importing Member(s) has made a notification to the Council for TRIPS, that:

(i) specifies the names and expected quantities of the product(s) needed;

(ii) confirms that the eligible importing Member in question, other than a least developed country Member, has established that it has insufficient or no manufacturing capacities in the pharmaceutical sector for the product(s) in question in one of the ways set out in the Annex to this Decision; and

(iii) confirms that, where a pharmaceutical product is patented in its territory, it has granted or intends to grant a compulsory licence in accordance with Article 31 of the TRIPS Agreement and the provisions of this Decision;

(b) the compulsory licence issued by the exporting Member under this Decision shall contain the following conditions:

(i) only the amount necessary to meet the needs of the eligible importing Member(s) may be manufactured under the licence and the entirety of this production shall be exported to the Member(s) which has notified its needs to the Council for TRIPS;

(ii) products produced under the licence shall be clearly identified as being produced under the system set out in this Decision through specific labelling or marking. Suppliers should distinguish such products through special packaging and/or special colouring/shaping of the products themselves, provided that such distinction is feasible and does not have a significant impact on price; and

(iii) before shipment begins, the licensee shall post on a website the following information:

• the quantities being supplied to each destination as referred to in indent (i) above; and

• the distinguishing features of the product(s) referred to in indent (ii) above;

(c) the exporting Member shall notify the Council for TRIPS of the grant of the licence, including the conditions attached to it. The information provided shall include the name and address of the licensee, the product(s) for which the licence has been granted, the quantity(ies) for which it has been granted, the country(ies) to which the product(s) is (are) to be supplied and the duration of the licence. The notification shall also indicate the address of the website referred to in subparagraph (b)(iii) above.

3. Where a compulsory licence is granted by an exporting Member under the system set out in this Decision, adequate remuneration pursuant to Article 31(h) of the TRIPS Agreement shall be paid in that Member taking into account the economic value to the importing Member of the use that has been authorized in the exporting Member. Where a compulsory licence is granted for the same products in the eligible importing Member, the obligation of that Member under Article 31(h) shall be waived in respect of those products for which remuneration in accordance with the first sentence of this paragraph is paid in the exporting Member.

4. In order to ensure that the products imported under the system set out in this Decision are used for the public health purposes underlying their importation, eligible importing Members shall take reasonable measures within their means, proportionate to their administrative capacities and to the risk of trade diversion to prevent re-exportation of the products that have actually been imported into their territories under the system. In the event that an eligible importing Member that is a developing country Member or a least-developed country Member experiences difficulty in implementing this provision, developed country Members shall provide, on request and on mutually agreed terms and conditions, technical and financial cooperation in order to facilitate its implementation.

5. Members shall ensure the availability of effective legal means to prevent the importation into, and sale in, their territories of products produced under the system set out in this Decision and diverted to their markets inconsistently with its provisions, using the means already required to be available under the TRIPS Agreement. If any Member considers that such measures are proving insufficient for this purpose, the matter may be re-

viewed in the Council for TRIPS at the request of that Member.

6. With a view to harnessing economies of scale for the purposes of enhancing purchasing power for, and facilitating the local production of, pharmaceutical products:

(i) where a developing or least-developed country WTO Member is a party to a regional trade agreement within the meaning of Article XXIV of the GATT 1994 and the Decision of 28 November 1979 on Differential and More Favourable Treatment Reciprocity and Fuller Participation of Developing Countries (L/4903), at least half of the current membership of which is made up of countries presently on the United Nations list of least developed countries, the obligation of that Member under Article 31(f) of the TRIPS Agreement shall be waived to the extent necessary to enable a pharmaceutical product produced or imported under a compulsory licence in that Member to be exported to the markets of those other developing or least developed country parties to the regional trade agreement that share the health problem in question. It is understood that this will not prejudice the territorial nature of the patent rights in question;

(ii) it is recognized that the development of systems providing for the grant of regional patents to be applicable in the above Members should be promoted. To this end, developed country Members undertake to provide technical cooperation in accordance with Article 67 of the TRIPS Agreement, including in conjunction with other relevant intergovernmental organizations.

7. Members recognize the desirability of promoting the transfer of technology and capacity building in the pharmaceutical sector in order to overcome the problem identified in paragraph 6 of the Declaration. To this end, eligible importing Members and exporting Members are encouraged to use the system set out in this Decision in a way which would promote this objective. Members undertake to cooperate in paying special attention to the transfer of technology and capacity building in the pharmaceutical sector in the work to be undertaken pursuant to Article 66.2 of the TRIPS Agreement, paragraph 7 of the Declaration and any other relevant work of the Council for TRIPS.

8. The Council for TRIPS shall review annually the functioning of the system set out in this Decision with a view to ensuring its effective operation and shall annually report on its operation to the General Council. This review shall be deemed to fulfil the review requirements of Article IX:4 of the WTO Agreement.

9. This Decision is without prejudice to the rights, obligations and flexibilities that Members have under the provisions of the TRIPS Agreement other than paragraphs (f) and (h) of Article 31, including those reaffirmed by the Declaration, and to their interpretation. It is also without prejudice to the extent to which pharmaceutical products produced under a compulsory licence can be exported under the present provisions of Article 31(f) of the TRIPS Agreement.

10. Members shall not challenge any measures taken in conformity with the provisions of the waivers contained in this Decision under subparagraphs 1(b) and 1(c) of Article XXIII of GATT 1994.

11. This Decision, including the waivers granted in it, shall terminate for each Member on the date on which an amendment to the TRIPS Agreement replacing its provisions takes effect for that Member. The TRIPS Council shall initiate by the end of 2003 work on the preparation of such an amendment with a view to its adoption within six months, on the understanding that the amendment will be based, where appropriate, on this Decision and on the further understanding that it will not be part of the negotiations referred to in paragraph 45 of the Doha Ministerial Declaration (WT/MIN(01)/DEC/1).

ANNEX

Assessment of Manufacturing Capacities in the Pharmaceutical Sector

Least-developed country Members are deemed to have insufficient or no manufacturing capacities in the pharmaceutical sector.

For other eligible importing Members insufficient or no manufacturing capacities for the product(s) in question may be established in either of the following ways:

(i) the Member in question has established that it

has no manufacturing capacity in the pharmaceutical sector;

OR

(ii) where the Member has some manufacturing capacity in this sector, it has examined this capacity and found that, excluding any capacity owned or controlled by the patent owner, it is currently insufficient for the purposes of meeting its needs. When it is established that such capacity has become sufficient to meet the Member's needs, the system shall no longer apply.

Norms on the Responsibilities of Transnational Corporations and Other Business Enterprises with Regard to Human Rights (2003)

Approved August 13, 2003, by U.N. Sub-Commission on the Promotion and Protection of Human Rights Resolution 2003/16. [Available in U.N. Doc. E/CN.4/Sub.2/2003/12/Rev.2 and at http://www.ap.ohchr.org/documents/dpage_e.aspx?s=58]

PREAMBLE

Bearing in mind the principles and obligations under the Charter of the United Nations, in particular the preamble and Articles 1, 2, 55 and 56, inter alia to promote universal respect for, and observance of, human rights and fundamental freedoms, Recalling that the Universal Declaration of Human Rights proclaims a common standard of achievement for all peoples and all nations, to the end that Governments, other organs of society and individuals shall strive, by teaching and education to promote respect for human rights and freedoms, and, by progressive measures, to secure universal and effective recognition and observance, including of equal rights of women and men and the promotion of social progress and better standards of life in larger freedom, Recognizing that even though States have the primary responsibility to promote, secure the fulfilment of, respect, ensure respect of and protect human rights, transnational corporations and other business enterprises, as organs of society, are also responsible for promoting and securing the human rights set forth in the Universal Declaration of Human Rights,

Realizing that transnational corporations and other business enterprises, their officers and persons working for them are also obligated to respect generally recognized responsibilities and norms contained in United Nations treaties and other international instruments such as the Convention on the Prevention and Punishment of the Crime of Genocide; the Convention Against Torture and Other Cruel, Inhuman or Degrading Treatment or Punishment; the Slavery Convention and the Supplementary Convention on the Abolition of Slavery, the Slave Trade, and Institutions and Practices Similar to Slavery; the International Convention on the Elimination of All Forms of Racial Discrimination; the Convention on the Elimination of All Forms of Discrimination against Women; the International Covenant on Economic, Social and Cultural Rights; the International Covenant on Civil and Political Rights; the Convention on the Rights of the Child; the International Convention on the Protection of the Rights of All Migrant Workers and Members of Their Families; the four Geneva Conventions of 12 August 1949 and two Additional Protocols thereto for the protection of victims of war; the Declaration on the Right and Responsibility of Individuals, Groups and Organs of Society to Promote and Protect Universally Recognized Human Rights and Fundamental Freedoms; the Rome Statute of the International Criminal Court; the United Nations Convention against Transnational Organized Crime; the Convention on Biological Diversity; the International Convention on Civil Liability for Oil Pollution Damage; the Convention on Civil Liability for Damage Resulting from Activities Dangerous to the Environment; the Declaration on the Right to Development; the Rio Declaration on the Environment and Development; the Plan of Implementation of the World Summit on Sustainable Development; the United Nations Millennium Declaration; the Universal Declaration on the Human Genome and Human

Rights; the International Code of Marketing of Breast-milk Substitutes adopted by the World Health Assembly; the Ethical Criteria for Medical Drug Promotion and the "Health for All in the Twenty-First Century" policy of the World Health Organization; the Convention against Discrimination in Education of the United Nations Educational, Scientific, and Cultural Organization; conventions and recommendations of the International Labour Organization; the Convention and Protocol relating to the Status of Refugees; the African Charter on Human and Peoples' Rights; the American Convention on Human Rights; the European Convention for the Protection of Human Rights and Fundamental Freedoms; the Charter of Fundamental Rights of the European Union; the Convention on Combating Bribery of Foreign Public Officials in International Business Transactions of the Organization for Economic Cooperation and Development; and other instruments,

Taking into account the standards set forth in the Tripartite Declaration of Principles Concerning Multinational Enterprises and Social Policy and the Declaration on Fundamental Principles and Rights at Work of the International Labour Organization,

Aware of the Guidelines for Multinational Enterprises and the Committee on International Investment and Multinational Enterprises of the Organization for Economic Cooperation and Development,

Aware also of the United Nations Global Compact initiative which challenges business leaders to "embrace and enact" nine basic principles with respect to human rights, including labour rights and the environment,

Conscious of the fact that the Governing Body Subcommittee on Multinational Enterprises and Social Policy, the Governing Body, the Committee of Experts on the Application of Standards, as well as the Committee on Freedom of Association of the International Labour Organization have named business enterprises implicated in States' failure to comply with Conventions No. 87 concerning the Freedom of Association and Protection of the Right to

Organize and No. 98 concerning the Application of the Principles of the Right to Organize and Bargain Collectively, and seeking to supplement and assist their efforts to encourage transnational corporations and other business enterprises to protect human rights,

Conscious also of the Commentary on the Norms on the responsibilities of transnational corporations and other business enterprises with regard to human rights, and finding it a useful interpretation and elaboration of the standards contained in the Norms,

Taking note of global trends which have increased the influence of transnational corporations and other business enterprises on the economies of most countries and in international economic relations, and of the growing number of other business enterprises which operate across national boundaries in a variety of arrangements resulting in economic activities beyond the actual capacities of any one national system,

Noting that transnational corporations and other business enterprises have the capacity to foster economic well-being, development, technological improvement and wealth as well as the capacity to cause harmful impacts on the human rights and lives of individuals through their core business practices and operations, including employment practices, environmental policies, relationships with suppliers and consumers, interactions with Governments and other activities,

Noting also that new international human rights issues and concerns are continually emerging and that transnational corporations and other business enterprises often are involved in these issues and concerns, such that further standard-setting and implementation are required at this time and in the future,

Acknowledging the universality, indivisibility, interdependence and interrelatedness of human rights, including the right to development, which entitles every human person and all peoples to participate in, contribute to and enjoy economic, social, cultural and political development in which all human rights and fundamental freedoms can be fully realized,

Reaffirming that transnational corporations and other business enterprises, their officers — including managers, members of corporate boards or directors and other executives — and persons working for them have, inter alia, human rights obligations and responsibilities and that these human rights norms will contribute to the making and development of international law as to those responsibilities and obligations,

Solemnly proclaims these Norms on the Responsibilities of Transnational Corporations and Other Business Enterprises with Regard to Human Rights and urges that every effort be made so that they become generally known and respected.

A. General Obligations

1. States have the primary responsibility to promote, secure the fulfilment of, respect, ensure respect of and protect human rights recognized in international as well as national law, including ensuring that transnational corporations and other business enterprises respect human rights. Within their respective spheres of activity and influence, transnational corporations and other business enterprises have the obligation to promote, secure the fulfilment of, respect, ensure respect of and protect human rights recognized in international as well as national law, including the rights and interests of indigenous peoples and other vulnerable groups.

B. Right to Equal Opportunity and Non-Discriminatory Treatment

2. Transnational corporations and other business enterprises shall ensure equality of opportunity and treatment, as provided in the relevant international instruments and national legislation as well as international human rights law, for the purpose of eliminating discrimination based on race, colour, sex, language, religion, political opinion, national or social origin, social status, indigenous status, disability, age — except for children, who may be given greater protection — or other status of the individual unrelated to the inherent requirements to perform the job, or of complying with special measures designed to overcome past discrimination against certain groups.

C. Right to Security of Persons

3. Transnational corporations and other business enterprises shall not engage in nor benefit from war crimes, crimes against humanity, genocide, torture, forced disappearance, forced or compulsory labour, hostage-taking, extrajudicial, summary or arbitrary executions, other violations of humanitarian law and other international crimes against the human person as defined by international law, in particular human rights and humanitarian law.

4. Security arrangements for transnational corporations and other business enterprises shall observe international human rights norms as well as the laws and professional standards of the country or countries in which they operate.

D. Rights of Workers

5. Transnational corporations and other business enterprises shall not use forced or compulsory labour as forbidden by the relevant international instruments and national legislation as well as international human rights and humanitarian law.

6. Transnational corporations and other business enterprises shall respect the rights of children to be protected from economic exploitation as forbidden by the relevant international instruments and national legislation as well as international human rights and humanitarian law.

7. Transnational corporations and other business enterprises shall provide a safe and healthy working environment as set forth in relevant international instruments and national legislation as well as international human rights and humanitarian law.

8. Transnational corporations and other business enterprises shall provide workers with remuneration that ensures an adequate standard of living for them and their families. Such remuneration shall take due account of their needs for adequate living conditions with a view towards progressive improvement.

9. Transnational corporations and other business enterprises shall ensure freedom of association and effective recognition of the right to collective bargaining by protecting the right to establish and,

subject only to the rules of the organization concerned, to join organizations of their own choosing without distinction, previous authorization, or interference, for the protection of their employment interests and for other collective bargaining purposes as provided in national legislation and the relevant conventions of the International Labour Organization.

E. Respect for National Sovereignty and Human Rights

10. Transnational corporations and other business enterprises shall recognize and respect applicable norms of international law, national laws and regulations, as well as administrative practices, the rule of law, the public interest, development objectives, social, economic and cultural policies including transparency, accountability and prohibition of corruption, and authority of the countries in which the enterprises operate.

11. Transnational corporations and other business enterprises shall not offer, promise, give, accept, condone, knowingly benefit from, or demand a bribe or other improper advantage, nor shall they be solicited or expected to give a bribe or other improper advantage to any Government, public official, candidate for elective post, any member of the armed forces or security forces, or any other individual or organization. Transnational corporations and other business enterprises shall refrain from any activity which supports, solicits, or encourages States or any other entities to abuse human rights. They shall further seek to ensure that the goods and services they provide will not be used to abuse human rights.

12. Transnational corporations and other business enterprises shall respect economic, social and cultural rights as well as civil and political rights and contribute to their realization, in particular the rights to development, adequate food and drinking water, the highest attainable standard of physical and mental health, adequate housing, privacy, education, freedom of thought, conscience, and religion and freedom of opinion and expression, and shall refrain from actions which obstruct or impede the realization of those rights.

F. Obligations with Regard to Consumer Protection

13. Transnational corporations and other business enterprises shall act in accordance with fair business, marketing and advertising practices and shall take all necessary steps to ensure the safety and quality of the goods and services they provide, including observance of the precautionary principle. Nor shall they produce, distribute, market, or advertise harmful or potentially harmful products for use by consumers.

G. Obligations with Regard to Environmental Protection

14. Transnational corporations and other business enterprises shall carry out their activities in accordance with national laws, regulations, administrative practices and policies relating to the preservation of the environment of the countries in which they operate, as well as in accordance with relevant international agreements, principles, objectives, responsibilities and standards with regard to the environment as well as human rights, public health and safety, bioethics and the precautionary principle, and shall generally conduct their activities in a manner contributing to the wider goal of sustainable development.

H. General Provisions of Implementation

15. As an initial step towards implementing these Norms, each transnational corporation or other business enterprise shall adopt, disseminate and implement internal rules of operation in compliance with the Norms. Further, they shall periodically report on and take other measures fully to implement the Norms and to provide at least for the prompt implementation of the protections set forth in the Norms. Each transnational corporation or other business enterprise shall apply and incorporate these Norms in their contracts or other arrangements and dealings with contractors, subcontractors, suppliers, licensees, distributors, or natural or other legal persons that enter into any agreement with the transnational corporation or business enterprise in order to ensure respect for and implementation of the Norms.

16. Transnational corporations and other business enterprises shall be subject to periodic monitoring

and verification by United Nations, other international and national mechanisms already in existence or yet to be created, regarding application of the Norms. This monitoring shall be transparent and independent and take into account input from stakeholders (including non-governmental organizations) and as a result of complaints of violations of these Norms. Further, transnational corporations and other business enterprises shall conduct periodic evaluations concerning the impact of their own activities on human rights under these Norms.

17. States should establish and reinforce the necessary legal and administrative framework for ensuring that the Norms and other relevant national and international laws are implemented by transnational corporations and other business enterprises.

18. Transnational corporations and other business enterprises shall provide prompt, effective and adequate reparation to those persons, entities and communities that have been adversely affected by failures to comply with these Norms through, inter alia, reparations, restitution, compensation and rehabilitation for any damage done or property taken. In connection with determining damages, in regard to criminal sanctions, and in all other respects, these Norms shall be applied by national courts and/or international tribunals, pursuant to national and international law.

19. Nothing in these Norms shall be construed as diminishing, restricting, or adversely affecting the human rights obligations of States under national and international law, nor shall they be construed as diminishing, restricting, or adversely affecting more protective human rights norms, nor shall they be construed as diminishing, restricting, or adversely affecting other obligations or responsibilities of transnational corporations and other business enterprises in fields other than human rights.

I. Definitions

20. The term "transnational corporation" refers to an economic entity operating in more than one country or a cluster of economic entities operating in two or more countries — whatever their legal form, whether in their home country or country of activity, and whether taken individually or collectively.

21. The phrase "other business enterprise" includes any business entity, regardless of the international or domestic nature of its activities, including a transnational corporation, contractor, subcontractor, supplier, licensee or distributor; the corporate, partnership, or other legal form used to establish the business entity; and the nature of the ownership of the entity. These Norms shall be presumed to apply, as a matter of practice, if the business enterprise has any relation with a transnational corporation, the impact of its activities is not entirely local, or the activities involve violations of the right to security as indicated in paragraphs 3 and 4.

22. The term "stakeholder" includes stockholders, other owners, workers and their representatives, as well as any other individual or group that is affected by the activities of transnational corporations or other business enterprises. The term "stakeholder" shall be interpreted functionally in the light of the objectives of these Norms and include indirect stakeholders when their interests are or will be substantially affected by the activities of the transnational corporation or business enterprise. In addition to parties directly affected by the activities of business enterprises, stakeholders can include parties which are indirectly affected by the activities of transnational corporations or other business enterprises such as consumer groups, customers, Governments, neighbouring communities, indigenous peoples and communities, non-governmental organizations, public and private lending institutions, suppliers, trade associations, and others.

23. The phrases "human rights" and "international human rights" include civil, cultural, economic, political and social rights, as set forth in the International Bill of Human Rights and other human rights treaties, as well as the right to development and rights recognized by international humanitarian law, international refugee law, international labour law, and other relevant instruments adopted within the United Nations system.

C. Occupational Health and Safety

Convention Concerning Occupational Safety and Health and the Working Environment (1981)

ILO Convention C155, adopted by the International Labour Conference at its 67th session on June 22 1981. Entered into force: 11 August 1983.
[Available at http://www.ilo.org/ilolex/english/subjlst.htm]

The General Conference of the International Labour Organisation,

Having been convened at Geneva by the Governing Body of the International Labour Office, and having met in its Sixty-seventh Session on 3 June 1981, and

Having decided upon the adoption of certain proposals with regard to safety and health and the working environment, which is the sixth item on the agenda of the session, and

Having determined that these proposals shall take the form of an international Convention,

Adopts this twenty-second day of June of the year one thousand nine hundred and eighty-one the following Convention, which may be cited as the Occupational Safety and Health Convention, 1981:

PART I
SCOPE AND DEFINITIONS

Article 1

1. This Convention applies to all branches of economic activity.

2. A Member ratifying this Convention may, after consultation at the earliest possible stage with the representative organisations of employers and workers concerned, exclude from its application, in part or in whole, particular branches of economic activity, such as maritime shipping or fishing, in respect of which special problems of a substantial nature arise.

3. Each Member which ratifies this Convention shall list, in the first report on the application of the

Convention submitted under Article 22 of the Constitution of the International Labour Organisation, any branches which may have been excluded in pursuance of paragraph 2 of this Article, giving the reasons for such exclusion and describing the measures taken to give adequate protection to workers in excluded branches, and shall indicate in subsequent reports any progress towards wider application.

Article 2

1. This Convention applies to all workers in the branches of economic activity covered.

2. A Member ratifying this Convention may, after consultation at the earliest possible stage with the representative organisations of employers and workers concerned, exclude from its application, in part or in whole, limited categories of workers in respect of which there are particular difficulties.

3. Each Member which ratifies this Convention shall list, in the first report on the application of the Convention submitted under Article 22 of the Constitution of the International Labour Organisation, any limited categories of workers which may have been excluded in pursuance of paragraph 2 of this Article, giving the reasons for such exclusion, and shall indicate in subsequent reports any progress towards wider application.

Article 3

For the purpose of this Convention —

(a) the term *branches of economic activity* covers all branches in which workers are employed, including the public service;

(b) the term *workers* covers all employed persons, including public employees;

(c) the term *workplace* covers all places where workers need to be or to go by reason of their work and which are under the direct or indirect control of the employer;

(d) the term *regulations* covers all provisions given force of law by the competent authority or authorities;

(e) the term *health*, in relation to work, indicates not merely the absence of disease or infirmity; it also includes the physical and mental elements affecting health which are directly related to safety and hygiene at work.

PART II
PRINCIPLES OF NATIONAL POLICY

Article 4

1. Each Member shall, in the light of national conditions and practice, and in consultation with the most representative organisations of employers and workers, formulate, implement and periodically review a coherent national policy on occupational safety, occupational health and the working environment.

2. The aim of the policy shall be to prevent accidents and injury to health arising out of, linked with or occurring in the course of work, by minimising, so far as is reasonably practicable, the causes of hazards inherent in the working environment.

Article 5

The policy referred to in Article 4 of this Convention shall take account of the following main spheres of action in so far as they affect occupational safety and health and the working environment:

(a) design, testing, choice, substitution, installation, arrangement, use and maintenance of the material elements of work (workplaces, working environment, tools, machinery and equipment, chemical, physical and biological substances and agents, work processes);

(b) relationships between the material elements of work and the persons who carry out or supervise the work, and adaptation of machinery, equipment, working time, organisation of work and work processes to the physical and mental capacities of the workers;

(c) training, including necessary further training, qualifications and motivations of persons involved, in one capacity or another, in the achievement of adequate levels of safety and health;

(d) communication and co-operation at the levels of the working group and the undertaking and at all other appropriate levels up to and including the national level;

(e) the protection of workers and their representatives from disciplinary measures as a result of actions properly taken by them in conformity with the policy referred to in Article 4 of this Convention.

Article 6

The formulation of the policy referred to in Article 4 of this Convention shall indicate the respective functions and responsibilities in respect of occupational safety and health and the working environment of public authorities, employers, workers and others, taking account both of the complementary character of such responsibilities and of national conditions and practice.

Article 7

The situation regarding occupational safety and health and the working environment shall be reviewed at appropriate intervals, either over-all or in respect of particular areas, with a view to identifying major problems, evolving effective methods for dealing with them and priorities of action, and evaluating results.

PART III
ACTION AT THE NATIONAL LEVEL

Article 8

Each Member shall, by laws or regulations or any other method consistent with national conditions and practice and in consultation with the representative organisations of employers and workers concerned, take such steps as may be necessary to give effect to Article 4 of this Convention.

Article 9

1. The enforcement of laws and regulations concerning occupational safety and health and the working environment shall be secured by an adequate and appropriate system of inspection.

HUMAN RIGHTS ASPECTS OF HEALTH POLICY

2. The enforcement system shall provide for adequate penalties for violations of the laws and regulations.

Article 10

Measures shall be taken to provide guidance to employers and workers so as to help them to comply with legal obligations.

Article 11

To give effect to the policy referred to in Article 4 of this Convention, the competent authority or authorities shall ensure that the following functions are progressively carried out:

(a) the determination, where the nature and degree of hazards so require, of conditions governing the design, construction and layout of undertakings, the commencement of their operations, major alterations affecting them and changes in their purposes, the safety of technical equipment used at work, as well as the application of procedures defined by the competent authorities;

(b) the determination of work processes and of substances and agents the exposure to which is to be prohibited, limited or made subject to authorisation or control by the competent authority or authorities; health hazards due to the simultaneous exposure to several substances or agents shall be taken into consideration;

(c) the establishment and application of procedures for the notification of occupational accidents and diseases, by employers and, when appropriate, insurance institutions and others directly concerned, and the production of annual statistics on occupational accidents and diseases;

(d) the holding of inquiries, where cases of occupational accidents, occupational diseases or any other injuries to health which arise in the course of or in connection with work appear to reflect situations which are serious;

(e) the publication, annually, of information on measures taken in pursuance of the policy referred to in Article 4 of this Convention and on occupational accidents, occupational diseases and other injuries to health which arise in the course of or in connection with work;

(f) the introduction or extension of systems, taking into account national conditions and possibilities, to examine chemical, physical and biological agents in respect of the risk to the health of workers.

Article 12

Measures shall be taken, in accordance with national law and practice, with a view to ensuring that those who design, manufacture, import, provide or transfer machinery, equipment or substances for occupational use —

(a) satisfy themselves that, so far as is reasonably practicable, the machinery, equipment or substance does not entail dangers for the safety and health of those using it correctly;

(b) make available information concerning the correct installation and use of machinery and equipment and the correct use of substances, and information on hazards of machinery and equipment and dangerous properties of chemical substances and physical and biological agents or products, as well as instructions on how known hazards are to be avoided;

(c) undertake studies and research or otherwise keep abreast of the scientific and technical knowledge necessary to comply with subparagraphs (a) and (b) of this Article.

Article 13

A worker who has removed himself from a work situation which he has reasonable justification to believe presents an imminent and serious danger to his life or health shall be protected from undue consequences in accordance with national conditions and practice.

Article 14

Measures shall be taken with a view to promoting in a manner appropriate to national conditions and practice, the inclusion of questions of occupational safety and health and the working environment at all levels of education and training, including higher technical, medical and professional education, in a manner meeting the training needs of all workers.

Occupational Health and Safety

Article 15

1. With a view to ensuring the coherence of the policy referred to in Article 4 of this Convention and of measures for its application, each Member shall, after consultation at the earliest possible stage with the most representative organisations of employers and workers, and with other bodies as appropriate, make arrangements appropriate to national conditions and practice to ensure the necessary co-ordination between various authorities and bodies called upon to give effect to Parts II and III of this Convention.

2. Whenever circumstances so require and national conditions and practice permit, these arrangements shall include the establishment of a central body.

PART IV
ACTION AT THE LEVEL
OF THE UNDERTAKING
Article 16

1. Employers shall be required to ensure that, so far as is reasonably practicable, the workplaces, machinery, equipment and processes under their control are safe and without risk to health.

2. Employers shall be required to ensure that, so far as is reasonably practicable, the chemical, physical and biological substances and agents under their control are without risk to health when the appropriate measures of protection are taken.

3. Employers shall be required to provide, where necessary, adequate protective clothing and protective equipment to prevent, so far is reasonably practicable, risk of accidents or of adverse effects on health.

Article 17

Whenever two or more undertakings engage in activities simultaneously at one workplace, they shall collaborate in applying the requirements of this Convention.

Article 18

Employers shall be required to provide, where necessary, for measures to deal with emergencies and accidents, including adequate first-aid arrangements.

Article 19

There shall be arrangements at the level of the undertaking under which —

(a) workers, in the course of performing their work, co-operate in the fulfilment by their employer of the obligations placed upon him;

(b) representatives of workers in the undertaking co-operate with the employer in the field of occupational safety and health;

(c) representatives of workers in an undertaking are given adequate information on measures taken by the employer to secure occupational safety and health and may consult their representative organisations about such information provided they do not disclose commercial secrets;

(d) workers and their representatives in the undertaking are given appropriate training in occupational safety and health;

(e) workers or their representatives and, as the case may be, their representative organisations in an undertaking, in accordance with national law and practice, are enabled to enquire into, and are consulted by the employer on, all aspects of occupational safety and health associated with their work; for this purpose technical advisers may, by mutual agreement, be brought in from outside the undertaking;

(f) a worker reports forthwith to his immediate supervisor any situation which he has reasonable justification to believe presents an imminent and serious danger to his life or health; until the employer has taken remedial action, if necessary, the employer cannot require workers to return to a work situation where there is continuing imminent and serious danger to life or health.

Article 20

Co-operation between management and workers and/or their representatives within the undertaking shall be an essential element of organisational and other measures taken in pursuance of Articles 16 to 19 of this Convention.

Article 21

Occupational safety and health measures shall not involve any expenditure for the workers.

PART V
FINAL PROVISIONS

Article 22

This Convention does not revise any international labour Conventions or Recommendations.

Article 23

The formal ratifications of this Convention shall be communicated to the Director-General of the International Labour Office for registration.

Article 24

1. This Convention shall be binding only upon those Members of the International Labour Organisation whose ratifications have been registered with the Director-General.

2. It shall come into force twelve months after the date on which the ratifications of two Members have been registered with the Director-General.

3. Thereafter, this Convention shall come into force for any Member twelve months after the date on which its ratification has been registered.

Article 25

1. A Member which has ratified this Convention may denounce it after the expiration of ten years from the date on which the Convention first comes into force, by an act communicated to the Director-General of the International Labour Office for registration. Such denunciation shall not take effect until one year after the date on which it is registered.

2. Each Member which has ratified this Convention and which does not, within the year following the expiration of the period of ten years mentioned in the preceding paragraph, exercise the right of denunciation provided for in this Article, will be bound for another period of ten years and, thereafter, may denounce this Convention at the expiration of each period of ten years under the terms provided for in this Article.

Article 26

1. The Director-General of the International Labour Office shall notify all Members of the International Labour Organisation of the registration of all ratifi-cations and denunciations communicated to him by the Members of the Organisation.

2. When notifying the Members of the Organisation of the registration of the second ratification communicated to him, the Director-General shall draw the attention of the Members of the Organisation to the date upon which the Convention will come into force.

Article 27

The Director-General of the International Labour Office shall communicate to the Secretary-General of the United Nations for registration in accordance with Article 102 of the Charter of the United Nations full particulars of all ratifications and acts of denunciation registered by him in accordance with the provisions of the preceding Articles.

Article 28

At such times as it may consider necessary the Governing Body of the International Labour Office shall present to the General Conference a report on the working of this Convention and shall examine the desirability of placing on the agenda of the Conference the question of its revision in whole or in part.

Article 29

1. Should the Conference adopt a new Convention revising this Convention in whole or in part, then, unless the new Convention otherwise provides:

a) the ratification by a Member of the new revising Convention shall ipso jure involve the immediate denunciation of this Convention, notwithstanding the provisions of Article 25 above, if and when the new revising Convention shall have come into force;

b) as from the date when the new revising Convention comes into force this Convention shall cease to be open to ratification by the Members.

2. This Convention shall in any case remain in force in its actual form and content for those Members which have ratified it but have not ratified the revising Convention.

Article 30

The English and French versions of the text of this Convention are equally authoritative.

Protocol of 2002 to the Occupational Safety and Health Convention (2002)

ILO Convention: P155, adopted by the International Labour Conference at its 90th session on 20 June 2002, to come into force on 9 February 2005. [Available at http://www.ilo.org/ilolex/cgi-lex/convde.pl?P155]

The General Conference of the International Labour Organization,

Having been convened at Geneva by the Governing Body of the International Labour Office, and having met in its 90th Session on 3 June 2002, and

Noting the provisions of Article 11 of the Occupational Safety and Health Convention, 1981, (hereinafter referred to as "the Convention"), which states in particular that:

"To give effect to the policy referred to in Article 4 of this Convention, the competent authority or authorities shall ensure that the following functions are progressively carried out:

* * *

(c) the establishment and application of procedures for the notification of occupational accidents and diseases, by employers and, when appropriate, insurance institutions and others directly concerned, and the production of annual statistics on occupational accidents and diseases;

* * *

(e) the publication, annually, of information on measures taken in pursuance of the policy referred to in Article 4 of this Convention and on occupational accidents, occupational diseases and other injuries to health which arise in the course of or in connection with work",

and

Having regard to the need to strengthen recording and notification procedures for occupational acci-

dents and diseases and to promote the harmonization of recording and notification systems with the aim of identifying their causes and establishing preventive measures, and

Having decided upon the adoption of certain proposals with regard to the recording and notification of occupational accidents and diseases, which is the fifth item on the agenda of the session, and

Having determined that these proposals shall take the form of a protocol to the Occupational Safety and Health Convention, 1981;

Adopts this twentieth day of June two thousand and two the following Protocol, which may be cited as the Protocol of 2002 to the Occupational Safety and Health Convention, 1981.

I. DEFINITIONS

Article 1

For the purpose of this Protocol:

(a) the term *occupational accident* covers an occurrence arising out of, or in the course of, work which results in fatal or non-fatal injury;

(b) the term *occupational disease* covers any disease contracted as a result of an exposure to risk factors arising from work activity;

(c) the term *dangerous occurrence* covers a readily identifiable event as defined under national laws and regulations, with potential to cause an injury or disease to persons at work or to the public;

(d) the term *commuting accident* covers an accident resulting in death or personal injury occurring on the direct way between the place of work and:

(i) the worker's principal or secondary residence; or

(ii) the place where the worker usually takes a meal; or

(iii) the place where the worker usually receives his or her remuneration.

II. SYSTEMS FOR RECORDING AND NOTIFICATION

Article 2

The competent authority shall, by laws or regulations or any other method consistent with national conditions and practice, and in consultation with the most representative organizations of employers and workers, establish and periodically review requirements and procedures for:

(a) the recording of occupational accidents, occupational diseases and, as appropriate, dangerous occurrences, commuting accidents and suspected cases of occupational diseases; and

(b) the notification of occupational accidents, occupational diseases and, as appropriate, dangerous occurrences, commuting accidents and suspected cases of occupational diseases.

Article 3

The requirements and procedures for recording shall determine:

(a) the responsibility of employers:

(i) to record occupational accidents, occupational diseases and, as appropriate, dangerous occurrences, commuting accidents and suspected cases of occupational diseases;

(ii) to provide appropriate information to workers and their representatives concerning the recording system;

(iii) to ensure appropriate maintenance of these records and their use for the establishment of preventive measures; and

(iv) to refrain from instituting retaliatory or disciplinary measures against a worker for reporting an occupational accident, occupational disease, dangerous occurrence, commuting accident or suspected case of occupational disease;

(b) the information to be recorded;

(c) the duration for maintaining these records; and

(d) measures to ensure the confidentiality of personal and medical data in the employer's possession, in accordance with national laws and regulations, conditions and practice.

Article 4

The requirements and procedures for the notification shall determine:

(a) the responsibility of employers:

(i) to notify the competent authorities or other designated bodies of occupational accidents, occupational diseases and, as appropriate, dangerous occurrences, commuting accidents and suspected cases of occupational diseases; and

(ii) to provide appropriate information to workers and their representatives concerning the notified cases;

(b) where appropriate, arrangements for notification of occupational accidents and occupational diseases by insurance institutions, occupational health services, medical practitioners and other bodies directly concerned;

(c) the criteria according to which occupational accidents, occupational diseases and, as appropriate, dangerous occurrences, commuting accidents and suspected cases of occupational diseases are to be notified; and

(d) the time limits for notification.

Article 5

The notification shall include data on:

(a) the enterprise, establishment and employer;

(b) if applicable, the injured persons and the nature of the injuries or disease; and

(c) the workplace, the circumstances of the accident or the dangerous occurrence and, in the case of an occupational disease, the circumstances of the exposure to health hazards.

III. NATIONAL STATISTICS

Article 6

Each Member which ratifies this Protocol shall, based on the notifications and other available information, publish annually statistics that are compiled in such a way as to be representative of the country as a whole, concerning occupational accidents, occupational diseases and, as appropriate, dangerous occurrences and commuting accidents, as well as the analyses thereof.

Article 7

The statistics shall be established following classification schemes that are compatible with the latest relevant international schemes established under the auspices of the International Labour Organization or other competent international organizations.

FINAL

IV. FINAL PROVISIONS

Article 8

1. A Member may ratify this Protocol at the same time as or at any time after its ratification of the Convention, by communicating its formal ratification to the Director-General of the International Labour Office for registration.

2. The Protocol shall come into force 12 months after the date on which ratifications of two Members have been registered by the Director-General. Thereafter, this Protocol shall come into force for a Member 12 months after the date on which its ratification has been registered by the Director-General and the Convention shall be binding on the Member concerned with the addition of Articles 1 to 7 of this Protocol.

Article 9

1. A Member which has ratified this Protocol may denounce it whenever the Convention is open to denunciation in accordance with its Article 25, by an act communicated to the Director-General of the International Labour Office for registration.

2. Denunciation of the Convention in accordance with its Article 25 by a Member which has ratified this Protocol shall ipso jure involve the denunciation of this Protocol.

3. Any denunciation of this Protocol in accordance with paragraphs 1 or 2 of this Article shall not take effect until one year after the date on which it is registered.

Article 10

1. The Director-General of the International Labour Office shall notify all Members of the International Labour Organization of the registration of all ratifications and acts of denunciation communicated by the Members of the Organization.

2. When notifying the Members of the Organization of the registration of the second ratification, the Director-General shall draw the attention of the Members of the Organization to the date upon which the Protocol shall come into force.

Article 11

The Director-General of the International Labour Office shall communicate to the Secretary-General of the United Nations, for registration in accordance with article 102 of the Charter of the United Nations, full particulars of all ratifications and acts of denunciation registered by the Director-General in accordance with the provisions of the preceding Articles.

Article 12

The English and French versions of the text of this Protocol are equally authoritative.

VII. BIOTECHNOLOGY

Universal Declaration on the Human Genome and Human Rights (1997)

Adopted by the General Conference of UNESCO at its 29th session on 11 November 1997.
UNESCO, Records of the General Conference, vol. 29, pp. 41-46 (1997).
[Available at http://www.unesco.org/shs/human_rights/hrbc.htm]

Recalling that the Preamble of UNESCO's Constitution refers to "the democratic principles of the dignity, equality and mutual respect of men", rejects any "doctrine of the inequality of men and races", stipulates "that the wide diffusion of culture, and the education of humanity for justice and liberty and peace are indispensable to the dignity of men and constitute a sacred duty which all the nations must fulfil in a spirit of mutual assistance and concern", proclaims that "peace must be founded upon the intellectual and moral solidarity of mankind", and states that the Organization seeks to advance "through the educational and scientific and cultural relations of the peoples of the world, the objectives of international peace and of the common welfare of mankind for which the United Nations Organization was established and which its Charter proclaims",

Solemnly recalling its attachment to the universal principles of human rights, affirmed in particular in the Universal Declaration of Human Rights of 10 December 1948 and in the two International United Nations Covenants on Economic, Social and Cultural Rights and on Civil and Political Rights of 16 December 1966, in the United Nations Convention on the Prevention and Punishment of the Crime of Genocide of 9 December 1948, the International United Nations Convention on the Elimination of All Forms of Racial Discrimination of 21 December 1965, the United Nations Declaration on the Rights of Mentally Retarded Persons of 20 December 1971, the United Nations Declaration on the Rights of Disabled Persons of 9 December 1975, the United Nations Convention on the Elimination of All Forms of Discrimination Against Women of 18 December 1979, the United Nations Declaration of Basic Principles of Justice for Victims of Crime and Abuse of Power of 29 November 1985, the United Nations Convention on the Rights of the

Child of 20 November 1989, the United Nations Standard Rules on the Equalization of Opportunities for Persons with Disabilities of 20 December 1993, the Convention on the Prohibition of the Development, Production and Stockpiling of Bacteriological (Biological) and Toxin Weapons and on their Destruction of 16 December 1971, the UNESCO Convention against Discrimination in Education of 14 December 1960, the UNESCO Declaration of the Principles of International Cultural Co-operation of 4 November 1966, the UNESCO Recommendation on the Status of Scientific Researchers of 20 November 1974, the UNESCO Declaration on Race and Racial Prejudice of 27 November 1978, the ILO Convention (No. 111) concerning Discrimination in Respect of Employment and Occupation of 25 June 1958 and the ILO Convention (No. 169) concerning Indigenous and Tribal Peoples in Independent Countries of 27 June 1989,

Bearing in mind, and without prejudice to, the international instruments which could have a bearing on the applications of genetics in the field of intellectual property, inter alia the Bern Convention for the Protection of Literary and Artistic Works of 9 September 1886 and the UNESCO Universal Copyright Convention of 6 September 1952, as last revised in Paris on 24 July 1971, the Paris Convention for the Protection of Industrial Property of 20 March 1883, as last revised at Stockholm on 14 July 1967, the Budapest Treaty of the WIPO on International Recognition of the Deposit of Micro-Organisms for the Purposes of Patent Procedures of 28 April 1977, and the Trade Related Aspects of Intellectual Property Rights Agreement (TRIPS) annexed to the Agreement establishing the World Trade Organization, which entered into force on 1st January 1995,

Bearing in mind also the United Nations Convention on Biological Diversity of 5 June 1992 and emphasizing in that connection that the recognition of the genetic diversity of humanity must not give rise to any interpretation of a social or political nature which could call into question "the inherent dignity and (...) the equal and inalienable rights of all members of the human family", in accordance with the Preamble to the Universal Declaration of Human Rights,

Recalling 22 C/Resolution 13.1, 23 C/Resolution 13.1, 24 C/Resolution 13.1, 25 C/Resolutions 5.2 and 7.3, 27 C/Resolution 5.15 and 28 C/Resolutions 0.12, 2.1 and 2.2, urging UNESCO to promote and develop ethical studies, and the actions arising out of them, on the consequences of scientific and technological progress in the fields of biology and genetics, within the framework of respect for human rights and fundamental freedoms,

Recognizing that research on the human genome and the resulting applications open up vast prospects for progress in improving the health of individuals and of humankind as a whole, but emphasizing that such research should fully respect human dignity, freedom and human rights, as well as the prohibition of all forms of discrimination based on genetic characteristics,

Proclaims the principles that follow and adopts the present Declaration.

A. HUMAN DIGNITY AND THE HUMAN GENOME

Article 1

The human genome underlies the fundamental unity of all members of the human family, as well as the recognition of their inherent dignity and diversity. In a symbolic sense, it is the heritage of humanity.

Article 2

(a) Everyone has a right to respect for their dignity and for their rights regardless of their genetic characteristics.

(b) That dignity makes it imperative not to reduce individuals to their genetic characteristics and to respect their uniqueness and diversity.

Article 3

The human genome, which by its nature evolves, is subject to mutations. It contains potentialities that are expressed differently according to each individual's natural and social environment including the individual's state of health, living conditions, nutrition and education.

Article 4

The human genome in its natural state shall not give rise to financial gains.

B. RIGHTS OF THE PERSONS CONCERNED

Article 5

(a) Research, treatment or diagnosis affecting an individual's genome shall be undertaken only after rigorous and prior assessment of the potential risks and benefits pertaining thereto and in accordance with any other requirement of national law.

(b) In all cases, the prior, free and informed consent of the person concerned shall be obtained. If the latter is not in a position to consent, consent or authorization shall be obtained in the manner prescribed by law, guided by the person's best interest.

(c) The right of each individual to decide whether or not to be informed of the results of genetic examination and the resulting consequences should be respected.

(d) In the case of research, protocols shall, in addition, be submitted for prior review in accordance with relevant national and international research standards or guidelines.

(e) If according to the law a person does not have the capacity to consent, research affecting his or her genome may only be carried out for his or her direct health benefit, subject to the authorization and the protective conditions prescribed by law. Research which does not have an expected direct health benefit may only be undertaken by way of exception, with the utmost restraint, exposing the person only to a minimal risk and minimal burden and if the research is intended to contribute to the health benefit of other persons in the same age category or with the same genetic condition, subject to the conditions prescribed by law, and provided such research is compatible with the protection of the individual's human rights.

Article 6

No one shall be subjected to discrimination based on genetic characteristics that is intended to infringe or has the effect of infringing human rights, fundamental freedoms and human dignity.

Article 7

Genetic data associated with an identifiable person and stored or processed for the purposes of research or any other purpose must be held confidential in the conditions set by law.

Article 8

Every individual shall have the right, according to international and national law, to just reparation for any damage sustained as a direct and determining result of an intervention affecting his or her genome.

Article 9

In order to protect human rights and fundamental freedoms, limitations to the principles of consent and confidentiality may only be prescribed by law, for compelling reasons within the bounds of public international law and the international law of human rights.

C. RESEARCH ON THE HUMAN GENOME

Article 10

No research or research applications concerning the human genome, in particular in the fields of biology, genetics and medicine, should prevail over respect for the human rights, fundamental freedoms and human dignity of individuals or, where applicable, of groups of people.

Article 11

Practices which are contrary to human dignity, such as reproductive cloning of human beings, shall not be permitted. States and competent international organizations are invited to co-operate in identifying such practices and in taking, at national or international level, the measures neces-

sary to ensure that the principles set out in this Declaration are respected.

Article 12

(a) Benefits from advances in biology, genetics and medicine, concerning the human genome, shall be made available to all, with due regard for the dignity and human rights of each individual.

(b) Freedom of research, which is necessary for the progress of knowledge, is part of freedom of thought. The applications of research, including applications in biology, genetics and medicine, concerning the human genome, shall seek to offer relief from suffering and improve the health of individuals and humankind as a whole.

D. CONDITIONS FOR THE EXERCISE OF SCIENTIFIC ACTIVITY

Article 13

The responsibilities inherent in the activities of researchers, including meticulousness, caution, intellectual honesty and integrity in carrying out their research as well as in the presentation and utilization of their findings, should be the subject of particular attention in the framework of research on the human genome, because of its ethical and social implications. Public and private science policy-makers also have particular responsibilities in this respect.

Article 14

States should take appropriate measures to foster the intellectual and material conditions favourable to freedom in the conduct of research on the human genome and to consider the ethical, legal, social and economic implications of such research, on the basis of the principles set out in this Declaration.

Article 15

States should take appropriate steps to provide the framework for the free exercise of research on the human genome with due regard for the principles set out in this Declaration, in order to safeguard respect for human rights, fundamental freedoms and human dignity and to protect public health. They should seek to ensure that research results are not used for non-peaceful purposes.

Article 16

States should recognize the value of promoting, at various levels, as appropriate, the establishment of independent, multidisciplinary and pluralist ethics committees to assess the ethical, legal and social issues raised by research on the human genome and its application.

E. SOLIDARITY AND INTERNATIONAL CO-OPERATION

Article 17

States should respect and promote the practice of solidarity towards individuals, families and population groups who are particularly vulnerable to or affected by disease or disability of a genetic character. They should foster, inter alia, research on the identification, prevention and treatment of genetically-based and genetically-influenced diseases, in particular rare as well as endemic diseases which affect large numbers of the world's population.

Article 18

States should make every effort, with due and appropriate regard for the principles set out in this Declaration, to continue fostering the international dissemination of scientific knowledge concerning the human genome, human diversity and genetic research and, in that regard, to foster scientific and cultural co-operation, particularly between industrialized and developing countries.

Article 19

(a) In the framework of international co-operation with developing countries, States should seek to encourage measures enabling:

(i) assessment of the risks and benefits pertaining to research on the human genome to be carried out and abuse to be prevented;

(ii) the capacity of developing countries to carry out research on human biology and genetics, taking into consideration their specific problems, to be developed and strengthened;

(iii) developing countries to benefit from the achievements of scientific and technological research so that their use in favour of economic and social progress can be to the benefit of all;

(iv) the free exchange of scientific knowledge and information in the areas of biology, genetics and medicine to be promoted.

(b) Relevant international organizations should support and promote the initiatives taken by States for the above-mentioned purposes.

F. PROMOTION OF THE PRINCIPLES SET OUT IN THE DECLARATION

Article 20

States should take appropriate measures to promote the principles set out in the Declaration, through education and relevant means, inter alia through the conduct of research and training in interdisciplinary fields and through the promotion of education in bioethics, at all levels, in particular for those responsible for science policies.

Article 21

States should take appropriate measures to encourage other forms of research, training and information dissemination conducive to raising the awareness of society and all of its members of their responsibilities regarding the fundamental issues relating to the defence of human dignity which may be raised by research in biology, in genetics and in medicine, and its applications. They should also undertake to facilitate on this subject an open international discussion, ensuring the free expression of various socio-cultural, religious and philosophical opinions.

G. IMPLEMENTATION OF THE DECLARATION

Article 22

States should make every effort to promote the principles set out in this Declaration and should, by means of all appropriate measures, promote their implementation.

Article 23

States should take appropriate measures to promote, through education, training and information dissemination, respect for the above-mentioned principles and to foster their recognition and effective application. States should also encourage exchanges and networks among independent ethics committees, as they are established, to foster full collaboration.

Article 24

The International Bioethics Committee of UNESCO should contribute to the dissemination of the principles set out in this Declaration and to the further examination of issues raised by their applications and by the evolution of the technologies in question. It should organize appropriate consultations with parties concerned, such as vulnerable groups. It should make recommendations, in accordance with UNESCO's statutory procedures, addressed to the General Conference and give advice concerning the follow-up of this Declaration, in particular regarding the identification of practices that could be contrary to human dignity, such as germ-line interventions.

Article 25

Nothing in this Declaration may be interpreted as implying for any State, group or person any claim to engage in any activity or to perform any act contrary to human rights and fundamental freedoms, including the principles set out in this Declaration.

* * *

Convention for the Protection of Human Rights and Dignity of the Human Being with Regard to the Application of Biology and Medicine: Convention on Human Rights and Biomedicine (1997)

Council of Europe Oviedo, 4.IV.1997. Reprinted in 36 ILM 821.
[Available at http://www.mpil.de/en/hp/embryo/regional/CPHR04041997.pdf]

PREAMBLE

The member States of the Council of Europe, the other States and the European Community, signatories hereto,

Bearing in mind the Universal Declaration of Human Rights proclaimed by the General Assembly of the United Nations on 10 December 1948;

Bearing in mind the Convention for the Protection of Human Rights and Fundamental Freedoms of 4 November 1950;

Bearing in mind the European Social Charter of 18 October 1961;

Bearing in mind the International Covenant on Civil and Political Rights and the International Covenant on Economic, Social and Cultural Rights of 16 December 1966;

Bearing in mind the Convention for the Protection of Individuals with regard to Automatic Processing of Personal Data of 28 January 1981;

Bearing also in mind the Convention on the Rights of the Child of 20 November 1989;

Considering that the aim of the Council of Europe is the achievement of a greater unity between its members and that one of the methods by which that aim is to be pursued is the maintenance and further realisation of human rights and fundamental freedoms;

Conscious of the accelerating developments in biology and medicine;

Convinced of the need to respect the human being both as an individual and as a member of the human species and recognising the importance of ensuring the dignity of the human being;

Conscious that the misuse of biology and medicine may lead to acts endangering human dignity;

Affirming that progress in biology and medicine should be used for the benefit of present and future generations;

Stressing the need for international co-operation so that all humanity may enjoy the benefits of biology and medicine;

Recognising the importance of promoting a public debate on the questions posed by the application of biology and medicine and the responses to be given thereto;

Wishing to remind all members of society of their rights and responsibilities;

Taking account of the work of the Parliamentary Assembly in this field, including Recommendation 1160 (1991) on the preparation of a convention on bioethics;

Resolving to take such measures as are necessary to safeguard human dignity and the fundamental rights and freedoms of the individual with regard to the application of biology and medicine,

Have agreed as follows:

CHAPTER I
GENERAL PROVISIONS

Article 1
Purpose and Object

Parties to this Convention shall protect the dignity and identity of all human beings and guarantee everyone, without discrimination, respect for their integrity and other rights and fundamental freedoms with regard to the application of biology and medicine. Each Party shall take in its internal law the necessary measures to give effect to the provisions of this Convention.

Article 2
Primacy of the Human Being

The interests and welfare of the human being shall prevail over the sole interest of society or science.

Article 3
Equitable Access to Health Care

Parties, taking into account health needs and available resources, shall take appropriate measures with a view to providing, within their jurisdiction, equitable access to health care of appropriate quality.

Article 4
Professional Standards

Any intervention in the health field, including research, must be carried out in accordance with relevant professional obligations and standards.

CHAPTER II
CONSENT

Article 5
General Rule

An intervention in the health field may only be carried out after the person concerned has given free and informed consent to it. This person shall beforehand be given appropriate information as to the purpose and nature of the intervention as well as on its consequences and risks. The person concerned may freely withdraw consent at any time.

Article 6
Protection of Persons Not
Able to Consent

1. Subject to Articles 17 and 20 below, an intervention may only be carried out on a person who does not have the capacity to consent, for his or her direct benefit.

2. Where, according to law, a minor does not have the capacity to consent to an intervention, the intervention may only be carried out with the authorisation of his or her representative or an authority or a person or body provided for by law. The opinion of the minor shall be taken into consideration as an increasingly determining factor in proportion to his or her age and degree of maturity.

3. Where, according to law, an adult does not have the capacity to consent to an intervention because of a mental disability, a disease or for similar reasons, the intervention may only be carried out with the authorisation of his or her representative or an authority or a person or body provided for by law. The individual concerned shall as far as possible take part in the authorisation procedure.

4. The representative, the authority, the person or the body mentioned in paragraphs 2 and 3 above shall be given, under the same conditions, the information referred to in Article 5.

5. The authorisation referred to in paragraphs 2 and 3 above may be withdrawn at any time in the best interests of the person concerned.

Article 7
Protection of Persons Who
Have a Mental Disorder

Subject to protective conditions prescribed by law, including supervisory, control and appeal procedures, a person who has a mental disorder of a serious nature may be subjected, without his or her consent, to an intervention aimed at treating his or her mental disorder only where, without such treatment, serious harm is likely to result to his or her health.

Article 8
Emergency Situation

When because of an emergency situation the appropriate consent cannot be obtained, any medically necessary intervention may be carried out immediately for the benefit of the health of the individual concerned.

Article 9
Previously Expressed Wishes

The previously expressed wishes relating to a medical intervention by a patient who is not, at the time of the intervention, in a state to express his or her wishes shall be taken into account.

CHAPTER III
PRIVATE LIFE AND RIGHT
TO INFORMATION

Article 10
Private Life and Right to Information

1. Everyone has the right to respect for private life in relation to information about his or her health.

2. Everyone is entitled to know any information collected about his or her health. However, the wishes of individuals not to be so informed shall be observed.

3. In exceptional cases, restrictions may be placed by law on the exercise of the rights contained in paragraph 2 in the interests of the patient.

CHAPTER IV
HUMAN GENOME

Article 11
Non-Discrimination

Any form of discrimination against a person on grounds of his or her genetic heritage is prohibited.

Article 12
Predictive Genetic Tests

Tests which are predictive of genetic diseases or which serve either to identify the subject as a carrier of a gene responsible for a disease or to detect a genetic predisposition or susceptibility to a disease may be performed only for health purposes or for scientific research linked to health purposes, and subject to appropriate genetic counselling.

Article 13
Interventions on the Human Genome

An intervention seeking to modify the human genome may only be undertaken for preventive, diagnostic or therapeutic purposes and only if its aim is not to introduce any modification in the genome of any descendants.

Article 14
Non-Selection of Sex

The use of techniques of medically assisted procreation shall not be allowed for the purpose of choosing a future child's sex, except where serious hereditary sex-related disease is to be avoided.

CHAPTER V
SCIENTIFIC RESEARCH

Article 15
General Rule

Scientific research in the field of biology and medicine shall be carried out freely, subject to the provisions of this Convention and the other legal provisions ensuring the protection of the human being.

Article 16
Protection of Persons
Undergoing Research

Research on a person may only be undertaken if all the following conditions are met:

i. there is no alternative of comparable effectiveness to research on humans;

ii. the risks which may be incurred by that person are not disproportionate to the potential benefits of the research;

iii. the research project has been approved by the competent body after independent examination of its scientific merit, including assessment of the importance of the aim of the research, and multidisciplinary review of its ethical acceptability;

iv. the persons undergoing research have been informed of their rights and the safeguards prescribed by law for their protection;

v. the necessary consent as provided for under Article 5 has been given expressly, specifically and is documented. Such consent may be freely withdrawn at any time.

Article 17
Protection of Persons Not Able
to Consent to Research

1. Research on a person without the capacity to consent as stipulated in Article 5 may be undertaken only if all the following conditions are met:

i. the conditions laid down in Article 16, sub-paragraphs i to iv, are fulfilled;

ii. the results of the research have the potential to produce real and direct benefit to his or her health;

iii. research of comparable effectiveness cannot be carried out on individuals capable of giving consent;

iv. the necessary authorisation provided for under Article 6 has been given specifically and in writing; and

v. the person concerned does not object.

2. Exceptionally and under the protective conditions prescribed by law, where the research has not the potential to produce results of direct benefit to the health of the person concerned, such research may be authorised subject to the conditions laid down in paragraph 1, sub-paragraphs i, iii, iv and v above, and to the following additional conditions:

i. the research has the aim of contributing, through significant improvement in the scientific understanding of the individual's condition, disease or disorder, to the ultimate attainment of results capable of conferring benefit to the person concerned or to other persons in the same age category or afflicted with the same disease or disorder or having the same condition;

ii. the research entails only minimal risk and minimal burden for the individual concerned.

Article 18
Research on Embryos in Vitro

1. Where the law allows research on embryos in vitro, it shall ensure adequate protection of the embryo.

2. The creation of human embryos for research purposes is prohibited.

CHAPTER VI
ORGAN AND TISSUE REMOVAL
FROM LIVING DONORS FOR
TRANSPLANTATION PURPOSES

Article 19
General Rule

1. Removal of organs or tissue from a living person for transplantation purposes may be carried out solely for the therapeutic benefit of the recipient and where there is no suitable organ or tissue available from a deceased person and no other alternative therapeutic method of comparable effectiveness.

2. The necessary consent as provided for under Article 5 must have been given expressly and specifically either in written form or before an official body.

Article 20
Protection of Persons Not Able to Consent to Organ Removal

1. No organ or tissue removal may be carried out on a person who does not have the capacity to consent under Article 5.

2. Exceptionally and under the protective conditions prescribed by law, the removal of regenerative tissue from a person who does not have the capacity to consent may be authorised provided the following conditions are met:

i. there is no compatible donor available who has the capacity to consent;

ii. the recipient is a brother or sister of the donor;

iii. the donation must have the potential to be life-saving for the recipient;

iv. the authorisation provided for under paragraphs 2 and 3 of Article 6 has been given specifically and in writing, in accordance with the law and with the approval of the competent body;

v. the potential donor concerned does not object.

CHAPTER VII
PROHIBITION OF FINANCIAL GAIN AND DISPOSAL OF A PART OF THE HUMAN BODY

Article 21
Prohibition of Financial Gain

The human body and its parts shall not, as such, give rise to financial gain.

Article 22
Disposal of a Removed Part of the Human Body

When in the course of an intervention any part of a human body is removed, it may be stored and used for a purpose other than that for which it was removed, only if this is done in conformity with appropriate information and consent procedures.

CHAPTER VIII
INFRINGEMENTS OF THE PROVISIONS OF THE CONVENTION

Article 23
Infringement of the Rights or Principles

The Parties shall provide appropriate judicial protection to prevent or to put a stop to an unlawful infringement of the rights and principles set forth in this Convention at short notice.

Article 24
Compensation for Undue Damage

The person who has suffered undue damage resulting from an intervention is entitled to fair compensation according to the conditions and procedures prescribed by law.

Article 25
Sanctions

Parties shall provide for appropriate sanctions to be applied in the event of infringement of the provisions contained in this Convention.

CHAPTER IX
RELATION BETWEEN THIS CONVENTION AND OTHER PROVISIONS

Article 26
Restrictions on the Exercise of the Rights

1. No restrictions shall be placed on the exercise of the rights and protective provisions contained in this Convention other than such as are prescribed by law and are necessary in a democratic society in the interest of public safety, for the prevention of crime, for the protection of public health or for the protection of the rights and freedoms of others.

2. The restrictions contemplated in the preceding paragraph may not be placed on Articles 11, 13, 14, 16, 17, 19, 20 and 21.

Article 27
Wider Protection

None of the provisions of this Convention shall be interpreted as limiting or otherwise affecting the possibility for a Party to grant a wider measure of protection with regard to the application of biology and medicine than is stipulated in this Convention.

CHAPTER X
PUBLIC DEBATE

Article 28
Public Debate

Parties to this Convention shall see to it that the fundamental questions raised by the developments of biology and medicine are the subject of appropriate public discussion in the light, in particular, of relevant medical, social, economic, ethical and legal implications, and that their possible application is made the subject of appropriate consultation.

CHAPTER XI
INTERPRETATION AND FOLLOW-UP OF THE CONVENTION

Article 29
Interpretation of the Convention

The European Court of Human Rights may give, without direct reference to any specific proceedings pending in a court, advisory opinions on legal questions concerning the interpretation of the present Convention at the request of:

• the Government of a Party, after having informed the other Parties;

• the Committee set up by Article 32, with membership restricted to the Representatives of the Parties to this Convention, by a decision adopted by a two thirds majority of votes cast.

Article 30
Reports on the Application of the Convention

On receipt of a request from the Secretary General of the Council of Europe any Party shall furnish an explanation of the manner in which its internal law ensures the effective implementation of any of the provisions of the Convention.

CHAPTER XII
PROTOCOLS

Article 31
Protocols

Protocols may be concluded in pursuance of Article 32, with a view to developing, in specific fields, the principles contained in this Convention. The Protocols shall be open for signature by Signatories of the Convention. They shall be subject to ratification, acceptance or approval. A Signatory may not ratify, accept or approve Protocols without previously or simultaneously ratifying accepting or approving the Convention.

Chapter XIII
Amendments to the Convention
* * *

Chapter XIV
Final Clauses
* * *

International Declaration on Human Genetic Data

Adopted by the General Conference of UNESCO on 16 October 2003.
UNESCO Records of the General Conference, 32nd Session Paris, 29 September to
17 October 2003, Volume 1. Resolutions, pp. 39-46.
[Available at http://portal.unesco.org/en/ev.php-
URL_ID=17720&URL_DO=DO_TOPIC&URL_SECTION=201.html]

The General Conference,

Recalling the Universal Declaration of Human Rights of 10 December 1948, the two United Nations International Covenants on Economic, Social and Cultural Rights and on Civil and Political Rights of 16 December 1966, the United Nations International Convention on the Elimination of All Forms of Racial Discrimination of 21 December 1965, the United Nations Convention on the Elimination of All Forms of Discrimination against Women of 18 December 1979, the United Nations Convention on the Rights of the Child of 20 November 1989, the United Nations Economic and Social Council resolutions 2001/39 on Genetic Privacy and Non-Discrimination of 26 July 2001 and 2003/232 on Genetic Privacy and Non-Discrimination of 22 July 2003, the ILO Convention (No. 111) concerning Discrimination in Respect of Employment and Occupation of 25 June 1958, the UNESCO Universal Declaration on Cultural Diversity of 2 November 2001, the Trade Related Aspects of Intellectual Property Rights Agreement (TRIPS) annexed to the Agreement establishing the World Trade Organization, which entered into force on 1 January 1995, the Doha Declaration on the TRIPS Agreement and Public Health of 14 November 2001 and the other international human rights instruments adopted by the United Nations and the specialized agencies of the United Nations system,

Recalling more particularly the Universal Declaration on the Human Genome and Human Rights which it adopted, unanimously and by acclamation, on 11 November 1997 and which was endorsed by the United Nations General Assembly on 9 December 1998 and the Guidelines for the implementation of the Universal Declaration on the Human Genome and Human Rights which it endorsed on 16 November 1999 by 30 C/Resolution 23,

Welcoming the broad public interest worldwide in the Universal Declaration on the Human Genome and Human Rights, the firm support it has received from the international community and its impact in Member States drawing upon it for their legislation, regulations, norms and standards, and ethical codes of conduct and guidelines,

Bearing in mind the international and regional instruments, national laws, regulations and ethical texts relating to the protection of human rights and fundamental freedoms and to respect for human dignity as regards the collection, processing, use and storage of scientific data, as well as of medical data and personal data,

Recognizing that genetic information is part of the overall spectrum of medical data and that the information content of any medical data, including genetic data and proteomic data, is highly contextual and dependent on the particular circumstances,

Also recognizing that human genetic data have a special status on account of their sensitive nature since they can be predictive of genetic predispositions concerning individuals and that the power of predictability can be stronger than assessed at the time of deriving the data; they may have a significant impact on the family, including offspring, extending over generations, and in some instances on the whole group; they may contain information the significance of which is not necessarily known at the time of the collection of biological samples; and they may have cultural significance for persons or groups, ·

Emphasizing that all medical data, including genetic data and proteomic data, regardless of their apparent information content, should be treated with the same high standards of confidentiality,

Noting the increasing importance of human genetic data for economic and commercial purposes,

Having regard to the special needs and vulnerabilities of developing countries and the need to reinforce international cooperation in the field of human genetics,

Considering that the collection, processing, use and storage of human genetic data are of paramount importance for the progress of life sciences and medicine, for their applications and for the use of such data for non-medical purposes,

Also considering that the growing amount of personal data collected makes genuine irretrievability increasingly difficult,

Aware that the collection, processing, use and storage of human genetic data have potential risks for the exercise and observance of human rights and fundamental freedoms and respect for human dignity,

Noting that the interests and welfare of the individual should have priority over the rights and interests of society and research,

Reaffirming the principles established in the Universal Declaration on the Human Genome and Human Rights and the principles of equality, justice, solidarity and responsibility as well as respect for human dignity, human rights and fundamental freedoms, particularly freedom of thought and expression, including freedom of research, and privacy and security of the person, which must underlie the collection, processing, use and storage of human genetic data,

Proclaims the principles that follow and adopts the present Declaration.

A. GENERAL PROVISIONS

Article 1
Aims and Scope

(a) The aims of this Declaration are: to ensure the respect of human dignity and protection of human rights and fundamental freedoms in the collection, processing, use and storage of human genetic data, human proteomic data and of the biological samples from which they are derived, referred to hereinafter as "biological samples", in keeping with the requirements of equality, justice and solidarity, while giving due consideration to freedom of thought and expression, including freedom of research; to set out the principles which should guide States in the formulation of their legislation and their policies on these issues; and to form the basis for guidelines of good practices in these areas for the institutions and individuals concerned.

(b) Any collection, processing, use and storage of human genetic data, human proteomic data and biological samples shall be consistent with the international law of human rights.

(c) The provisions of this Declaration apply to the collection, processing, use and storage of human genetic data, human proteomic data and biological samples, except in the investigation, detection and prosecution of criminal offences and in parentage testing that are subject to domestic law that is consistent with the international law of human rights.

Article 2
Use of Terms

For the purposes of this Declaration, the terms used have the following meanings:

(i) Human genetic data: Information about heritable characteristics of individuals obtained by analysis of nucleic acids or by other scientific analysis;

(ii) Human proteomic data: Information pertaining to an individual's proteins including their expression, modification and interaction;

(iii) Consent: Any freely given specific, informed and express agreement of an individual to his or her genetic data being collected, processed, used and stored;

(iv) Biological samples: Any sample of biological material (for example blood, skin and bone cells or blood plasma) in which nucleic acids are present and which contains the characteristic genetic make-up of an individual;

(v) Population-based genetic study: A study which aims at understanding the nature and extent of genetic variation among a population or individuals within a group or between individuals across different groups;

(vi) Behavioural genetic study: A study that aims at establishing possible connections between genetic characteristics and behaviour;

(vii) Invasive procedure: Biological sampling using a method involving intrusion into the human body, such as obtaining a blood sample by using a needle and syringe;

(viii) Non-invasive procedure: Biological sampling using a method which does not involve intrusion into the human body, such as oral smears;

(ix) Data linked to an identifiable person: Data that contain information, such as name, birth date and address, by which the person from whom the data were derived can be identified;

(x) Data unlinked to an identifiable person: Data that are not linked to an identifiable person, through the replacement of, or separation from, all identifying information about that person by use of a code;

(xi) Data irretrievably unlinked to an identifiable person: Data that cannot be linked to an identifiable person, through destruction of the link to any identifying information about the person who provided the sample;

(xii) Genetic testing: A procedure to detect the presence or absence of, or change in, a particular gene or chromosome, including an indirect test for a gene product or other specific metabolite that is primarily indicative of a specific genetic change;

(xiii) Genetic screening: Large-scale systematic genetic testing offered in a programme to a population or subsection thereof intended to detect genetic characteristics in asymptomatic people;

(xiv) Genetic counselling: A procedure to explain the possible implications of the findings of genetic testing or screening, its advantages and risks and where applicable to assist the individual in the long-term handling of the consequences; It takes place before and after genetic testing and screening;

(xv) Cross-matching: Matching of information about an individual or a group contained in various data files set up for different purposes.

Article 3
Person's Identity

Each individual has a characteristic genetic make-up. Nevertheless, a person's identity should not be reduced to genetic characteristics, since it involves complex educational, environmental and personal factors and emotional, social, spiritual and cultural bonds with others and implies a dimension of freedom.

Article 4
Special Status

(a) Human genetic data have a special status because:

(i) they can be predictive of genetic predispositions concerning individuals;

(ii) they may have a significant impact on the family, including offspring, extending over generations, and in some instances on the whole group to which the person concerned belongs;

(iii) they may contain information the significance of which is not necessarily known at the time of the collection of the biological samples;

(iv) they may have cultural significance for persons or groups.

(b) Due consideration should be given to the sensitivity of human genetic data and an appropriate level of protection for these data and biological samples should be established.

Article 5
Purposes

Human genetic data and human proteomic data may be collected, processed, used and stored only for the purposes of:

(i) diagnosis and health care, including screening and predictive testing;

(ii) medical and other scientific research, including epidemiological, especially population-based genetic studies, as well as anthropological or archaeological studies, collectively referred to hereinafter as "medical and scientific research";

(iii) forensic medicine and civil, criminal and other legal proceedings, taking into account the provisions of Article 1(c);

(iv) or any other purpose consistent with the Universal Declaration on the Human Genome and Human Rights and the international law of human rights.

Article 6
Procedures

(a) It is ethically imperative that human genetic data and human proteomic data be collected, processed, used and stored on the basis of transparent and ethically acceptable procedures. States should endeavour to involve society at large in the decision-making process concerning broad policies for the collection, processing, use and storage of human genetic data and human proteomic data and the evaluation of their management, in particular in the case of population-based genetic studies. This decision-making process, which may benefit from international experience, should ensure the free expression of various viewpoints.

(b) Independent, multidisciplinary and pluralist ethics committees should be promoted and established at national, regional, local or institutional levels, in accordance with the provisions of Article 16 of the Universal Declaration on the Human Genome and Human Rights. Where appropriate, ethics committees at national level should be consulted with regard to the establishment of standards, regulations and guidelines for the collection, processing, use and storage of human genetic data, human proteomic data and biological samples. They should also be consulted concerning matters where there is no domestic law. Ethics committees at institutional or local levels should be consulted with regard to their application to specific research projects.

(c) When the collection, processing, use and storage of human genetic data, human proteomic data or biological samples are carried out in two or more States, the ethics committees in the States concerned, where appropriate, should be consulted and the review of these questions at the appropriate level should be based on the principles set out in this Declaration and on the ethical and legal standards adopted by the States concerned.

(d) It is ethically imperative that clear, balanced, adequate and appropriate information shall be provided to the person whose prior, free, informed and express consent is sought. Such information shall, alongside with providing other necessary details, specify the purpose for which human genetic data and human proteomic data are being derived from biological samples, and are used and stored. This information should indicate, if necessary, risks and consequences. This information should also indicate that the person concerned can withdraw his or her consent, without coercion, and this should entail neither a disadvantage nor a penalty for the person concerned.

Article 7
Non-Discrimination and
Non-Stigmatization

(a) Every effort should be made to ensure that human genetic data and human proteomic data are not used for purposes that discriminate in a way that is intended to infringe, or has the effect of infringing human rights, fundamental freedoms or human dignity of an individual or for purposes that lead to the stigmatization of an individual, a family, a group or communities.

(b) In this regard, appropriate attention should be paid to the findings of population-based genetic studies and behavioural genetic studies and their interpretations.

B. COLLECTION

Article 8
Consent

(a) Prior, free, informed and express consent, without inducement by financial or other personal gain, should be obtained for the collection of human genetic data, human proteomic data or biological samples, whether through invasive or non-invasive procedures, and for their subsequent processing, use and storage, whether carried out by public or private institutions. Limitations on this principle of consent should only be prescribed for compelling reasons by domestic law consistent with the international law of human rights.

(b) When, in accordance with domestic law, a person is incapable of giving informed consent, authorization should be obtained from the legal representative, in accordance with domestic law. The legal representative should have regard to the best interest of the person concerned.

(c) An adult not able to consent should as far as possible take part in the authorization procedure. The opinion of a minor should be taken into consideration as an increasingly determining factor in proportion to age and degree of maturity.

(d) In diagnosis and health care, genetic screening and testing of minors and adults not able to consent will normally only be ethically acceptable when they have important implications for the health of the person and have regard to his or her best interest.

Article 9
Withdrawal of Consent

(a) When human genetic data, human proteomic data or biological samples are collected for medical and scientific research purposes, consent may be withdrawn by the person concerned unless such data are irretrievably unlinked to an identifiable person. In accordance with the provisions of Article 6(d), withdrawal of consent should entail neither a disadvantage nor a penalty for the person concerned.

(b) When a person withdraws consent, the person's genetic data, proteomic data and biological samples should no longer be used unless they are irretrievably unlinked to the person concerned.

(c) If not irretrievably unlinked, the data and biological samples should be dealt with in accordance with the wishes of the person. If the person's wishes cannot be determined or are not feasible or are unsafe, the data and biological samples should either be irretrievably unlinked or destroyed.

Article 10
The Right to Decide Whether or Not to Be Informed About Research Results

When human genetic data, human proteomic data or biological samples are collected for medical and scientific research purposes, the information provided at the time of consent should indicate that the person concerned has the right to decide whether or not to be informed of the results. This does not apply to research on data irretrievably unlinked to identifiable persons or to data that do not lead to individual findings concerning the persons who have participated in such a research. Where appropriate, the right not to be informed should be extended to identified relatives who may be affected by the results.

Article 11
Genetic Counseling

It is ethically imperative that when genetic testing that may have significant implications for a person's health is being considered, genetic counselling should be made available in an appropriate manner. Genetic counselling should be non-directive, culturally adapted and consistent with the best interest of the person concerned.

Article 12
Collection of Biological Samples for Forensic Medicine or in Civil, Criminal and Other Legal Proceedings

When human genetic data or human proteomic data are collected for the purposes of forensic medicine or in civil, criminal and other legal proceedings, including parentage testing, the collection of biological samples, in vivo or post-mortem, should be made only in accordance with domestic law consistent with the international law of human rights.

C. PROCESSING

Article 13
Access

No one should be denied access to his or her own genetic data or proteomic data unless such data are irretrievably unlinked to that person as the identifiable source or unless domestic law limits such access in the interest of public health, public order or national security.

Article 14
Privacy and Confidentiality

(a) States should endeavour to protect the privacy of individuals and the confidentiality of human genetic data linked to an identifiable person, family or, where appropriate, group, in accordance with domestic law consistent with the international law of human rights.

(b) Human genetic data, human proteomic data and biological samples linked to an identifiable person should not be disclosed or made accessible to third parties, in particular, employers, insurance companies, educational institutions and the family, except for an important public interest reason in cases restrictively provided for by domestic law consistent with the international law of human rights or where the prior, free, informed and express consent of the person concerned has been obtained provided that such consent is in accordance with domestic law and the international law of human rights. The privacy of an individual participating in a study using human genetic data, human proteomic data or biological samples should be protected and the data should be treated as confidential.

(c) Human genetic data, human proteomic data and biological samples collected for the purposes of scientific research should not normally be linked to an identifiable person. Even when such data or biological samples are unlinked to an identifiable person, the necessary precautions should be taken to ensure the security of the data or biological samples.

(d) Human genetic data, human proteomic data and biological samples collected for medical and scientific research purposes can remain linked to an identifiable person, only if necessary to carry out the research and provided that the privacy of the individual and the confidentiality of the data or biological samples concerned are protected in accordance with domestic law.

(e) Human genetic data and human proteomic data should not be kept in a form which allows the data subject to be identified for any longer than is necessary for achieving the purposes for which they were collected or subsequently processed.

Article 15
Accuracy, Reliability, Quality and Security

The persons and entities responsible for the processing of human genetic data, human proteomic data and biological samples should take the necessary measures to ensure the accuracy, reliability, quality and security of these data and the processing of biological samples. They should exercise rigour, caution, honesty and integrity in the processing and interpretation of human genetic data, human proteomic data or biological samples, in view of their ethical, legal and social implications.

D. USE

Article 16
Change of Purpose

(a) Human genetic data, human proteomic data and the biological samples collected for one of the purposes set out in Article 5 should not be used for a different purpose that is incompatible with the original consent, unless the prior, free, informed and express consent of the person concerned is obtained according to the provisions of Article 8(a) or unless the proposed use, decided by domestic law, corresponds to an important public interest reason and is consistent with the international law of human rights. If the person concerned lacks the capacity to consent, the provisions of Article 8(b) and (c) should apply mutatis mutandis.

(b) When prior, free, informed and express consent cannot be obtained or in the case of data irretrievably unlinked to an identifiable person, human genetic data may be used in accordance with domestic law or following the consultation procedures set out in Article 6(b).

Article 17
Stored Biological Sample

(a) Stored biological samples collected for purposes other than set out in Article 5 may be used to produce human genetic data or human proteomic data with the prior, free, informed and express consent of the person concerned. However, domestic law may provide that if such data have significance for medical and scientific research purposes e.g. epidemiological studies, or public health purposes, they may be used for those purposes, following the consultation procedures set out in Article 6(b).

(b) The provisions of Article 12 should apply mutatis mutandis to stored biological samples used to produce human genetic data for forensic medicine.

Article 18
Circulation and International Cooperation

(a) States should regulate, in accordance with their domestic law and international agreements, the cross-border flow of human genetic data, human proteomic data and biological samples so as to foster international medical and scientific cooperation and ensure fair access to these data. Such a system should seek to ensure that the receiving party provides adequate protection in accordance with the principles set out in this Declaration.

(b) States should make every effort, with due and appropriate regard for the principles set out in this Declaration, to continue fostering the international dissemination of scientific knowledge concerning human genetic data and human proteomic data and, in that regard, to foster scientific and cultural cooperation, particularly between industrialized and developing countries.

(c) Researchers should endeavour to establish cooperative relationships, based on mutual respect with regard to scientific and ethical matters and, subject to the provisions of Article 14, should encourage the free circulation of human genetic data and human proteomic data in order to foster the sharing of scientific knowledge, provided that the principles set out in this Declaration are observed by the parties concerned. To this end, they should also endeavour to publish in due course the results of their research.

Article 19
Sharing of Benefits

(a) In accordance with domestic law or policy and international agreements, benefits resulting from the use of human genetic data, human proteomic data or biological samples collected for medical and scientific research should be shared with the society as a whole and the international community. In giving effect to this principle, benefits may take any of the following forms:

(i) special assistance to the persons and groups that have taken part in the research;

(ii) access to medical care;

(iii) provision of new diagnostics, facilities for

new treatments or drugs stemming from the research;

(iv) support for health services;

(v) capacity-building facilities for research purposes;

(vi) development and strengthening of the capacity of developing countries to collect and process human genetic data, taking into consideration their specific problems;

(vii) any other form consistent with the principles set out in this Declaration.

(b) Limitations in this respect could be provided by domestic law and international agreements.

E. STORAGE
Article 20
Monitoring and Management Framework

States may consider establishing a framework for the monitoring and management of human genetic data, human proteomic data and biological samples based on the principles of independence, multidisciplinarity, pluralism and transparency as well as the principles set out in this Declaration. This framework could also deal with the nature and purposes of the storage of these data.

Article 21
Destruction

(a) The provisions of Article 9 apply mutatis mutandis in the case of stored human genetic data, human proteomic data and biological samples.

(b) Human genetic data, human proteomic data and the biological samples collected from a suspect in the course of a criminal investigation should be destroyed when they are no longer necessary, unless otherwise provided for by domestic law consistent with the international law of human rights.

(c) Human genetic data, human proteomic data and biological samples should be available for forensic purposes and civil proceedings only for as long as they are necessary for those proceedings, unless otherwise provided for by domestic law consistent with the international law of human rights.

Article 22
Cross-Matching

Consent should be essential for the cross-matching of human genetic data, human proteomic data or biological samples stored for diagnostic and health care purposes and for medical and other scientific research purposes, unless otherwise provided for by domestic law for compelling reasons and consistent with the international law of human rights.

F. PROMOTION AND IMPLEMENTATION

Article 23
Implementation

(a) States should take all appropriate measures, whether of a legislative, administrative or other character, to give effect to the principles set out in this Declaration, in accordance with the international law of human rights. Such measures should be supported by action in the sphere of education, training and public information.

(b) In the framework of international cooperation, States should endeavour to enter into bilateral and multilateral agreements enabling developing countries to build up their capacity to participate in generating and sharing scientific knowledge concerning human genetic data and the related know-how.

Article 24
Ethics Education, Training
and Information

In order to promote the principles set out in this Declaration, States should endeavour to foster all forms of ethics education and training at all levels as well as to encourage information and knowledge dissemination programmes about human genetic data. These measures should aim at specific audiences, in particular researchers and members of ethics committees, or be addressed to the public at large. In this regard, States should encourage the participation of international and regional intergovernmental organizations and international, regional and national non-governmental organizations in this endeavour.

Article 25
Roles of the International
Bioethics Committee (IBC)
and the Intergovernmental
Bioethics Committee (IGBC)

The International Bioethics Committee (IBC) and the Intergovernmental Bioethics Committee (IGBC) shall contribute to the implementation of this Declaration and the dissemination of the principles set out therein. On a collaborative basis, the two Committees should be responsible for its monitoring and for the evaluation of its implementation, inter alia, on the basis of reports provided by States. The two Committees should be responsible in particular for the formulation of any opinion or proposal likely to further the effectiveness of this Declaration. They should make recommendations in accordance with UNESCO's statutory procedures, addressed to the General Conference.

Article 26
Follow-up Action by UNESCO

UNESCO shall take appropriate action to follow up this Declaration so as to foster progress of the life sciences and their applications through technologies, based on respect for human dignity and the exercise and observance of human rights and fundamental freedoms.

Article 27
Denial of Acts Contrary to Human
Rights, Fundamental Freedoms and
Human Dignity

Nothing in this Declaration may be interpreted as implying for any State, group or person any claim to engage in any activity or to perform any act contrary to human rights, fundamental freedoms and human dignity, including, in particular, the principles set out in this Declaration.

Draft International Convention on the Prohibition of All Forms of Human Cloning (2004)

Draft negotiating text under consideration in 2004.
Annex I to the letter dated 2 April 2003 from the Permanent Representative of Costa Rica
to the United Nations addressed to the Secretary-General, contained in UN doc. A/58/73
of 17 April 2003. [Available at http://ods-dds-
ny.un.org/doc/UNDOC/GEN/N03/330/84/PDF/N0333084.pdf?OpenElement]

[Footnotes omitted.]

PREAMBLE

The States Parties to this Convention,

Recalling the Universal Declaration on the Human Genome and Human Rights adopted by the General Conference of the United Nations Educational, Scientific and Cultural Organization on 11 November 1997, in particular article 11 thereof, in which the Conference specified that practices which are contrary to human dignity, such as reproductive cloning of human beings, shall not be permitted,

Recalling also General Assembly resolution 53/152 of 9 December 1998, by which the Assembly endorsed the Universal Declaration on the Human Genome and Human Rights,

Bearing in mind resolution 2001/71 of the Commission on Human Rights of 25 April 2001 entitled "Human rights and bioethics", adopted by the Commission at its fifty-seventh session,

Recalling that, in accordance with the Universal Declaration of Human Rights, recognition of the inherent dignity and of the equal and inalienable rights of all members of the human family is the foundation of freedom, justice and peace in the world,

Convinced that the cloning of human beings, whether carried out on an experimental basis, in the context of fertility treatments or pre-implantation diagnosis, for tissue transplantation or for any other purpose whatsoever, is morally repugnant, unethical and contrary to respect for the person and constitutes a grave violation of fundamental human rights which cannot under any circumstances be justified or accepted,

Seeking to promote scientific and technical progress in the fields of biology and genetics in a manner respectful of fundamental human rights and for the benefit of all,

Concerned at recently disclosed information on research into and attempts at the creation of human beings through cloning processes,

Conscious of widespread preoccupations that the human body and its parts should not, as such, give rise to financial gain,

Have agreed as follows:

Article 1
Definitions

For the purposes of this Convention:

1. "Somatic cell nuclear transfer" means introduction of nuclear material from a somatic cell into a fertilized or unfertilized oocyte whose nuclear material has been removed or inactivated;

2. "Somatic cell" means a cell containing a complete set of chromosomes;

3. "Genetically virtually identical organism" means an organism containing the same complete set of chromosomes as another organism;

4. "Victim" means both the person whose genetic material or oocyte is used without permission to commit an offence set forth in article 2, paragraph 1, and the living organism created by the commission of the offence set forth in article 2, paragraph 1.

Article 2
Scope of Application
(Definition of the Crime)

1. Any person commits an offence within the

299

meaning of this Convention if that person intentionally engages in an action, such as somatic cell nuclear transfer or embryo-splitting, resulting in the creation of a living organism, at any stage of physical development, that is genetically virtually identical to an existing or previously existing human organism.

2. Any person also commits an offence if that person attempts to commit an offence set forth in paragraph 1 of this article.

3. Any person also commits an offence if that person:

(a) Participates as an accomplice in an offence set forth in paragraph 1 or 2 of this article;

(b) Organizes or directs others to commit an offence set forth in paragraph 1 or 2 of this article;

(c) Contributes to the commission of one or more of the offences set forth in paragraph 1 or 2 of this article by a group of persons acting with a common purpose. Such contribution shall be intentional and shall either:

(i) Be made with the aim of furthering the criminal activity or criminal purpose of the group, where such activity or purpose involves the commission of an offence as set forth in paragraph 1 of this article; or

(ii) Be made in the knowledge of the intention of the group to commit an offence set forth in paragraph 1 of this article.

Article 3
Obligation to Criminalize

Each State Party shall adopt such measures as may be necessary:

(a) To establish as criminal offences under its domestic law the offences set forth in article 2;

(b) To make those offences punishable by appropriate penalties which take into account the grave nature of the offences.

Article 4
Liability of Legal Persons

1. Each State Party, in accordance with its domestic legal principles, shall take the necessary measures to enable a legal entity located in its territory or organized under its laws to be held liable when a person responsible for the management or control of that legal entity has, in that capacity, committed an offence set forth in article 2. Such liability may be criminal, civil or administrative.

2. Such liability is incurred without prejudice to the criminal liability of individuals who have committed the offences.

3. Each State Party shall ensure, in particular, that legal entities liable in accordance with paragraph 1 above are subject to effective, proportionate and dissuasive criminal, civil or administrative sanctions. Such sanctions may include monetary sanctions.

Article 5
Jurisdiction

1. Each State Party shall take such measures as may be necessary to establish its jurisdiction over the offences set forth in article 2 when:

(a) The offence is committed in the territory of that State;

(b) The offence is committed on board a vessel flying the flag of that State or an aircraft registered under the laws of that State at the time the offence is committed;

(c) The offence is committed by a national of that State.

2. A State Party may also establish its jurisdiction over any such offence when:

(a) The offence was directed towards or resulted in the carrying out of an offence referred to in article 2, paragraph 1, in the territory of or against a national of that State;

(b) The victim of one of the offences set forth in article 2, paragraph 1, is a national of that State;

(c) The offence is committed by a stateless person who has his or her habitual residence in the territory of that State.

3. Upon ratifying, accepting, approving or acceding to this Convention, each State Party shall notify the Secretary-General of the United Nations of the jurisdiction it has established in accordance with its domestic law in accordance with paragraph 2. Should any change take place, the State Party concerned shall immediately notify the Secretary-General.

4. Each State Party shall likewise take such measures as may be necessary to establish its jurisdiction over the offences set forth in article 2 in cases where the alleged offender is present in its territory and it does not extradite that person to any of the States Parties that have established their jurisdiction in accordance with paragraph 1 or 2.

5. When more than one State Party claims jurisdiction over one of the offences set forth in article 2, the relevant States Parties shall strive to coordinate their actions appropriately, in particular concerning the conditions for prosecution and the modalities for mutual legal assistance.

6. Without prejudice to the norms of general international law, this Convention does not exclude the exercise of any criminal jurisdiction established by a State Party in accordance with its domestic law.

Article 6
Seizure of Funds

1. Each State Party shall take appropriate measures, in accordance with its domestic legal principles, for the identification, detection and freezing or seizure of any funds used or allocated for the purpose of committing the offences set forth in article 2 as well as the proceeds derived from such offences, for purposes of possible forfeiture.

2. Each State Party shall take appropriate measures, in accordance with its domestic legal principles, for the forfeiture of funds used or allocated for the purpose of committing the offences set forth in article 2 and the proceeds derived from such offences.

3. Each State Party concerned may give consideration to concluding agreements on the sharing with other States Parties, on a regular or case-by-case basis, of the funds derived from the forfeitures referred to in this article.

4. Each State Party shall consider establishing mechanisms whereby the funds derived from the forfeitures referred to in this article are utilized to compensate the victims of offences referred to in article 2 or their families.

5. The provisions of this article shall be implemented without prejudice to the rights of third parties acting in good faith.

Article 7
Duty to Investigate

1. Upon receiving information that a person who has committed or who is alleged to have committed an offence set forth in article 2 may be present in its territory, the State Party concerned shall immediately take such measures as may be necessary under its domestic law to investigate the facts contained in the information.

2. Upon being satisfied that the circumstances so warrant, the State Party in whose territory the offender or alleged offender is present shall take the appropriate measures under its domestic law so as to ensure that person's presence for the purpose of prosecution or extradition.

3. Any person regarding whom the measures referred to in paragraph 2 are being taken shall be entitled to:

(a) Communicate without delay with the nearest appropriate representative of the State of which that person is a national or which is otherwise entitled to protect that person's rights or, if that person is a stateless person, the State in the territory of which that person habitually resides;

(b) Be visited by a representative of that State;

(c) Be informed of that person's rights under subparagraphs (a) and (b).

4. The rights referred to in paragraph 3 shall be exercised in conformity with the laws and regulations of the State in the territory of which the offender or alleged offender is present, subject to the provision that the said laws and regulations must

enable full effect to be given to the purposes for which the rights accorded under paragraph 3 are intended.

Article 8
Obligation to Prosecute or Extradite

1. The State Party in the territory of which the alleged offender is present shall, in cases to which article 5 applies, if it does not extradite that person, be obliged, without exception whatsoever and whether or not the offence was committed in its territory, to submit the case without undue delay to its competent authorities for the purpose of prosecution, through proceedings in accordance with the laws of that State. Those authorities shall take their decision in the same manner as in the case of any other offence of a grave nature under the law of that State.

2. Whenever a State Party is permitted under its domestic law to extradite or otherwise surrender one of its nationals only upon the condition that the person will be returned to that State to serve the sentence imposed as a result of the trial or proceeding for which the extradition or surrender of the person was sought, and this State and the State seeking the extradition of the person agree with this option and any other terms they may deem appropriate, such a conditional extradition or surrender shall be sufficient to discharge the obligation set forth in paragraph 1.

Article 9
Existing Extradition Treaties

1. The offences set forth in article 2 shall be deemed to be included as extraditable offences in any extradition treaty existing between any of the States Parties before the entry into force of this Convention. States Parties undertake to include such offences as extraditable offences in every extradition treaty to be subsequently concluded between them.

2. When a State Party which makes extradition conditional on the existence of a treaty receives a request for extradition from another State Party with which it has no extradition treaty, the requested State Party may, at its option, consider this Convention as a legal basis for extradition in respect of the offences set forth in article 2.

Extradition shall be subject to the other conditions provided by the law of the requested State.

3. States Parties which do not make extradition conditional on the existence of a treaty shall recognize the offences set forth in article 2 as extraditable offences between themselves, subject to the conditions provided by the law of the requested State.

4. If necessary the offences set forth in article 2 shall be treated, for the purposes of extradition between States Parties, as if they had been committed not only in the place in which they occurred but also in the territory of the States that have established jurisdiction in accordance with article 7, paragraphs 1 and 2.

5. The provisions of all extradition treaties and arrangements in force between States Parties with regard to the offences set forth in article 2 shall be deemed to be modified as between States Parties to the extent that they are incompatible with this Convention.

Article 10
Judicial Cooperation

1. States Parties shall afford one another the greatest measure of assistance in connection with criminal investigations or criminal or extradition proceedings in respect of the offences set forth in article 2, including assistance in obtaining evidence in their possession necessary for the proceedings.

2. The requesting State Party shall not use nor transmit information or evidence furnished by the requested State Party for investigations, prosecutions or proceedings other than those stated in the request without the prior consent of the requested State Party.

3. Each State Party may give consideration to establishing mechanisms to share with other States Parties information or evidence needed to establish criminal, civil or administrative liability pursuant to article 4.

4. States Parties shall carry out their obligations under paragraphs 1 and 2 in conformity with any treaties or other arrangements on mutual legal assistance or infor-

mation exchange that may exist between them. In the absence of such treaties or arrangements, States Parties shall afford one another assistance in accordance with their domestic law.

Article 11
Rights of the Accused

Any person who is taken into custody or regarding whom any other measures are taken or proceedings are carried out pursuant to this Convention shall be guaranteed fair treatment, including enjoyment of all rights and guarantees in conformity with the law of the State in the territory of which that person is present and applicable provisions of international law, including international human rights law.

Article 12
Preventive Measures

1. States Parties shall cooperate in the prevention of the offences set forth in article 2 by taking all practicable measures, inter alia, by adapting their domestic legislation, if necessary, to prevent and counter preparations in their respective territories for the commission of those offences within or outside their territories, including:

(a) Measures to prohibit in their territories illegal activities of persons and organizations that knowingly encourage, instigate, organize or engage in the commission of offences set forth in article 2;

(b) Measures requiring any research project involving human genetic material to be duly authorized by the competent authorities or, as appropriate, by a multidisciplinary national organ entrusted with that task;

(c) Measures requiring centres and establishments where research or activities are conducted that use gene technology to be previously registered, approved and authorized for such purposes by the health or scientific authorities or, as appropriate, by a multidisciplinary national organ.

2. States Parties shall further cooperate in the prevention of offences set forth in article 2 by exchanging accurate and verified information in accordance with their domestic law and coordinating administrative and other measures taken, as appropriate, to prevent the commission of offences set forth in article 2, in particular by:

(a) Establishing and maintaining channels of communication between their competent agencies and services to facilitate the secure and rapid exchange of information concerning all aspects of offences set forth in article 2;

(b) Cooperating with one another in conducting inquiries, with respect to the offences set forth in article 2, concerning:

(i) The identity, whereabouts and activities of persons in respect of whom reasonable suspicion exists that they are involved in such offences;

(ii) The movement of funds relating to the commission of such offences.

3. States Parties may exchange information through the International Criminal Police Organization (Interpol).

Article 13
Safeguard Clause

None of the provisions of this Convention shall be interpreted as limiting or otherwise affecting the possibility for each State Party to grant a wider measure of protection with regard to the applications of biology and medicine than is stipulated in this Convention.

Article 14
Settlement of Disputes

1. Any disputes between two or more States Parties concerning the interpretation or application of this Convention which cannot be settled through negotiation within a reasonable time shall, at the request of one of them, be submitted to arbitration. If, within six months from the date of the request for arbitration, the parties are unable to agree on the organization of the arbitration, any one of those parties may refer the dispute to the International Court of Justice, by application, in conformity with the Statute of the Court.

2. Each State may at the time of signature, ratification, acceptance or approval of this Convention or accession thereto declare that it does not consider itself bound by paragraph 1 of this article. The other States Parties shall not be bound by paragraph 1 with respect to any State Party which has made such a reservation.

3. Any State which has made a reservation in accordance with paragraph 2 may at any time withdraw that reservation by notification to the Secretary-General of the United Nations.

Article 15
Signature and Ratification

1. This Convention shall be open for signature by all States from ... to ... at United Nations Headquarters in New York.

2. This Convention is subject to ratification, acceptance or approval. The instruments of ratification, acceptance or approval shall be deposited with the Secretary-General of the United Nations.

3. This Convention shall be open to accession by any State. The instruments of accession shall be deposited with the Secretary-General of the United Nations.

Article 16
Reservations

No reservations shall be permitted to articles 1, 2 and 3 of this Convention.

Article 17
Entry into Force

1. This Convention shall enter into force on the thirtieth day following the date of the deposit of the twenty-second instrument of ratification, acceptance, approval or accession with the Secretary-General of the United Nations.

2. For each State ratifying, accepting, approving or acceding to the Convention after the deposit of the twenty-second instrument of ratification, acceptance, approval or accession, the Convention shall enter into force on the thirtieth day after deposit by such State of its instrument of ratification, acceptance, approval or accession.

Article 18
Denunciation

1. Any State Party may denounce this Convention by written notification to the Secretary-General of the United Nations.

2. Denunciation shall take effect one year following the date on which notification is received by the Secretary-General of the United Nations.

Article 19
Authentic Texts

The original of this Convention, of which the Arabic, Chinese, English, French, Russian and Spanish texts are equally authentic, shall be deposited with the Secretary-General of the United Nations, who shall send certified copies thereof to all States.

VIII. Protection of the Environment

African [Banjul] Charter on Human and Peoples' Rights

Adopted 27 June 1981. Entered into force 21 October 1986.
[Available in OAU Doc. CAB/LEG/67/3 rev. 5, 21 I.L.M. 58 (1982) and at
http://www.umn.edu/humanrts/instree/z1afchar.htm]

* * *

Article 24

All peoples shall have the right to a general satisfactory environment favorable to their development.

* * *

Additional Protocol to the American Convention on Human Rights in the Area of Economic, Social and Cultural Rights

Adopted on 17 November 1988. Entered into force on 16 November 1999.
[Available in O.A.S. Treaty Series No. 69 (1988), Basic Documents Pertaining to Human
Rights in the Inter-American System, OEA/Ser.L.V/II.82 doc.6 rev.1 at 67 (1992)
and at http://www.oas.org/main/main.asp?sLang=E&sLink=http://
www.oas.org/documents/eng/documents.asp]

* * *

Article 11
Right to a Healthy Environment

1. Everyone shall have the right to live in a healthy environment and to have access to basic public services.

2. States Parties shall promote the protection, preservation, and improvement of the enviroment.

* * *

ILO Convention (No. 169) Concerning Indigenous and Tribal Peoples in Independent Countries

Adopted on 27 June 1989 by the General Conference of the International Labour
Organisation at its seventy-sixth session. Entered into force 5 September 1991.
[Available at http://www.ilo.org/ilolex/cgi-lex/convde.pl?c169]

The General Conference of the International Labour Organisation,

Having been convened at Geneva by the Governing Body of the International Labour Office, and having met in its seventy-sixth session on 7 June 1989, and

Noting the international standards contained in the Indigenous and Tribal Populations Convention and Recommendation, 1957, and

Recalling the terms of the Universal Declaration of Human Rights, the International Covenant on Economic, Social and Cultural Rights, the

International Covenant on Civil and Political Rights, and the many international instruments on the prevention of discrimination, and

Considering that the developments which have taken place in international law since 1957, as well as developments in the situation of indigenous and tribal peoples in all regions of the world, have made it appropriate to adopt new international standards on the subject with a view to removing the assimilationist orientation of the earlier standards, and

Recognising the aspirations of these peoples to exercise control over their own institutions, ways of life and economic development and to maintain and develop their identities, languages and religions, within the framework of the States in which they live, and

Noting that in many parts of the world these peoples are unable to enjoy their fundamental human rights to the same degree as the rest of the population of the States within which they live, and that their laws, values, customs and perspectives have often been eroded, and

Calling attention to the distinctive contributions of indigenous and tribal peoples to the cultural diversity and social and ecological harmony of humankind and to international co-operation and understanding, and

Noting that the following provisions have been framed with the co-operation of the United Nations, the Food and Agriculture Organization of the United Nations, the United Nations Educational, Scientific and Cultural Organization and the World Health Organization, as well as of the Inter-American Indian Institute, at appropriate levels and in their respective fields, and that it is proposed to continue this co-operation in promoting and securing the application of these provisions, and

Having decided upon the adoption of certain proposals with regard to the partial revision of the Indigenous and Tribal Populations Convention, 1957 (No. 107), which is the fourth item on the agenda of the session, and

Having determined that these proposals shall take the form of an international Convention revising the Indigenous and Tribal Populations Convention, 1957,

Adopts this twenty-seventh day of June of the year one thousand nine hundred and eighty-nine the following Convention, which may be cited as the Indigenous and Tribal Peoples Convention, 1989.

PART I.
GENERAL POLICY
Article 1

1. This Convention applies to:

(a) Tribal peoples in independent countries whose social, cultural and economic conditions distinguish them from other sections of the national community, and whose status is regulated wholly or partially by their own customs or traditions or by special laws or regulations;

(b) Peoples in independent countries who are regarded as indigenous on account of their descent from the populations which inhabited the country, or a geographical region to which the country belongs, at the time of conquest or colonisation or the establishment of present State boundaries and who, irrespective of their legal status, retain some or all of their own social, economic, cultural and political institutions.

2. Self-identification as indigenous or tribal shall be regarded as a fundamental criterion for determining the groups to which the provisions of this Convention apply.

3. The use of the term "peoples" in this Convention shall not be construed as having any implications as regards the rights which may attach to the term under international law.

Article 2

1. Governments shall have the responsibility for developing, with the participation of the peoples concerned, co-ordinated and systematic action to protect the rights of these peoples and to guarantee respect for their integrity.

2. Such action shall include measures for:

(a) Ensuring that members of these peoples benefit on an equal footing from the rights and opportunities which national laws and regulations grant to other members of the population;

(b) Promoting the full realisation of the social, economic and cultural rights of these peoples with respect for their social and cultural identity, their customs and traditions and their institutions;

(c) Assisting the members of the peoples concerned to eliminate socio-economic gaps that may exist between indigenous and other members of the national community, in a manner compatible with their aspirations and ways of life.

Article 3

1. Indigenous and tribal peoples shall enjoy the full measure of human rights and fundamental freedoms without hindrance or discrimination. The provisions of the Convention shall be applied without discrimination to male and female members of these peoples.

2. No form of force or coercion shall be used in violation of the human rights and fundamental freedoms of the peoples concerned, including the rights contained in this Convention.

Article 4

1. Special measures shall be adopted as appropriate for safeguarding the persons, institutions, property, labour, cultures and environment of the peoples concerned.

2. Such special measures shall not be contrary to the freely-expressed wishes of the peoples concerned.

3. Enjoyment of the general rights of citizenship, without discrimination, shall not be prejudiced in any way by such special measures.

Article 5

In applying the provisions of this Convention:

(a) The social, cultural, religious and spiritual values and practices of these peoples shall be recognised and protected, and due account shall be taken of the nature of the problems which face them both as groups and as individuals;

(b) The integrity of the values, practices and institutions of these peoples shall be respected;

(c) Policies aimed at mitigating the difficulties experienced by these peoples in facing new conditions of life and work shall be adopted, with the participation and co-operation of the peoples affected.

Article 6

1. In applying the provisions of this Convention, Governments shall:

(a) Consult the peoples concerned, through appropriate procedures and in particular through their representative institutions, whenever consideration is being given to legislative or administrative measures which may affect them directly;

(b) Establish means by which these peoples can freely participate, to at least the same extent as other sectors of the population, at all levels of decision-making in elective institutions and administrative and other bodies responsible for policies and programmes which concern them;

(c) Establish means for the full development of these peoples' own institutions and initiatives, and in appropriate cases provide the resources necessary for this purpose.

2. The consultations carried out in application of this Convention shall be undertaken, in good faith and in a form appropriate to the circumstances, with the objective of achieving agreement or consent to the proposed measures.

Article 7

1. The peoples concerned shall have the right to decide their own priorities for the process of development as it affects their lives, beliefs, institutions and spiritual well-being and the lands they occupy or otherwise use, and to exercise control, to the extent possible, over their own economic, social and cultural development. In addition, they shall participate in the formulation, implementation and evaluation of plans and programmes for national and regional development which may affect them directly.

2. The improvement of the conditions of life and work and levels of health and education of the

peoples concerned, with their participation and co-operation, shall be a matter of priority in plans for the overall economic development of areas they inhabit. Special projects for development of the areas in question shall also be so designed as to promote such improvement.

3. Governments shall ensure that, whenever appropriate, studies are carried out, in co-operation with the peoples concerned, to assess the social, spiritual, cultural and environmental impact on them of planned development activities. The results of these studies shall be considered as fundamental criteria for the implementation of these activities.

4. Governments shall take measures, in co-operation with the peoples concerned, to protect and preserve the environment of the territories they inhabit.

Article 8

1. In applying national laws and regulations to the peoples concerned, due regard shall be had to their customs or customary laws.

2. These peoples shall have the right to retain their own customs and institutions, where these are not incompatible with fundamental rights defined by the national legal system and with internationally recognized human rights. Procedures shall be established, whenever necessary, to resolve conflicts which may arise in the application of this principle.

3. The application of paragraphs 1 and 2 of this Article shall not prevent members of these peoples from exercising the rights granted to all citizens and from assuming the corresponding duties.

Article 9

1. To the extent compatible with the national legal system, and internationally recognised human rights. the methods customarily practised by the peoples concerned for dealing with offences committed by their members shall be respected.

2. The customs of these peoples in regard to penal matters shall be taken into consideration by the authorities and courts dealing with such cases.

Article 10

1. In imposing penalties laid down by general law on members of these peoples account shall be taken of their economic, social and cultural characteristics.

2. Preference shall be given to methods of punishment other than confinement in prison.

Article 11

The exaction from members of the peoples concerned of compulsory personal services in any form, whether paid or unpaid, shall be prohibited and punishable by law, except in cases prescribed by law for all citizens.

Article 12

The peoples concerned shall be safeguarded against the abuse of their rights and shall be able to take legal proceedings, either individually or through their representative bodies, for the effective protection of these rights. Measures shall be taken to ensure that members of these peoples can understand and be understood in legal proceedings, where necessary through the provision of interpretation or by other effective means.

PART II.
LAND

Article 13

1. In applying the provisions of this Part of the Convention governments shall respect the special importance for the cultures and spiritual values of the peoples concerned of their relationship with the lands or territories, or both as applicable, which they occupy or otherwise use, and in particular the collective aspects of this relationship.

2. The use of the term "lands" in Articles 15 and 16 shall include the concept of territories, which covers the total environment of the areas which the peoples concerned occupy or otherwise use.

Article 14

1. The rights of ownership and possession of the peoples concerned over the lands which they traditionally occupy shall be recognised. In addition, measures shall be taken in appropriate cases to safeguard the right of the peoples concerned to use lands not exclusively occupied by them, but to which they have traditionally had access for their subsistence and traditional activities. Particular at-

tention shall be paid to the situation of nomadic peoples and shifting cultivators in this respect.

2. Governments shall take steps as necessary to identify the lands which the peoples concerned traditionally occupy, and to guarantee effective protection of their rights of ownership and possession.

3. Adequate procedures shall be established within the national legal system to resolve land claims by the peoples concerned.

Article 15

1. The rights of the peoples concerned to the natural resources pertaining to their lands shall be specially safeguarded. These rights include the right of these peoples to participate in the use, management and conservation of these resources.

2. In cases in which the State retains the ownership of mineral or sub-surface resources or rights to other resources pertaining to lands, governments shall establish or maintain procedures through which they shall consult these peoples, with a view to ascertaining whether and to what degree their interests would be prejudiced, before undertaking or permitting any programmes for the exploration or exploitation of such resources pertaining to their lands. The peoples concerned shall wherever possible participate in the benefits of such activities, and shall receive fair compensation for any damages which they may sustain as a result of such activities.

Article 16

1. Subject to the following paragraphs of this Article, the peoples concerned shall not be removed from the lands which they occupy.

2. Where the relocation of these peoples is considered necessary as an exceptional measure, such relocation shall take place only with their free and informed consent. Where their consent cannot be obtained, such relocation shall take place only following appropriate procedures established by national laws and regulations, including public inquiries where appropriate, which provide the opportunity for effective representation of the peoples concerned.

3. Whenever possible, these peoples shall have the right to return to their traditional lands, as soon as the grounds for relocation cease to exist.

4. When such return is not possible, as determined by agreement or, in the absence of such agreement, through appropriate procedures, these peoples shall be provided in all possible cases with lands of quality and legal status at least equal to that of the lands previously occupied by them, suitable to provide for their present needs and future development. Where the peoples concerned express a preference for compensation in money or in kind, they shall be so compensated under appropriate guarantees.

5. Persons thus relocated shall be fully compensated for any resulting loss or injury.

Article 17

1. Procedures established by the peoples concerned for the transmission of land rights among members of these peoples shall be respected.

2. The peoples concerned shall be consulted whenever consideration is being given to their capacity to alienate their lands or otherwise transmit their rights outside their own community.

3. Persons not belonging to these peoples shall be prevented from taking advantage of their customs or of lack of understanding of the laws on the part of their members to secure the ownership, possession or use of land belonging to them.

Article 18

Adequate penalties shall be established by law for unauthorised intrusion upon, or use of, the lands of the peoples concerned, and governments shall take measures to prevent such offences.

Article 19

National agrarian programmes shall secure to the peoples concerned treatment equivalent to that accorded to other sectors of the population with regard to:

(a) The provision of more land for these peoples when they have not the area necessary for providing the essentials of a normal existence, or for any possible increase in their numbers;

(b) The provision of the means required to promote the development of the lands which these peoples already possess.

PART III. RECRUITMENT AND CONDITIONS OF EMPLOYMENT
* * *

PART IV. VOCATIONAL TRAINING, HANDICRAFTS AND RURAL INDUSTRIES
* * *

PART V. SOCIAL SECURITY AND HEALTH

Article 24

Social security schemes shall be extended progressively to cover the peoples concerned, and applied without discrimination against them.

Article 25

1. Governments shall ensure that adequate health services are made available to the peoples concerned, or shall provide them with resources to allow them to design and deliver such services under their own responsibility and control, so that they may enjoy the highest attainable standard of physical and mental health.

2. Health services shall, to the extent possible, be community-based. These services shall be planned and administered in co-operation with the peoples concerned and take into account their economic, geographic, social and cultural conditions as well as their traditional preventive care, healing practices and medicines.

3. The health care system shall give preference to the training and employment of local community health workers, and focus on primary health care while maintaining strong links with other levels of health care services.

4. The provision of such health services shall be co-ordinated with other social, economic and cultural measures in the country.

PART VI. EDUCATION AND MEANS OF COMMUNICATION
* * *

PART VII. CONTACTS AND CO-OPERATION ACROSS BORDERS
* * *

PART VIII. ADMINISTRATION
* * *

PART IX. GENERAL PROVISIONS

Article 34

The nature and scope of the measures to be taken to give effect to this Convention shall be determined in a flexible manner, having regard to the conditions characteristic of each country.

Article 35

The application of the provisions of this Convention shall not adversely affect rights and benefits of the peoples concerned pursuant to other Conventions and Recommendations, international instruments, treaties, or national laws, awards, custom or agreements.

PART X. FINAL PROVISIONS
* * *

PROTECTION OF THE ENVIRONMENT

Convention on Access to Information, Public Participation in Decision-Making and Access to Justice in Environmental Matters

Done at Aarhus, Denmark, on 25 June 1998 at the Fourth Ministerial Conference on the Environment for Europe Process. Entered into force on 30 October 2001.
[Available at http://www.unece.org/env/pp/documents/cep43e.pdf]

The Parties to this Convention,

Recalling principle l of the Stockholm Declaration on the Human Environment,

Recalling also principle 10 of the Rio Declaration on Environment and Development,

Recalling further General Assembly resolutions 37/7 of 28 October 1982 on the World Charter for Nature and 45/94 of 14 December 1990 on the need to ensure a healthy environment for the well-being of individuals,

Recalling the European Charter on Environment and Health adopted at the First European Conference on Environment and Health of the World Health Organization in Frankfurt-am-Main, Germany, on 8 December 1989,

Affirming the need to protect, preserve and improve the state of the environment and to ensure sustainable and environmentally sound development,

Recognizing that adequate protection of the environment is essential to human well-being and the enjoyment of basic human rights, including the right to life itself,

Recognizing also that every person has the right to live in an environment adequate to his or her health and well-being, and the duty, both individually and in association with others, to protect and improve the environment for the benefit of present and future generations,

Considering that, to be able to assert this right and observe this duty, citizens must have access to information, be entitled to participate in decision-making and have access to justice in environmental matters, and acknowledging in this regard that citizens may need assistance in order to exercise their rights,

Recognizing that, in the field of the environment, improved access to information and public participation in decision-making enhance the quality and the implementation of decisions, contribute to public awareness of environmental issues, give the public the opportunity to express its concerns and enable public authorities to take due account of such concerns,

Aiming thereby to further the accountability of and transparency in decision-making and to strengthen public support for decisions on the environment,

Recognizing the desirability of transparency in all branches of government and inviting legislative bodies to implement the principles of this Convention in their proceedings,

Recognizing also that the public needs to be aware of the procedures for participation in environmental decision-making, have free access to them and know how to use them,

Recognizing further the importance of the respective roles that individual citizens, non-governmental organizations and the private sector can play in environmental protection,

Desiring to promote environmental education to further the understanding of the environment and sustainable development and to encourage widespread public awareness of, and participation in, decisions affecting the environment and sustainable development,

Noting, in this context, the importance of making use of the media and of electronic or other, future forms of communication,

Recognizing the importance of fully integrating environmental considerations in governmental decision-making and the consequent need for public authorities to be in possession of accurate, comprehensive and up-to date environmental information,

Acknowledging that public authorities hold environmental information in the public interest,

Concerned that effective judicial mechanisms should be accessible to the public, including organizations, so that its legitimate interests are protected and the law is enforced,

Noting the importance of adequate product information being provided to consumers to enable them to make informed environmental choices,

Recognizing the concern of the public about the deliberate release of genetically modified organisms into the environment and the need for increased transparency and greater public participation in decision-making in this field,

Convinced that the implementation of this Convention will contribute to strengthening democracy in the region of the United Nations Economic Commission for Europe (ECE),

Conscious of the role played in this respect by ECE and recalling, inter alia, the ECE Guidelines on Access to Environmental Information and Public Participation in Environmental Decision-making endorsed in the Ministerial Declaration adopted at the Third Ministerial Conference "Environment for Europe" in Sofia, Bulgaria, on 25 October 1995,

Bearing in mind the relevant provisions in the Convention on Environmental Impact Assessment in a Transboundary Context, done at Espoo, Finland, on 25 February 1991, and the Convention on the Transboundary Effects of Industrial Accidents and the Convention on the Protection and Use of Transboundary Watercourses and International Lakes, both done at Helsinki on 17 March 1992, and other regional conventions,

Conscious that the adoption of this Convention will have contributed to the further strengthening of the "Environment for Europe" process and to the results of the Fourth Ministerial Conference in Aarhus, Denmark, in June 1998,

Have agreed as follows:

Article 1

Objective

In order to contribute to the protection of the right of every person of present and future generations to live in an environment adequate to his or her health and well-being, each Party shall guarantee the rights of access to information, public participation in decision-making, and access to justice in environmental matters in accordance with the provisions of this Convention.

Article 2

Definitions

For the purposes of this Convention,

1. "Party" means, unless the text otherwise indicates, a Contracting Party to this Convention;

2. "Public authority" means:

(a) Government at national, regional and other level;

(b) Natural or legal persons performing public administrative functions under national law, including specific duties, activities or services in relation to the environment;

(c) Any other natural or legal persons having public responsibilities or functions, or providing public services, in relation to the environment, under the control of a body or person falling within subparagraphs (a) or (b) above;

(d) The institutions of any regional economic integration organization referred to in article 17 which is a Party to this Convention. This definition does not include bodies or institutions acting in a judicial or legislative capacity;

3. "Environmental information" means any information in written, visual, aural, electronic or any other material form on:

(a) The state of elements of the environment, such as air and atmosphere, water, soil, land, landscape and natural sites, biological diversity and its components, including genetically modified organisms, and the interaction among these elements;

(b) Factors, such as substances, energy, noise and radiation, and activities or measures, including administrative measures, environmental agreements, policies, legislation, plans and programmes, affecting or likely to affect the elements of the environment within the scope of subparagraph (a) above, and cost-benefit and other economic analyses and assumptions used in environmental decision-making;

(c) The state of human health and safety, conditions of human life, cultural sites and built structures, inasmuch as they are or may be affected by the state of the elements of the environment or, through these elements, by the factors, activities or measures referred to in subparagraph (b) above;

4. "The public" means one or more natural or legal persons, and, in accordance with national legislation or practice, their associations, organizations or groups;

5. "The public concerned" means the public affected or likely to be affected by, or having an interest in, the environmental decision-making; for the purposes of this definition, non-governmental organizations promoting environmental protection and meeting any requirements under national law shall be deemed to have an interest.

Article 3

General Provisions

1. Each Party shall take the necessary legislative, regulatory and other measures, including measures to achieve compatibility between the provisions implementing the information, public participation and access-to-justice provisions in this Convention, as well as proper enforcement measures, to establish and maintain a clear, transparent and consistent framework to implement the provisions of this Convention.

2. Each Party shall endeavour to ensure that officials and authorities assist and provide guidance to the public in seeking access to information, in facilitating participation in decision-making and in seeking access to justice in environmental matters.

3. Each Party shall promote environmental education and environmental awareness among the public, especially on how to obtain access to information, to participate in decision-making and to obtain access to justice in environmental matters.

4. Each Party shall provide for appropriate recognition of and support to associations, organizations or groups promoting environmental protection and ensure that its national legal system is consistent with this obligation.

5. The provisions of this Convention shall not affect the right of a Party to maintain or introduce measures providing for broader access to information, more extensive public participation in decision-making and wider access to justice in environmental matters than required by this Convention.

6. This Convention shall not require any derogation from existing rights of access to information, public participation in decision-making and access to justice in environmental matters.

7. Each Party shall promote the application of the principles of this Convention in international environmental decision-making processes and within the framework of international organizations in matters relating to the environment.

8. Each Party shall ensure that persons exercising their rights in conformity with the provisions of this Convention shall not be penalized, persecuted or harassed in any way for their involvement. This provision shall not affect the powers of national courts to award reasonable costs in judicial proceedings.

9. Within the scope of the relevant provisions of this Convention, the public shall have access to information, have the possibility to participate in decision-making and have access to justice in environmental matters without discrimination as to citizenship, nationality or domicile and, in the case of a legal person, without discrimination as to where it has its registered seat or an effective centre of its activities.

Article 4

Access to Environmental Information

1. Each Party shall ensure that, subject to the following paragraphs of this article, public authorities,

in response to a request for environmental information, make such information available to the public, within the framework of national legislation, including, where requested and subject to subparagraph (b) below, copies of the actual documentation containing or comprising such information:

(a) Without an interest having to be stated;

(b) In the form requested unless:

(i) It is reasonable for the public authority to make it available in another form, in which case reasons shall be given for making it available in that form; or

(ii) The information is already publicly available in another form.

2. The environmental information referred to in paragraph 1 above shall be made available as soon as possible and at the latest within one month after the request has been submitted, unless the volume and the complexity of the information justify an extension of this period up to two months after the request. The applicant shall be informed of any extension and of the reasons justifying it.

3. A request for environmental information may be refused if:

(a) The public authority to which the request is addressed does not hold the environmental information requested;

(b) The request is manifestly unreasonable or formulated in too general a manner; or

(c) The request concerns material in the course of completion or concerns internal communications of public authorities where such an exemption is provided for in national law or customary practice, taking into account the public interest served by disclosure.

4. A request for environmental information may be refused if the disclosure would adversely affect:

(a) The confidentiality of the proceedings of public authorities, where such confidentiality is provided for under national law;

(b) International relations, national defence or public security;

(c) The course of justice, the ability of a person to receive a fair trial or the ability of a public authority to conduct an enquiry of a criminal or disciplinary nature;

(d) The confidentiality of commercial and industrial information, where such confidentiality is protected by law in order to protect a legitimate economic interest. Within this framework, information on emissions which is relevant for the protection of the environment shall be disclosed;

(e) Intellectual property rights;

(f) The confidentiality of personal data and/or files relating to a natural person where that person has not consented to the disclosure of the information to the public, where such confidentiality is provided for in national law;

(g) The interests of a third party which has supplied the information requested without that party being under or capable of being put under a legal obligation to do so, and where that party does not consent to the release of the material; or

(h) The environment to which the information relates, such as the breeding sites of rare species. The aforementioned grounds for refusal shall be interpreted in a restrictive way, taking into account the public interest served by disclosure and taking into account whether the information requested relates to emissions into the environment.

5. Where a public authority does not hold the environmental information requested, this public authority shall, as promptly as possible, inform the applicant of the public authority to which it believes it is possible to apply for the information requested or transfer the request to that authority and inform the applicant accordingly.

6. Each Party shall ensure that, if information exempted from disclosure under paragraphs 3 (c) and 4 above can be separated out without prejudice to the confidentiality of the information exempted, public authorities make available the remainder of the environmental information that has been requested.

7. A refusal of a request shall be in writing if the request was in writing or the applicant so requests. A refusal shall state the reasons for the refusal and

PROTECTION OF THE ENVIRONMENT

give information on access to the review procedure provided for in accordance with article 9. The refusal shall be made as soon as possible and at the latest within one month, unless the complexity of the information justifies an extension of this period up to two months after the request. The applicant shall be informed of any extension and of the reasons justifying it.

8. Each Party may allow its public authorities to make a charge for supplying information, but such charge shall not exceed a reasonable amount. Public authorities intending to make such a charge for supplying information shall make available to applicants a schedule of charges which may be levied, indicating the circumstances in which they may be levied or waived and when the supply of information is conditional on the advance payment of such a charge.

Article 5
Collection and Dissemination of Environmental Information
** *

Article 6
Public Participation in Decisions on Specific Activities
** *

Article 7
Public Participation Concerning Plans, Programmes and Policies Relating to the Environment
* * *

Article 8
Public Participation During the Preparation of Executive Regulations and/or Generally Applicable Legally Binding Normative Instruments
* * *

Article 9
Access to Justice
* * *

Article 10
Meeting of the Parties
* * *

Article 11
Right to Vote
* * *

Article 12
Secretariat
* * *

Article 13
Annexes
* * *

Article 14
Amendments to the Convention
* * *

Article 15
Review of Compliance
* * *

Article 16
Settlement of Disputes
* * *

Article 17
Signature
* * *

Article 18
Depository
* * *

Article 19
Ratification, Acceptance, Approval and Accession
* * *

Article 20
Entry into Office
* * *

Article 21
Withdrawl
* * *

Article 22
Authentic Texts
* * *

IN WITNESS WHEREOF the undersigned, being duly authorized thereto, have signed this Convention.

DONE at Aarhus (Denmark), this twenty-fifth day of June, one thousand nine hundred and ninety-eight.

Draft Declaration of Principles on Human Rights and the Environment

*Drafted on 16 May 1994 by an international group of experts on human rights
and environmental protection convened at the United Nations in Geneva
at the invitation of the Sierra Club Legal Defense Fund — in cooperation with the
Association Mondiale pour L'école Instrument de Paix and the Société Suisse pour la
Protection de l'Environnement, on behalf of Madame Fatma Zohra Ksentini,
Special Rapporteur on Human Rights and the Environment for the United Nations
Sub-Commission on Prevention of Discrimination and Protection of Minorities.
[Available in UN Doc. E/CN.4/Sub.2/1994/9 (1994), annex 1 and
at http://www.anped.org/docs/ER%20UN%20Draft%20Principles.doc]*

PREAMBLE

Guided by the United Nations Charter, the Universal Declaration of Human Rights, the International Covenant on Economic, Social and Cultural Rights, the International Covenant on Civil and Political Rights, the Vienna Declaration and Program of Action of the World Conference of Human Rights, and other relevant international human rights instruments,

Guided also by the Stockholm Declaration of the United Nations Conference on the Human Environment, the World Charter for Nature, the Rio Declaration on Environment and Development, Agenda 21: Programme of Action for Sustainable Development, and other relevant instruments of international environmental law,

Guided also by the Declaration on the Right to Development, which recognizes that the right to development is an essential human right and that the human person is the central subject of development,

Guided further by fundamental principles of international humanitarian law,

Reaffirming the universality, indivisibility and interdependence of all human rights,

Recognizing that sustainable development links the right to development and the right to a secure, healthy and ecologically sound environment,

Recalling the right of peoples to self-determination by virtue of which they have the right freely to determine their political status and to pursue their economic, social and cultural development,

Deeply concerned by the severe human rights consequences of environmental harm caused by poverty, structural adjustment and debt programmes and by international trade and intellectual property regimes,

Convinced that the potential irreversibility of environmental harm gives rise to special responsibility to prevent such harm,

Concerned that human rights violations lead to environmental degradation and that environmental degradation leads to human rights violations,

The following principles are declared:

PART I

1. Human rights, an ecologically sound environment, sustainable development and peace are interdependent and indivisible.

2. All persons have the right to a secure, healthy and ecologically sound environment. This right and other human rights, including civil, cultural, economic, political and social rights, are universal, interdependent and indivisible.

3. All persons shall be free from any form of discrimination in regard to actions and decisions that affect the environment.

4. All persons have the right to an environment adequate to meet equitably the needs of present generations and that does not impair the rights of future generations to meet equitably their needs.

PART II

5. All persons have the right to freedom from pollution, environmental degradation and activities

PROTECTION OF THE ENVIRONMENT

that adversely affect the environment, threaten life, health, livelihood, well-being or sustainable development within, across or outside national boundaries.

6. All persons have the right to protection and preservation of the air, soil, water, sea-ice, flora and fauna, and the essential processes and areas necessary to maintain biological diversity and ecosystems.

7. All persons have the right to the highest attainable standard of health free from environmental harm.

8. All persons have the right to safe and healthy food and water adequate to their well-being.

9. All persons have the right to a safe and healthy working environment.

10. All persons have the right to adequate housing, land tenure and living conditions in a secure, healthy and ecologically sound environment.

11. All persons have the right not to be evicted from their homes or land for the purpose of, or as a consequence of, decisions or actions affecting the environment, except in emergencies or due to a compelling purpose benefiting society as a whole and not attainable by other means. All persons have the right to participate effectively in decisions and to negotiate concerning their eviction and the right, if evicted, to timely and adequate restitution, compensation and/or appropriate and sufficient accommodation or land.

12. All persons have the right to timely assistance in the event of natural or technological or other human-caused catastrophes.

13. Everyone has the right to benefit equitably from the conservation and sustainable use of nature and natural resources for cultural, ecological, educational, health, livelihood, recreational, spiritual or other purposes. This includes ecologically sound access to nature. Everyone has the right to preservation of unique sites, consistent with the fundamental rights of persons or groups living in the area.

14. Indigenous peoples have the right to control their lands, territories and natural resources and to maintain their traditional way of life. This includes the right to security in the enjoyment of their means of subsistence.

Indigenous peoples have the right to protection against any action or course of conduct that may result in the destruction or degradation of their territories, including land, air, water, sea-ice, wildlife or other resources.

PART III

15. All persons have the right to information concerning the environment. This includes information, howsoever compiled, on actions and courses of conduct that may affect the environment and information necessary to enable effective public participation in environmental decision-making. The information shall be timely, clear, understandable and available without undue financial burden to the applicant.

16. All persons have the right to hold and express opinions and to disseminate ideas and information regarding the environment.

17. All persons have the right to environmental and human rights education.

18. All persons have the right to active, free, and meaningful participation in planning and decision-making activities and processes that may have an impact on the environment and development. This includes the right to a prior assessment of the environmental, developmental and human rights consequences of proposed actions.

19. All persons have the right to associate freely and peacefully with others for purposes of protecting the environment or the rights of persons affected by environmental harm.

20. All persons have the right to effective remedies and redress in administrative or judicial proceedings for environmental harm or the threat of such harm.

PART IV

21. All persons, individually and in association with others, have a duty to protect and preserve the environment.

22. All States shall respect and ensure the right to a secure, healthy and ecologically sound environment. Accordingly, they shall adopt the administrative, legislative and other measures necessary to effectively implement the rights in this Declaration.

These measures shall aim at the prevention of environmental harm, at the provision of adequate remedies, and at the sustainable use of natural resources and shall include, inter alia,

• collection and dissemination of information concerning the environment;

• prior assessment and control, licensing, regulation or prohibition of activities and substances potentially harmful to the environment;

• public participation in environmental decision-making;

• effective administrative and judicial remedies and redress for environmental harm and the threat of such harm;

• monitoring, management and equitable sharing of natural resources;

• measures to reduce wasteful processes of production and patterns of consumption;

• measures aimed at ensuring that transnational corporations, wherever they operate, carry out

their duties of environmental protection, sustainable development and respect for human rights; and

• measures aimed at ensuring that the international organizations and agencies to which they belong observe the rights and duties in this Declaration.

23. States and all other parties shall avoid using the environment as a means of war or inflicting significant, long-term or widespread harm on the environment, and shall respect international law providing protection for the environment in times of armed conflict and cooperate in its further development.

24. All international organizations and agencies shall observe the rights and duties in this Declaration.

PART V

25. In implementing the rights and duties in this Declaration, special attention shall be given to vulnerable persons and groups.

26. The rights in this Declaration may be subject only to restrictions provided by law and which are necessary to protect public order, health and the fundamental rights and freedoms of others.

27. All persons are entitled to a social and international order in which the rights in this Declaration can be fully realized.